Perinatal Cardiology
Part 2

Edited by

Edward Araujo Júnior

*Department of Obstetrics, Discipline of Fetal Medicine,
Paulista School of Medicine,
Federal University of São Paulo (EPM-UNIFESP),
São Paulo-SP,
Brazil*

Nathalie Jeanne M. Bravo-Valenzuela

*Department of Obstetrics, Discipline of Fetal Medicine,
Paulista School of Medicine,
Federal University of São Paulo (EPM-UNIFESP),
São Paulo-SP,
Brazil*

Alberto Borges Peixoto

*Discipline of Gynecology and Obstetrics,
University of Uberaba (UNIUBE), Uberaba-MG,
Brazil*

Perinatal Cardiology

Part # 2.

Editors: Edward Araujo Júnior, Nathalie Jeanne M. Bravo-Valenzuela and Alberto Borges Peixoto

ISBN (Online): 978-981-14-6655-7

ISBN (Print): 978-981-14-6653-3

ISBN (Paper Back): 978-981-14-6654-0

need for a court order if at any point you breach any terms of this License Agreement. In no event will any delay or failure by Bentham Science Publishers in enforcing your compliance with this License Agreement constitute a waiver of any of its rights.

3. You acknowledge that you have read this License Agreement, and agree to be bound by its terms and conditions. To the extent that any other terms and conditions presented on any website of Bentham Science Publishers conflict with, or are inconsistent with, the terms and conditions set out in this License Agreement, you acknowledge that the terms and conditions set out in this License Agreement shall prevail.

Bentham Science Publishers Pte. Ltd.
80 Robinson Road #02-00
Singapore 068898
Singapore
Email: subscriptions@benthamscience.net

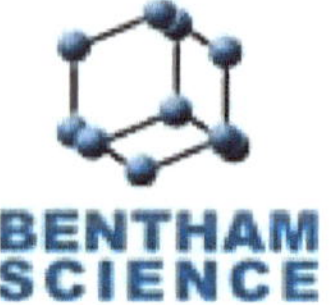

CONTENTS

FOREWORD

In *Perinatal Cardiology*, Edward Araujo Júnior, Nathalie Jeanne M. Bravo-Valenzuela, and Alberto Borges Peixoto have compiled a concise textbook, encompassing the fascinating, and demanding, study of the developing human heart. Malformations and disorders affecting the cardiovascular system are both the most commonly occurring in fetuses and neonates, and the most frequently missed in prenatal scanning. They contribute significantly to neonatal morbidity and mortality and impact on all stages of obstetric and neonatal management. Prenatal diagnosis of congenital heart disease (CHD) can improve neonatal and later outcomes. With the ongoing improvements in perinatal and pediatric care of patients with congenital heart defects, their impact will be evinced in later life stages, in reproductive care of women with CHD as well as genetic counseling for affected families.

Perinatal Cardiology comprises all these aspects of CHD, not overlooking the development of the uteroplacental circulation and the placenta itself, integral parts of the fetal cardiovascular system. The editors have enlisted an international cast of contributing authors who offer their expert guidance on fetal echocardiographic evaluation, and the particular nuances of fetal echocardiography performed early in gestation. Chapters are also devoted to the genetic investigation necessary in CHD, as well as the environmental factors that may be associated with CHD. This volume provides an overview of the anatomic malformations and disordered cardiovascular function that clinicians might encounter, and the pre- and post-natal interventions that can be offered.

Perinatal Cardiology will be of interest to everyone, including obstetricians, midwives, maternal-fetal medicine specialists, pediatric cardiologists, sonographers, and others dedicated to improve health and wellness of mothers and their babies.

Prof. Simcha Yagel
Division of Obstetrics and Gynecology
Hadassah-Hebrew University Medical Centers
Jerusalem
Israel

PREFACE

This first edition of the *Perinatal Cardiology* book is the culmination of concerted efforts of experts in the field of fetal cardiology. Congenital heart disease (CHD) accounts for the most common birth defects and is the leading cause of mortality associated with birth defects in infants. Critical CHD is defined as a condition that necessitates surgical intervention during the first year of life and accounts for approximately 25% of all CHD cases. Advances in prenatal diagnosis and surgical interventions/therapeutic *in utero* have improved the management and outcomes of CHD. Rapid technological advances in fetal echocardiography and prenatal cardiac ultrasonography (US) screening facilitate the early and accurate diagnosis of CHD, thereby ensuring prompt and optimal treatment. In accordance with the concepts and themes associated with this field, *Perinatal Cardiology* provides a comprehensive overview of the key learning points with regard to CHD. The authors have outlined strategies to improve prenatal diagnosis and management of this condition, which would benefit the following specialties: obstetricians, perinatal and pediatric cardiologists, general cardiologists, sonographers, and other allied health professionals. This book highlights the features of cardiac development, fetal cardiovascular hemodynamics, genetic factors associated with CHD, and fetal echocardiography/cardiac US evaluation, focusing on the prenatal diagnosis and perinatal management of CHD. The introductory chapters describe in detail the development of the cardiovascular and uteroplacental circulation, beginning with early gestation. This anatomical background will provide a better understanding of the pathogenesis/pathophysiology of cardiac malformations. The authors have described the US/echocardiographic features that would aid in the prenatal diagnosis of CHD and also highlighted features of fetal cardiac dysfunction correlated with their clinical applicability. Environmental exposures that can lead to cardiovascular malformations and the genetic aspects of CHD, including chromosomal abnormalities and extracardiac anomalies are discussed, for enhancing parental counseling. Additionally, this book provides updated information regarding *in utero* management and treatment of CHD, as well as postnatal clinical and surgical approaches to the management of most commonly occurring conditions categorized as CHD. Furthermore, the book describes interesting aspects of the cardiac rhythm *in utero* following the development of the cardiac conduction system, the characteristics of regular and irregular heart rhythms, and the important features of the different types of arrhythmias observed in these patients, as well as their perinatal management. The chapters in this book have been added after careful consideration and are subdivided into sections after thoughtful deliberation. These include various topics such as fetal cardiology, including the classification of prenatal CHD, cardiovascular and uteroplacental circulation development, fetal echocardiography evaluation, normal cardiac rhythm and arrhythmias, structural and functional defects, prenatal cardiac interventions, extracardiac cardiac defects in fetuses with CHD, genetic and environmental factors associated with cardiac defects, parental genetic counseling in cases of CHD, prenatal management and planned delivery of a fetus with CHD, and a systematic postnatal approach to the management of CHD. The anatomical classification of CHD is subdivided into the following topics: malpositions and abnormal situs, septal defects, right heart malformations, left heart malformations, conotruncal anomalies, aortic arch anomalies, myocardial and pericardial diseases, fetal cardiac tumors, and ventricular inflow anomalies. In recent years, significant technological progress in fetal echocardiography has enabled the diagnosis of various types of CHD, and it is possible to evaluate cardiac function in fetuses with CHD and in those without anatomical malformations. The following conditions (among several others) may affect fetal cardiac function: functional cardiac malformations such as premature closure of ductus arteriosus and foramen ovale and extracardiac conditions, such as maternal diseases (diabetes mellitus and chronic hypertension), fetal tumors, twin-to-twin transfusion syndrome, and fetal anemia. The Cardiovascular Profile Score is a useful tool for the assessment of fetuses with heart failure (HF). This tool utilizes US markers to monitor fetal cardiovascular unwellness based on univariate parameters, which are correlated with perinatal mortality. This instrument is used to record the "heart failure score" and is potentially useful in much the same way and in combination with the biophysical profile score. The chapters discussing fetal heart function comprise one of the differential topics of this book in the field of fetal cardiology. These chapters describe objective and important information regarding the clinical parameters for the evaluation of cardiac function. Chapters explaining the analysis of cardiac function discuss hemodynamic and cardiovascular fetal adaptations that enable optimization of outcomes and prediction of the risk in a fetus with HF or the one at risk of HF. Currently, the role of contemporary fetal cardiologists is not limited to the diagnosis and management of CHD *in utero*. These specialists also predict the risk of CHD in the newborn after delivery and participate in planning potential treatment after birth. Thus, a new classification system of prenatal CHD has been proposed based on risk stratification to identify an appropriate level of care. Critical CHD may progress *in utero*, and fetal echocardiography is an important tool to identify high-risk fetuses of mothers who require obstetric care at specialized centers to ensure optimal perinatal, obstetric, cardiology, and cardiothoracic surgery services. In conclusion, we hope this book serves as a comprehensive compendium of the latest optimal clinical approaches to the diagnosis, management and delivery planning for fetuses with CHD.

Edward Araujo Júnior
Department of Obstetrics, Discipline of Fetal Medicine, Paulista School of Medicine
Federal University of São Paulo (EPM-UNIFESP)
São Paulo-SP
Brazil

Nathalie Jeanne M. Bravo-Valenzuela
Department of Obstetrics, Discipline of Fetal Medicine, Paulista School of Medicine
Federal University of São Paulo (EPM-UNIFESP)
São Paulo-SP
Brazil

&

Alberto Borges Peixoto
Discipline of Gynecology and Obstetrics
University of Uberaba (UNIUBE)
Uberaba-MG
Brazil

List of Contributors

Ana B. Bianchi	Maternal-Fetal Medicine Unit, Hospital Center "Pereira Rossell", Montevideo, Uruguay
Alberto Borges Peixoto	Discipline of Gynecology and Obstetrics, University of Uberaba (UNIUBE), Uberaba-MG, Brazil Department of Gynecology and Obstetrics, Federal University of Triângulo Mineiro (UFTM), Uberaba-MG, Brazil
Ana Luisa Neves	Department of Pediatric Cardiology, Faculty of Medicine, University of Porto, Porto, Portugal
Ana Carolina Buso Faccinetto	Discipline of Cardiology, Department of Medicine, Paulista School of Medicine Federal University of São Paulo (EPM-UNIFESP), São Paulo-SP, Brazil
Carla Verona Barreto Farias	Department of Pediatrics, Fernandes Figueira Institute, Oswaldo Cruz Foundation (IFF-FIOCRUZ), Rio de Janeiro-RJ, Brazil Discipline of Pediatrics (Pediatric Cardiology), Department of Medicine, Federal University of Rio de Janeiro (UFRJ), Rio de Janeiro-RJ, Brazil
Christiane Simioni	Discipline of Fetal Medicine, Department of Obstetrics, Paulista School of Medicine, Federal University of São Paulo (EPM-UNIFESP), São Paulo-SP, Brazil
Célia Maria Camelo	Discipline of Cardiology, Department of Medicine, Paulista School of Medicine Federal University of São Paulo (EPM-UNIFESP), São Paulo-SP, Brazil
Edward Araujo Júnior	Discipline of Fetal Medicine, Department of Obstetrics, Paulista School of Medicine, Federal University of São Paulo (EPM-UNIFESP), São Paulo-SP, Brazil Medical Course, Municipal University of São Caetano do Sul (USCS), Bela Vista Campus, São Paulo-SP, Brazil
Eliane Lucas	Department of Pediatrics, Bonsucesso Federal Hospital (HFB-MS), Rio de Janeiro-RJ, Brazil Department of Pediatrics, University Center Organ Mountains (UNIFESO), Teresópolis-RJ, Brazil
Emma Bertucci	Prenatal Medicine Unit, Obstetrics and Gynaecology Unit, Department of Medical and Surgical Sciences for Mother, Child, and Adult, University of Modena and Reggio Emilia, Modena, Italy
Filomena Sileo	Prenatal Medicine Unit, Obstetrics and Gynaecology Unit, Department of Medical and Surgical Sciences for Mother, Child, and Adult, University of Modena and Reggio Emilia, Modena, Italy
Francesco D'Antonio	Department of Clinical Medicine, Faculty of Health Sciences, UiT - The Arctic University of Norway, Tromsø, Norway Department of Obstetrics and Gynaecology, University Hospital of Northern Norway, Tromsø, Norway
Ihosvanny Gonzalez	Maternal-Fetal Medicine Unit, Hospital Center "Pereira Rossell", Montevideo, Uruguay

James C. Huhta	Perinatal Cardiology, Mednax, St. Joseph Hospital, Tampa, FL, United States of America
Jose Pedro Da Silva	Department of Cardiothoracic Surgery, UPMC Children's Hospital of Pittsburgh, PA, United States of America
Luciana Fonseca Da Silva	Department of Cardiothoracic Surgery, UPMC Children's Hospital of Pittsburgh, PA, United States of America
Luciano Marcondes Machado Nardozza	Discipline of Fetal Medicine, Department of Obstetrics, Paulista School of Medicine, Federal University of São Paulo (EPM-UNIFESP), São Paulo-SP, Brazil
Lucas Otãno	Pediatric Cardiology Department, Hospital Italiano de Buenos Aires, Buenos Aires, Argentina
Maria Respondek-Liberska	Department of Prenatal Cardiology, Polish Mother's Memorial Hospital Research Institute, Lodz, Poland Department of Diagnoses and Prevention of Fetal Malformations, Medical University of Lodz, Lodz, Poland
Milene Carvalho Carrilho	Discipline of Fetal Medicine, Department of Obstetrics, Paulista School of Medicine, Federal University of São Paulo (EPM-UNIFESP), São Paulo-SP, Brazil
Nathalie J Magioli Bravo-Valenzuela	Department of Obstetrics, Discipline of Fetal Medicine, Paulista School of Medicine, Federal University of São Paulo (EPM-UNIFESP), São Paulo-SP, Brazil Discipline of Pediatrics (Pediatric Cardiology), Department of Medicine, Federal University of Rio de Janeiro (UFRJ), Rio de Janeiro-RJ, Brazil
Pablo Marantz	Pediatric Cardiology Department, Hospital Italiano de Buenos Aires, Buenos Aires, Argentina
Patricia Santana Correia	Department of Medical Genetics, Fernandes Figueira, Institute, Oswaldo Cruz Foundation (IFF-FIOCRUZ), Rio de Janeiro-RJ, Brazil Department of Pediatrics, Bonsucesso Federal Hospital (HFB-MS), Rio de Janeiro-RJ, Brazil
Sofía Grinenco	Pediatric Cardiology Department, Hospital Italiano de Buenos Aires, Buenos Aires, Argentina

CHAPTER 1

Fetal Ventricular Inflow Anomalies

Nathalie J. Magioli Bravo-Valenzuela[1,2,*]

[1] Department of Obstetrics, Discipline of Fetal Medicine, Paulista School of Medicine, Federal University of São Paulo (EPM-UNIFESP), São Paulo-SP, Brazil

[2] Discipline of Pediatrics (Pediatric Cardiology), Department of Medicine, Federal University of Rio de Janeiro (UFRJ), Rio de Janeiro-RJ, Brazil

Abstract: Congenital heart diseases (CHDs) are largely known as an important cause of fetal perinatal mortality. Currently, the accuracy of fetal echocardiography enables the detailed diagnosis of a significant variety of congenital cardiac anomalies, and it has also been demonstrated that prenatal outcomes may improve in critical CHDs. Accordingly, this chapter provides a detailed overview of the important anatomic aspects of some of the ventricular inflow anomalies, focusing on currently available information, to enable the prenatal diagnosis of such CHDs by ultrasound or echocardiography. Information regarding prenatal management, delivery plan strategies, and differential diagnosis of such anomalies is presented. The chapter also discusses the parental counseling and fetal and neonatal therapeutic management of such congenital cardiac anomalies. Univentricular atrioventricular (AV) connections, straddling and overriding of AV valves, and crisscross hearts are described in the current chapter. The concept of "functionally single ventricle" encompasses a group of CHDs in which the dominant ventricular chamber is responsible for maintaining the systemic and pulmonary circulations and not suitable for a biventricular repair. The central feature of such hearts is the univentricular AV connection. Regarding the type of the straddling of an inlet valve, it is based on the insertion of the tension apparatus of the AV valve into the crest of the ventricular septum or in the contralateral ventricle. Meanwhile, overriding of an inlet valve is related to the annulus of the AV valve and may interfere in the AV connection. Depending on the degree of the overriding of the straddled valve, the ventricles are in a dominant and rudimentary relationship, and a double-inlet AV connection, primarily the double-inlet left ventricle is the most frequent type of AV connection. In general, straddling and overriding of an AV valve requires a ventricular septal defect, and straddling may occur alone or in the presence of an overriding. In "crisscross" hearts, the ventricular inlet flows are in a cross shape and the ventricles are arranged in a superoinferior relationship. During an ultrasound examination, the crossed AV valves produce false images of the mitral valve or tricuspid atresia in a standard 4-chamber view, which makes the diagnosis difficult. In fact, the knowledge about the detailed anatomy, the assessment of the ventricular outflow tracts, and the identification of other possible associated cardiac anomalies are

*** Corresponding author Nathalie J. M. Bravo-valenzuela:** Department of Obstetrics, Discipline of Fetal Medicine, Paulista School of Medicine, Federal University of São Paulo (EPM-UNIFESP), R. Napoleão de Barros, 871/875 - Vila Clementino, 04024-002, São Paulo-SP, Brazil; Tel/Fax: +55 11 5571-0761; E-mail: njmbravo@cardiol.br

Edward Araujo Júnior, Nathalie Jeanne M. Bravo-Valenzuela and Alberto Borges Peixoto (Eds.)

important for improving *In Utero* and postnatal management in ventricular inlet anomalies described in the current chapter.

Keywords: Cardiac valves, Chordae Tendineae, Congenital heart disease, Crisscross Hearts, Double-inlet ventricle, Echocardiography, Mitral valve, Prenatal diagnosis, Single ventricle, Tricuspid valve, Univentricular heart, Ventricular morphology.

INTRODUCTION

Congenital heart diseases (CHDs) are an important cause of perinatal morbidity and mortality around the world; however, the risks of complications may vary according to the type of cardiopathy and health care assessment. Among CHDs, 50%–60% of them will require surgical correction, of which 25% are critical [1, 2]. In this setting, the survival, extensive medical care, and developmental disabilities depend on the time of the diagnosis, the delay of the treatment, and the severity of the CHD. Therefore, it has been observed that prenatal diagnosis of a treatable CHD reduces the risk of perinatal morbidity and mortality [3, 4]. Currently, fetal echocardiography allows an accurate diagnosis of univentricular atrioventricular (AV) connections and more complex ventricular inflow anomalies, which may influence prenatal and postnatal management and outcomes [4].

Traditionally known as a "single ventricle," the term univentricular heart is a generic term that includes a group of cardiac abnormalities in which there is only one "functionally single ventricle" [3]. Considering this concept of "functionally single ventricle," the following CHDs may be considered in such group: tricuspid atresia, hypoplastic left heart syndrome (HLHS), and unbalanced AV septal defect. However, it has been generally agreed that tricuspid atresia and HLHS are preferably described independently. In fact, stenoses of AV valves (mitral and tricuspid) among some other valve anomalies are not discussed in this chapter as they are included in the topics on right and left heart malformations.

UNIVENTRICULAR ATRIOVENTRICULAR CONNECTION

Univentricular atrioventricular connection is a rare cardiac anomaly that occurs in 2.3 cases per 10,000 live births with CHDs [5]. It has been believed that a "single ventricle" results from a failure of the development of the trabecular component at the bulboventricular loop stage. It has been previously known as "univentricular heart" or "single" or "common ventricle" in the 1960s and 1970s [6]. It is a condition in which one of the ventricular chambers is a large dominant ventricle and the other one is a small rudimentary chamber and functionally inadequate ventricle. Therefore, the term "single ventricle" is polemic as it alludes to the presence of a solitary ventricular chamber, which theoretically should exclude a second ventricular chamber even if it is rudimentary. Despite the controversy, the term "single ventricle" encompasses hearts in which there is a small nonfunctional ventricle with only one functional ventricle (dominant ventricle). It has been generally agreed that the univentricular atrioventricular connection is central in defining univentricular hearts. Consequently, in such cases, the dominant ventricle is responsible for maintaining the systemic and pulmonary circulations and not suitable for a biventricular repair.

Van Praagh *et al.* described a "single ventricle" as the heart with one ventricular chamber that receives a common or both AV valves, excluding mitral or tricuspid atresia [6]. Subsequently, Anderson *et al.* unified the criteria of univentricular heart by including all cases in which the AV junction is connected to one ventricular chamber [7]. Therefore, absent AV connections, double-inlet AV connections, and common AV valve such as an unbalanced atrioventricular septal defect in which one ventricle is hypoplastic and not suitable for biventricular repair could be considered as a "functionally single ventricle" (Fig. **1**). In this setting, other complex CHDs in which one of the ventricles is hypoplastic or absent may also be considered as a "functionally single ventricle." However, in cases of HLHS, in addition to the rudimentary left ventricle chamber, the other left-sided cardiac structures are also hypoplastic, and such cardiac malformation is classified separately (Fig. **2**).

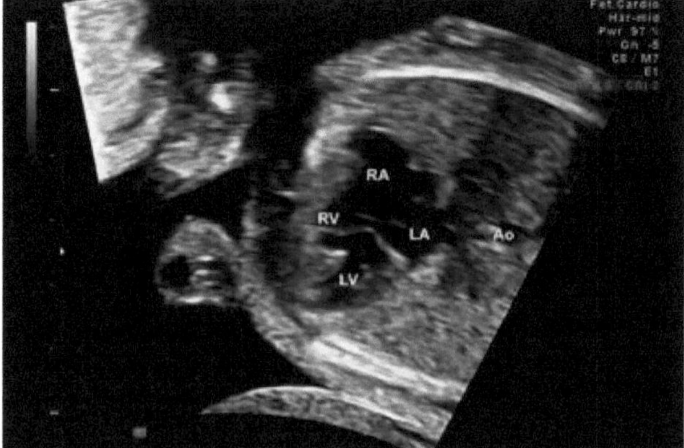

Fig. (1).   Fetal echocardiogram at 27 weeks of gestation demonstrating an unbalanced complete atrioventricular septal defect. In this fetus, the right morphologically right dominant ventricle is the dominant and the left ventricle is the rudimentary one. LA: left atrium; LV: left ventricle; RA: right atrium; RV: right ventricle; Ao: aorta.

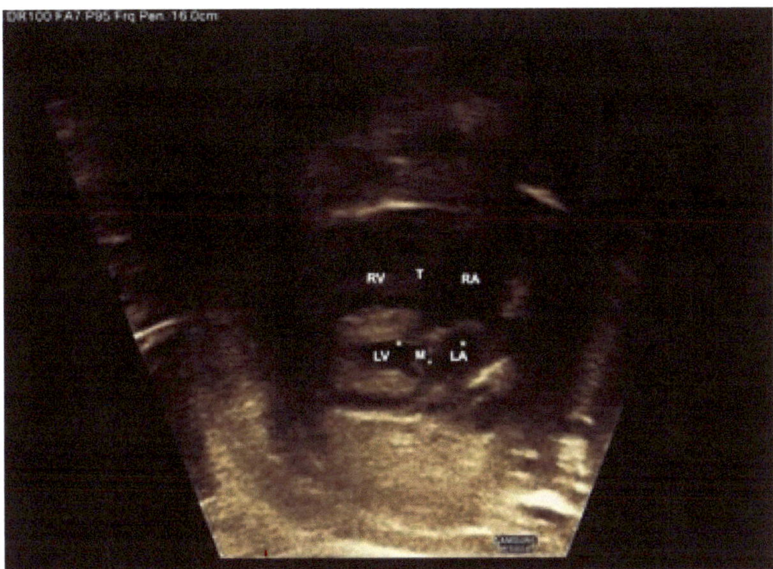

Fig. (2). Fetal echocardiogram at 27 weeks of gestation demonstrating a fetus with hypoplastic left heart syndrome (HLHS) with mitral stenosis and aortic atresia (*) The structures of the left heart (LA, mitral valve and LV) are hypoplastic. LA: left atrium; M: mitral valve; LV: left ventricle; RA: right atrium; RV: right ventricle; T: tricuspid valve.

Morphology

In the 2000s, authors described the features of a normal ventricle, focusing on the nomenclature of univentricular hearts [8, 9]. Normal ventricles have three components as follows: 1- inlet component that contains the AV valve and its tension apparatus, 2- outlet component with the VA valves, and 3- trabecular component that constitutes the space between the papillary muscles and the outlet component (apical trabecular part). In hearts described as a "functionally single ventricle," one of the ventricles is hypoplastic or even more rarely could be absent. The rudimentary (hypoplastic) ventricle may have one or more components absent, which renders it unable to function.

Considering the characteristics of the dominant ventricular chamber, four categories of a "functionally single ventricle" were described as follow: type A–single left ventricle, type B - single right ventricle, type C - common ventricle, and type D - indeterminate ventricle [10]. Hitherto, three of them are used to describe the dominant ventricle: dominant morphologically left ventricle, dominant morphologically right ventricle and single indeterminate ventricle (mixed or indeterminate ventricular morphology) [9, 11] (Fig. **3**). Posteriorly, Anderson *et al.* subclassified the types of univentricular AV connections as follows: 1- double-inlet ventricle (both valves connect to a main chamber), 2- single-inlet or absent AV connection (complete obstruction to the flow from the left atrium or from the right atrium to the ventricular chamber), and 3- common AV connection or common inlet (single AV valve) [12] (Figs. **4** and **5**). Focusing on the relationship among the great arteries, Van Praagh *et al.* included the following four subgroups of double-inlet LV: I- normally related great arteries, II- right anterior aorta, III- left anterior aorta, and IV- left posterior aorta (inverted great artery relationship) [10].

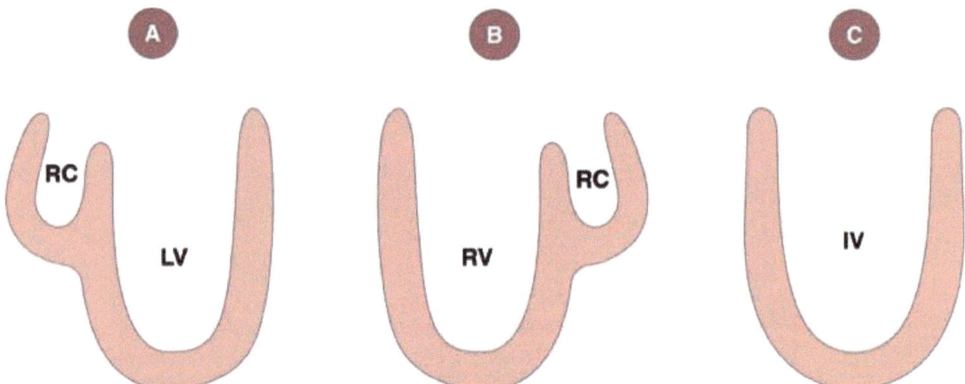

Fig. (3).   This figure shows the types of "univentricular AV connection" hearts considering the morphological characteristics of the dominant chamber: **A-** dominant left ventricle, **B-** dominant right ventricle and **C-** solitary ventricular chamber (indeterminate ventricle). RC: rudimentary chamber; LV: left ventricle; RV: right ventricle; IV: indeterminate ventricle.

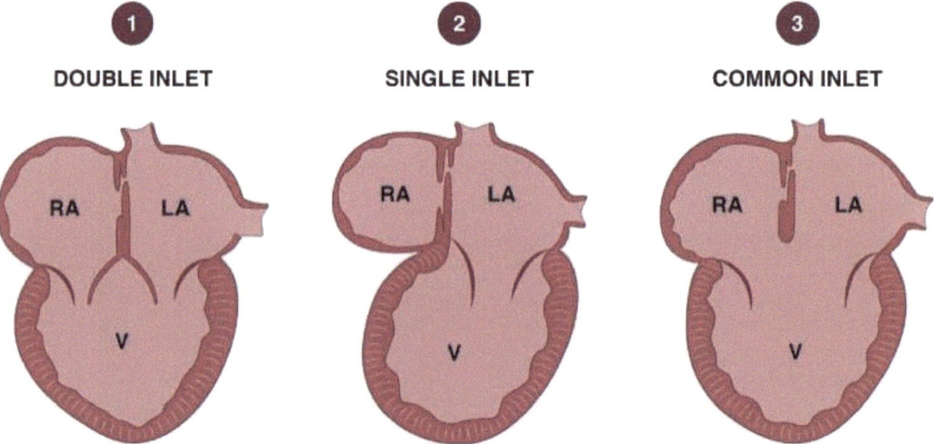

Fig. (4). Types of univentricular atrioventricular (AV) connection: 1- double-inlet (both valves connect to a main ventricular chamber); 2- single-inlet (absent left AV connection or absent right AV connection, the latter one is demonstrated in this figure); 3- common inlet (single AV valve). LA: left atrium; RA: right atrium; V: dominant ventricle.

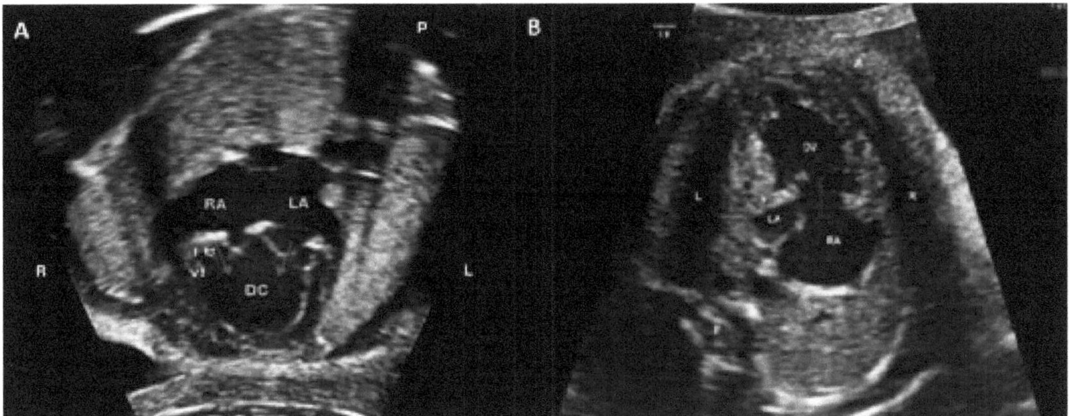

Fig. (5). Fetal echocardiogram demonstrating: **(A)** an univentricular AV connection with double-inlet LV in a fetus with 34 weeks of gestation and **(B)** an univentricular AV connection with single-inlet RV at 28 weeks' gestation. DC: dominant chamber; LA: left atrium; RA: right atrium; DV: dominant ventricle; *: rudimentary ventricle; R: right; L: left: P: posterior; A: anterior.

In univentricular hearts, any type of the following ventriculoarterial connections can exist: concordant connection, discordant connection, double-outlet from the dominant chamber or from the rudimentary chamber, and single outflow. In the setting of univentricular hearts with LV morphology, the double-inlet ventricle is almost always associated with a dominant morphologic LV. In such situation, the double-inlet LV with the discordant ventriculoarterial connection is the most common type (classical form of a "functional single ventricle") [13]. Subaortic obstruction, pulmonary outflow tract obstruction, and conduction abnormalities are common associations with double-inlet LV. In rare cases of double-inlet LV, the ventriculoarterial connection is concordant, which is known as "Holmes's heart" as it was first published by Andrew F. Holmes in 1901 [14]. In univentricular hearts with RV morphology, the double-inlet right ventricle is extremely rare and the double-outlet is instead common. In hearts with a common-inlet AV connection, the dominant ventricle is almost always of right ventricular morphology. Common-inlet right ventricle occurs much less frequently (12%) than double-inlet LV (88%) [15]. In cases of an absent (single-inlet) AV connection, the most frequent type is the tricuspid atresia in which the pulmonary artery arises from the morphologically right chamber and the left ventricle gives origin to the aorta.

Prenatal Diagnosis

For diagnosing the univentricular heart by an ultrasound, the four-chamber view is the most important plane. In normal hearts, the size of the left and right chambers is similar; however, in the third trimester, mild right–left asymmetry can be a normal variant (RV/LV ratio < 1.5). In cases of a "functionally single ventricle," the ventricles are asymmetric, one being dominant and the other being small and unfunctional. In rare cases, there is only one ventricular chamber (classically a "single ventricle"). The ventricular septum is absent or rudimentary.

Using the four-chamber view, the morphological characteristics of each ventricular chamber can be analyzed, enabling the assessment of the morphological characteristics of the dominant ventricle (LV, RV, or indeterminate) and the type of atrioventricular connection (double-inlet, single-inlet or absent AV connection, and common inlet). The best morphological criteria for identifying the dominant ventricle as an RV chamber is the presence of the moderator band crossing the ventricular cavity. The LV has fine trabeculations and in general is positioned posteroinferiorly. Rarely, the ventricular mass is a truly solitary chamber with indeterminate morphology [16, 17]. Qualitative assessment of the AV valve(s) should be done using the four-chamber view. In addition, the cardiac axis can be calculated on such view of the fetal heart during the first trimester of gestation and is considered as normal at 45+/−20° (Fig. **6**). An abnormal axis is associated with several CHDs, especially in univentricular hearts and conotruncal anomalies [18].

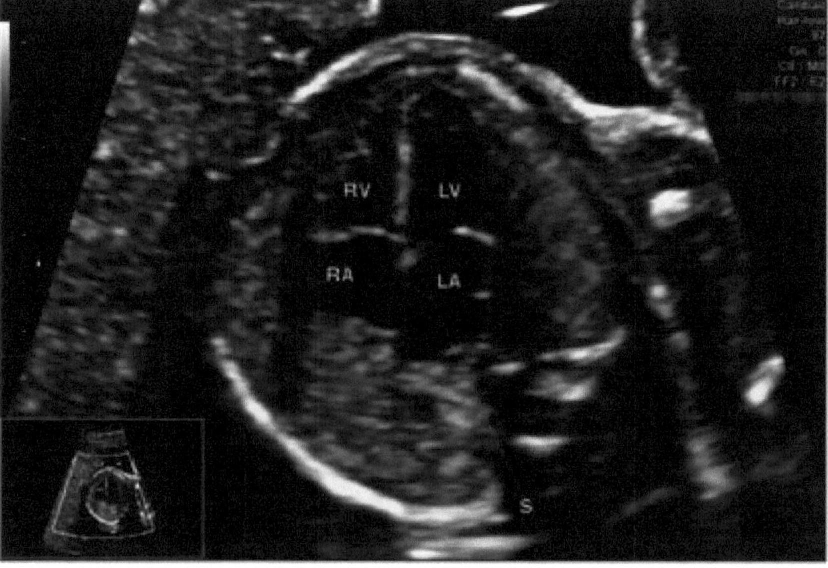

Fig. (6). Image showing how to measure the cardiac axis in the four-chamber view by fetal echocardiogram. The cardiac axis is obtained by measuring the angle between a line drawn from the spine (S) to the anterior chest wall and a second line drawn through the interventricular septum. LA: left atrium; LV: left ventricle; RA: right atrium; RV: right ventricle.

Identifying the type of ventriculoarterial connections is possible by the outflow tract view, and PW and/or color Doppler should be used to detect if there is any outflow tract obstruction (aortic or pulmonary atresia or of stenosis). If the great arteries are normally related, the pulmonary artery crosses over the ascending aorta. However, when the great arteries are in a transposed or a malposed relationship, the aorta and pulmonary arteries run in parallel. In addition, the three-vessel view (3VV) may demonstrate the relationship and the size of the pulmonary artery, the aorta, and the superior vena cava. The presence of two vessels instead of three in the 3VV should draw attention to a transposed relationship of the great arteries (anterior aorta) or some forms of double-outlet RV with malposed great arteries [19, 20]. In normal hearts, the pulmonary artery trunk is larger than the aorta and the superior vena cava (SVC) is smaller than the latter; therefore, the reduced caliber of the pulmonary artery or the aorta should raise the suspicion of stenosis or even hypoplasia if the diameter expressed by Z-score is below −2.0 (Fig. **7**). The presence of a reversed flow in the pulmonary trunk or the aorta shown by a color Doppler in 3VV indicates critical stenosis or atresia [20, 21] (Fig. **8**).

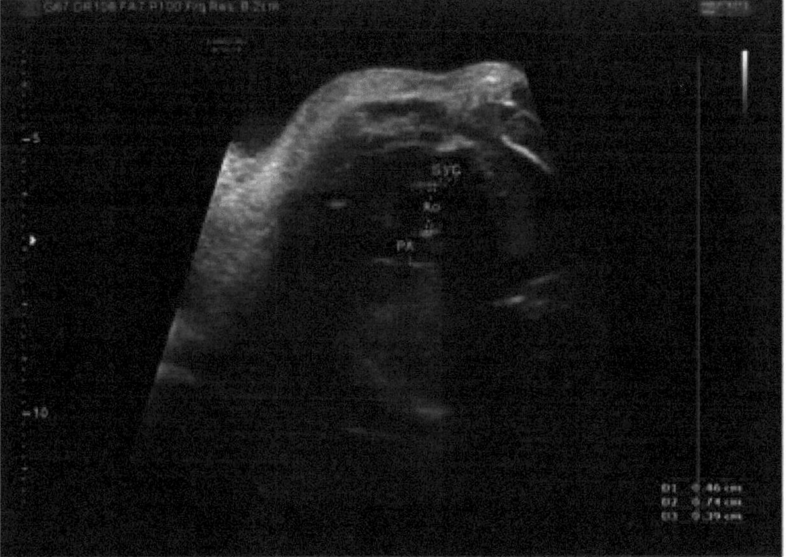

Fig. (7). The three-vessels view showing the relationship and the size of pulmonary artery, aorta and superior vena cava (three vessels). The pulmonary artery, to the left is smaller than aorta and the size of superior vena cava is smaller than aorta in case of univentricular connection with pulmonary stenosis and a normal relationship of the great arteries. SVC: superior vena cava; Ao: aorta; PA: pulmonary artery.

The Z-scores are in fact a very helpful tool to screen RV or LV hypoplasia and outflow tract anomalies, with values < −2.0 being considered as hypoplasia. The RV and LV widths and lengths should be measured at the end of diastole in a four-chamber cardiac view and can be expressed as Z-scores for gestational age. The maximal ventricular width should be measured from the inner edge-to- inner edge of such ventricle at the end of diastole. The maximal length of a ventricle is measured from the AV valve to the apex of such ventricle (Fig. **9**) [22, 23].

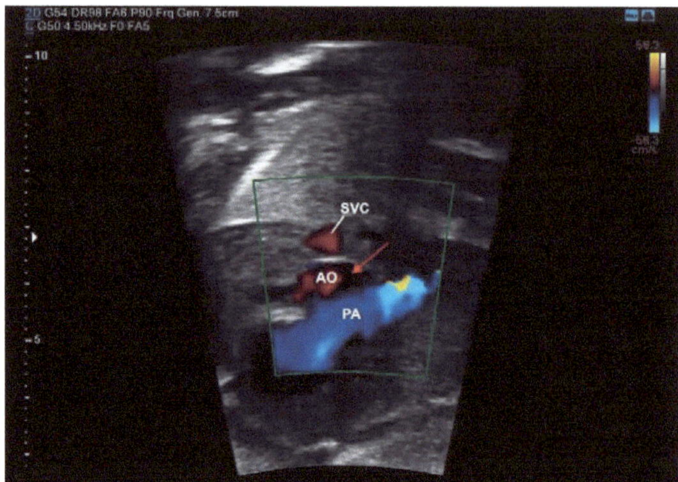

Fig. (8). Image showing by color Doppler the presence of reversed flow (red arrow) in aorta (critical aortic stenosis) and a with small size of such vessel in 3VV view. SVC: superior vena cava; AO: aorta; PA: pulmonary artery.

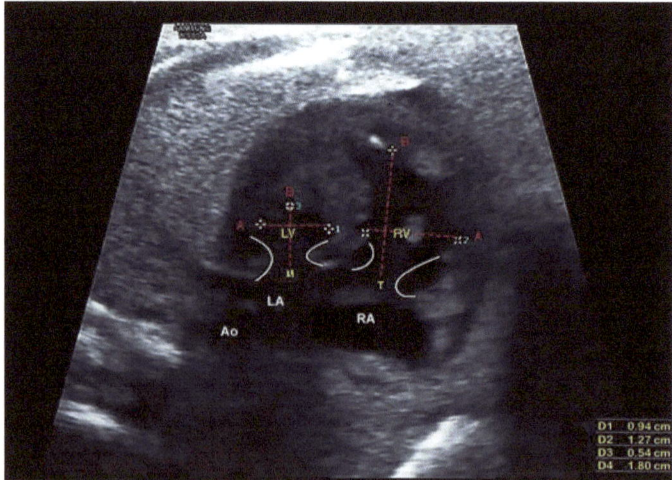

Fig. (9). Image demonstrating how to measure the ventricular chamber width and the ventricle length in the four-chamber view at the late diastole. Note the hypoplastic LV in this figure. A- ventricle width: from the inner edge to inner edge of each ventricle at the end of diastole. B- ventricle length: from the midpoint of the atrioventricular (AV) valve to the endocardial border at the apex of each ventricle at the end of diastole. LA: left atrium; LV: left ventricle; RA: right atrium; RV: right ventricle; M; mitral valve; T: tricuspid valve; Ao: aorta.

Advanced sonographic technologies such as three- and four-dimensional spatiotemporal image correlation (STIC) acquisition or fetal intelligent navigation echocardiography (FINE or 5D-heart) may improve the prenatal diagnosis of such complex CHDs. The novel method FINE automatically generates nine standard fetal echocardiography views from volume datasets obtained by spatiotemporal image correlation that reduces operator dependency. In both techniques, the cardiac volumes can be obtained and reanalyzed offline or even by consulting experts using the internet [24, 25].

In Utero and Postnatal Management

In utero, the existence of a "single ventricle" per se generally does not present a significant hemodynamic change in the fetus. If the diagnosis of univentricular AV connection is made during the first trimester, termination of pregnancy may be chosen in countries where legal abortions can be performed. The parental counseling should include the steps of planning of postnatal surgical procedures that are performed for such fetuses. However, some of the ventricular inflow anomalies may be progressive *in utero*, resulting in hypoplasia of the AV valve and consequently ventricular hypoplasia, which will result in a univentricular circulation after birth.

After birth, the hemodynamics of the univentricular heart depends on other associated anomalies. Perinatal cardiologists not only diagnose CHDs, but should be able to plan the delivery management of newborns with a prenatal diagnosis of cardiac malformations [26 - 28]. Depending on the outflow tracts, the newborns may require palliative surgery with PA banding or systemic-pulmonary shunt (Blalock–Taussig operation) (Fig. **10** and **11**). A surgical anastomosis between the SVC and pulmonary arteries (the Glenn operation) is performed between 3 and 6 months of age, and the final stage is completed by directing the flow of the inferior vena cava to the pulmonary circulation (the Fontan operation), generally at 2–4 years of age (Fig. **12** and **13**) [29].

ATRIOVENTRICULAR VALVES: STRADDLING AND OVERRIDING

Straddling is the condition in which the tension apparatus of the AV valve is attached to the crest of the ventricular septum or crosses the ventricular septal defect to attach the septum or the papillary muscle of the opposite ventricle. The classification of the anatomic severity of straddling is based on the chordal insertions in the contralateral ventricle as follows: A- into the crest of the ventricular septum, B- along the body of the ventricular septum, and C- onto the ventricular free wall (Fig. **14**). In general, the straddling of the AV valve requires a malalignment or an inlet ventricular septal defect.

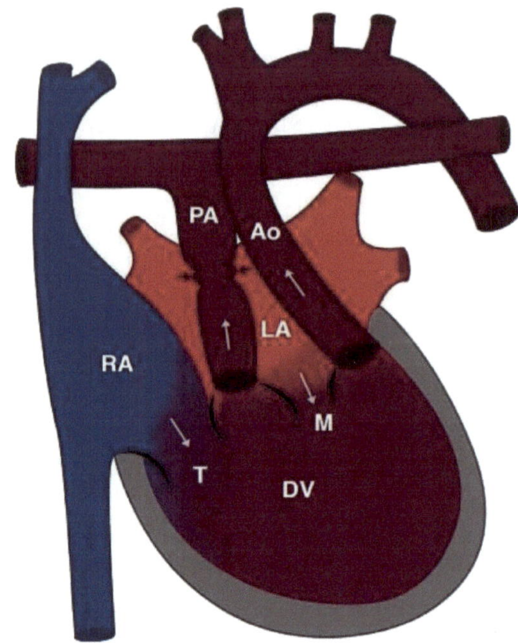

Fig. (10). Pulmonary artery banding is a palliative surgical procedure that involves the insertion of a band around the pulmonary artery (black arrows) to reduce blood flow in lungs in cases of "univentricular AV connection" in which the pulmonary flow is unrestricted. RA: right atrium; LA: left atrium; PA: pulmonary artery; Ao: aorta; M: mitral valve; T: tricuspid valve; DV: dominant ventricle.

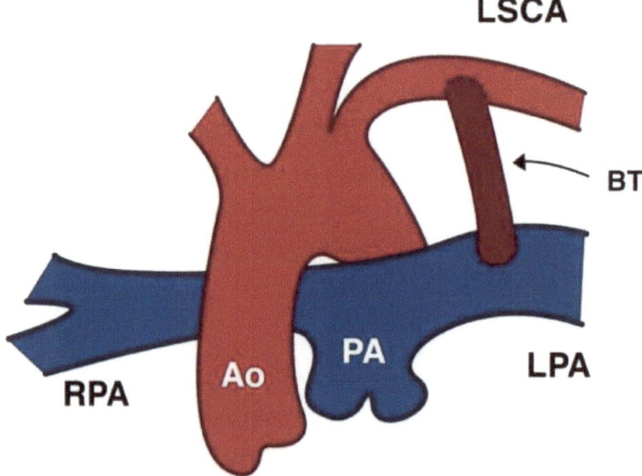

Fig. (11). Modified Blalock–Taussig surgical procedure is shown in black arrow (systemic-pulmonary shunt: anastomosis between the left subclavian artery and the pulmonary artery with a polytetrafluoroethylene graft). LSCA: left subclavian artery; Ao: aorta; PA; pulmonary artery; LPA: left pulmonary artery; RPA: right pulmonary artery; BT: Blalock–Taussig.

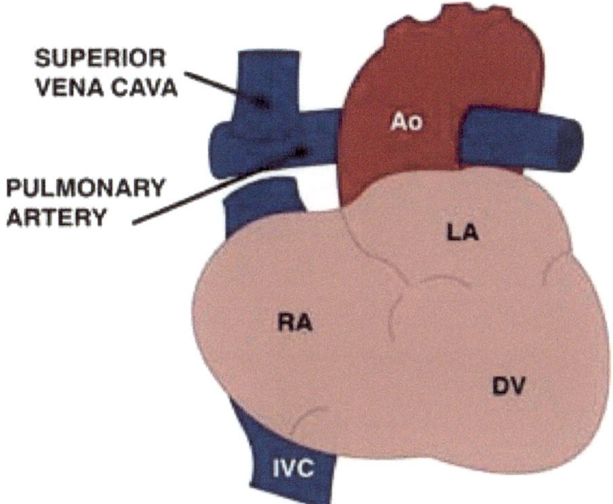

Fig. (12). Glenn procedure: an end-to-side anastomosis of the divided superior vena cava to the undivided pulmonary artery. IVC: inferior vena cava; Ao: aorta; PA; pulmonary artery; RA: right atrium; LA: left atrium; DV: dominant ventricle.

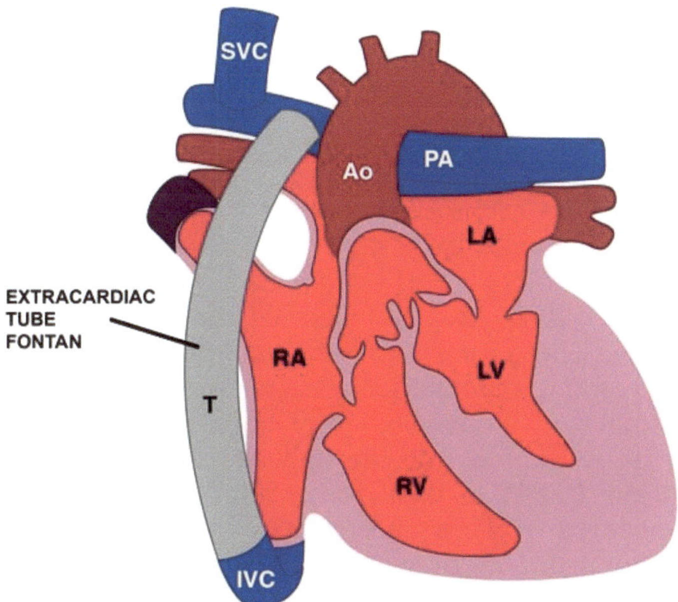

Fig. (13). Fontan operation (anastomosis between the inferior vena cava and pulmonary circulation) by an extracardiac tube. T: extracardiac tube; SVC: superior vena cava; Ao: aorta; PA: pulmonary artery; IVC: inferior vena cava; RA: right atrium; LA: left atrium; RV: right ventricle; LV: left ventricle.

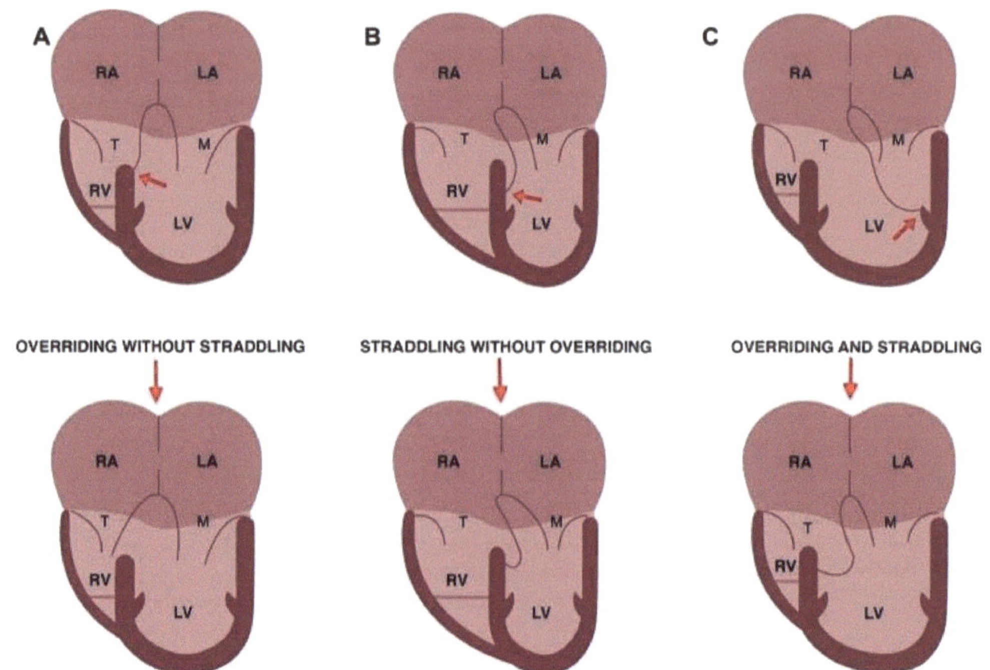

Fig. (14). Schematic illustration of the types of straddling of an atrioventricular (AV) valve based on the chordal insertions (red arrows): **A-** into the crest of the ventricular septum; **B-** along the septum of the contralateral ventricle and **C-** onto the opposite ventricle (papillary muscle). The other three figures show examples of: overriding of an AV valve without straddling, straddling without overriding and overriding with straddling. RA: right atrium; LA: left atrium; M: mitral valve; T: tricuspid valve; LV: left dominant ventricle; RV: right rudimentary ventricle.

Overriding of inlet valves may be defined as a condition in which an atrioventricular valve opens astride the septum with biventricular emptying. In this condition, the atrium and ventricular septa are misaligned due to a lateral shift, a rotational shift, or a combination of both. Depending on the degree of commitment of the AV valve with the opposite ventricle, overriding may be minor (<50%), major (50%), or double-inlet left or right ventricle (>50%). For determining the atrioventricular connections, an atrium is considered to join the ventricle when more than 50% of an AV valve empties in only one of the both ventricles (double-inlet AV connection) [30, 31]. However, in cases of a common AV valve, the double-inlet ventricle is considered when the atrioventricular junction is shared by >75% to one ventricle [30, 31]. Although hearts with a double-inlet ventricle have some relationships between the dominant and rudimentary ventricles, the most frequent pattern is a double-inlet to a dominant LV with rudimentary RV. Double-inlet LV with concordant ventriculoarterial connection is an important pattern, namely Holmes's heart [14, 31].

The ultrasound diagnosis of straddling and overriding of an AV valve in fetuses is based on the four chamber view and the features are as follows: 1- atrial and ventricular septa malalignment (no linear relationship between atrial and ventricular septa), 2- overriding: AV valve cusps are connected to both ventricles with a large inlet ventricular septal defect, 3- ventricular asymmetry, 4- straddling: anomalous insertions of the chordae tendineae of an AV wave into the ventricular septum or the papillary muscle of the contralateral ventricle, and 5- color Doppler enables the assessment of the emptying mode of the atrium into ventricles (Fig. **15**).

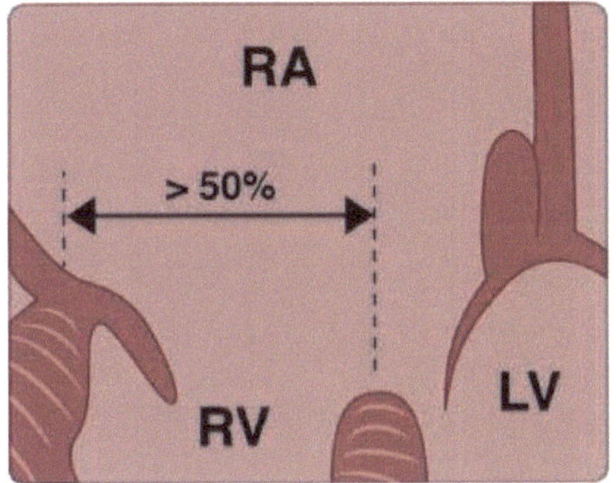

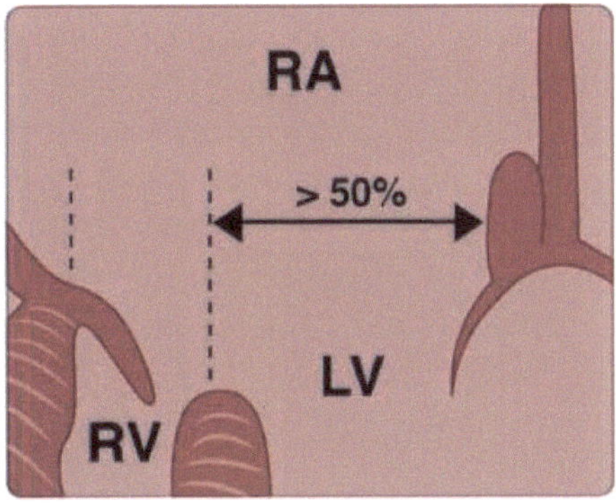

Fig. (15). Illustration of the determination of the atrioventricular (AV) connection based on the 50% rule. When an AV valve overrides >50% there is a double-inlet AV connection. RA: right atrium; RV: right ventricle; LV: left ventricle.

The cardiac anomalies most frequently associated with the straddling of an AV valve are ventricular double-outlet, malposition of great arteries, and L- or D-transposition of great arteries. In addition, overriding may or may not coexist with straddling.

Sequential fetal cardiac ultrasound or echocardiogram evaluation is recommended due to the hypoplastic left or right ventricle depending on which AV valve has straddling and/or overriding. After delivery, patients with straddling and/or overriding of an AV valve may require surgery, and the delivery must be planned at term in a hospital with pediatric cardiology and cardiac surgery team [26 - 28, 30]. Depending on the severity of the hypoplasia of the left or right ventricle chamber and the degree of obstruction of the ventricular outflow tract, these patients will require catheter or surgical intervention during the neonatal period. Commonly, patients with straddling of the left or right AV valve into the contralateral ventricle and/or major overriding are subjected to a univentricular surgical approach.

CRISSCROSS HEART

Crisscross heart is a rare CHD occurring in <0.1% of full-term live births [32, 33]. It results from an abnormal rotation of the ventricular mass along its longitudinal axis, during early cardiogenesis [32, 33]. As a result, the ventricles have a superoinferior relationship, in which the right morphologically ventricle (RMV) is often the superior ventricle and the left morphologically ventricle (LMV) is the inferior one, resulting in a crossing flow through the AV valves [32 - 34]. In normal hearts, the ventricular inlet flows are in a parallel relationship, whereas crisscross hearts are characterized by a crossing through the AV valves. In patients with atrial situs solitus and D-looped ventricles, the right atrium opens into the RMV (superior) and the left atrium opens into the LMV (inferior) with AV concordance. In contrast, in patients with situs solitus of the atria with L-looped ventricles, the systemic venous return (right atrium) is related to a LMV that is located superiorly, and the pulmonary venous return (left atrium) drains into the RMV (AV discordance). As the ventricles are arranged in a superoinferior relationship, it produces a crossed spatial atrioventricular arrangement (Fig. **16**). The VA connections may be discordant, double-outlet right ventricle, and discordant. In general, the subpulmonary infundibulum is deficient and the subaortic infundibulum is present when the great arteries are transposed [35].

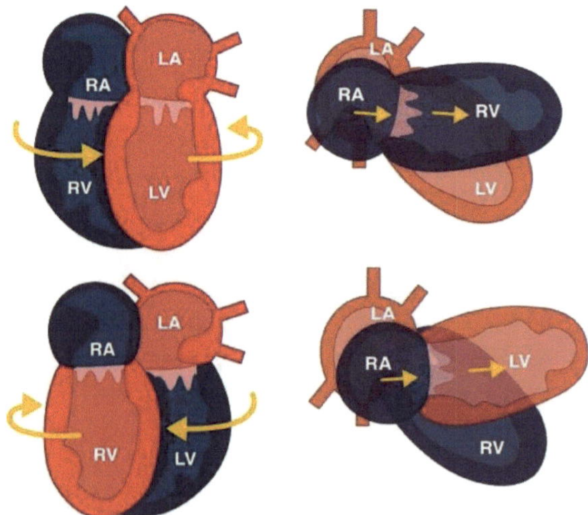

Fig. (16). In "criss-cross hearts" the ventricular inlet flows are crisscrossed and the ventricles are arranged in a superoinferior relationship. In D-looped ventricles: the right ventricle is superior and the left one is the inferior. In contrast, in L-lopped ventricles, there is atrioventricular (AV) discordance as the left ventricle is located superiorly. RA: right atrium; RV: right ventricle; LA: left atrium; LV: left ventricle.

This anomaly was first described by Lev and Rowaltt; however, the term crisscross heart was introduced subsequently [34, 36]. The cause of such complex

CHD remains unknown; however, some studies have demonstrated a link between Cx43 gene mutation and its pathogenesis [37]. In general, this complex CHD is associated with other cardiac anomalies such as large ventricular septal defect, straddling of mitral or tricuspid valve, subaortic stenosis, arch aortic obstruction, mitral stenosis, and ventriculoarterial (VA) connection abnormalities (such as discordant VA connection or double right ventricular outflow tract) [38, 39]. In rare cases, the great arteries are normally related and even more rarely the ventricular septum is intact [40]. Conversely, hypoplasia of the tricuspid valve and the right ventricle associated with pulmonary stenosis are common associated cardiac anomalies [41].

The differential diagnosis of crisscross hearts includes severe forms of Ebstein's anomaly of the tricuspid valve, in which the tricuspid valve opens into the infundibulum, some forms of straddling of the AV valves, and double-outlet of the atrium where one AV valve appears to cross the other one. In addition, superoinferior ventricles and crisscross are not synonymous. Although the ventricles are in a superoinferior relationship in crisscross hearts, the atrioventricular connections are crisscrossed.

Prenatal diagnosis of crisscross hearts is possible using fetal echocardiography. An inability to visualize simultaneously the tricuspid and the mitral valves in the standard 4-chamber plane with a transverse section should draw attention of the sonographer to suspect such a diagnosis. When the AV valves are not on the same level, the diagnosis becomes difficult, producing false images of the mitral valve or tricuspid atresia (Fig. **17**). By tilting the transducer from the upper abdomen to the chest of the fetus, the four-chamber view can be obtained only with a sagittal section of the fetal chest. Sequentially, the identification of the ventricles' inlet in a superior–inferior relationship, the horizontal interventricular septum, and the ventricular inlet flow in a cross shape enable making this diagnosis. In addition, the use of color Doppler facilitates better spatial visualization of the two ventricular inflow tracts in a cross shape [42]. Furthermore, the 3- or 4-dimensional ultrasound with color Doppler (HD live flow) shows simultaneously the crossing bloodstreams of the two ventricular inlets in the four-chamber view, facilitating the prenatal diagnosis of "crisscross heart" [43, 44].

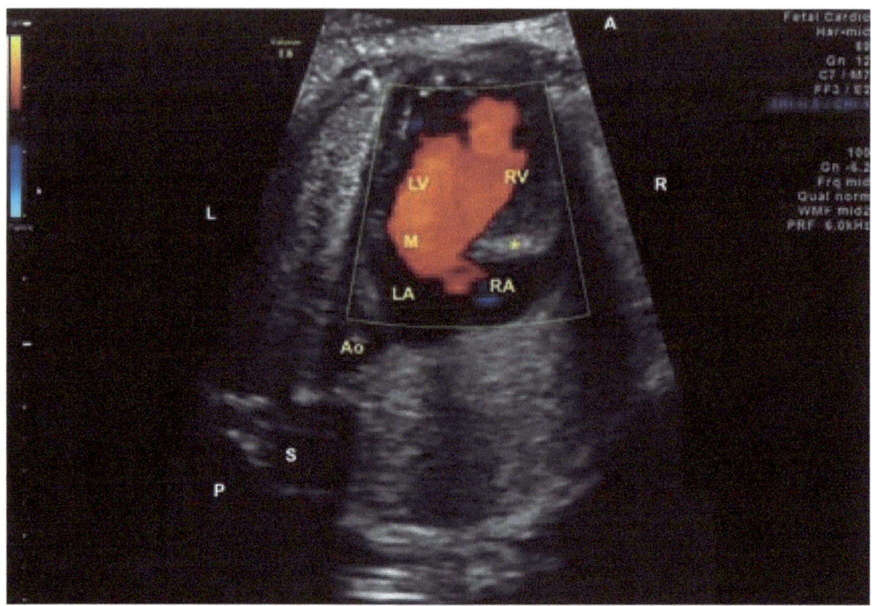

Fig. (17). Fetal echocardiogram showing a crisscross heart. Note the inability to visualize simultaneously tricuspid and mitral valve in the 4-chamber view. RA: right atrium; RV: right ventricle; LA: left atrium; LV: left ventricle; M: mitral valve; *: "false tricuspid atresia"; Ao: aorta; S: spine; P: posterior; A: anterior; L: left; R: right.

In Utero and postnatal management depends on the associated cardiac anomalies. Several cases with pulmonary stenosis may progress to pulmonary atresia during fetal life, and sequential fetal echocardiograms must be performed. After birth, magnetic resonance imaging could add to the anatomic details of echocardiography. Depending on the associated cardiac anomalies, neonates with crossed ventricles may present with cyanosis and a systolic murmur. Postnatally, only a small minority of these patients are suitable for a two-ventricle repair due to the hypoplasia of the tricuspid valve and the right ventricle. In cases of critical pulmonary stenosis or atresia, prostaglandin E1 should be given at birth until the surgical systemic-pulmonary shunt (Blalock–Taussig procedure) is performed because pulmonary blood perfusion is ductal-dependent [26 - 28, 45]. If biventricular repair is possible, ventricular septal defect can be closed. If the great arteries are transposed, an atrial switch or an arterial switch (Jatene's procedure) should be added the surgical repair of the ventricular septal defect. In fact, in cases with an intact interventricular septum and in the absence of other associated cardiac anomalies, there will be no symptoms and surgical treatment will not be required [35, 40].

CONCLUSION

- Univentricular atrioventricular connections: 1- one dominant ventricle (RV or LV) and one rudimentary ventricular chamber, rarely solitary (indeterminate ventricle); 2- the types of univentricular AV connections are: double-inlet ventricle (both valves connect to a main chamber), single-inlet or absent AV connection (complete obstruction to the flow from the atrium to the ventricular chamber) and a common AV connection (single AV valve); 3- the double-inlet LV with discordant ventriculoarterial connection is the most common type, in which the LV is located inferiorly and posteriorly; and 5- the four-chamber view is the most important plane for making a prenatal diagnosis, thereby enabling the assessment of the morphological characteristics of the dominant ventricle and the type of the atrioventricular connection.

- Straddling and overriding: 1- Straddling is the condition in which the tension apparatus of the AV valve straddles the ventricular septum; 2- Overriding of inlet valves is the condition in which an atrioventricular valve opens astride the septum with biventricular emptying. The overriding valve is assigned to the same ventricle (double-inlet ventricle: 50% or >75% in cases of common AV valve); and 3- ultrasound diagnosis of straddling and overriding of an AV valve in fetuses is based on the 4- chamber view.

- Crisscross: 1- Crisscross hearts are characterized by crossing flow through the AV valves as the ventricles are in a superoinferior relationship; 2- an inability to visualize simultaneously the tricuspid and mitral valves in the standard 4-chamber plane with a transverse section should raise the suspicion of such diagnosis; and 3- ventricles in a superoinferior relationship and the two ventricular inflow tracts (color Doppler) in a cross shape are the clues for this diagnosis.

CONSENT FOR PUBLICATION

Not applicable.

CONFLICT OF INTEREST

The authors confirm that the contents of this chapter have no conflict of interest.

ACKNOWLEDGEMENT

I acknowledge Liana Bravo-Valenzuela e Silva graphic designer at Pedicor Pediatric Cardiology center in Brazil for editing figures to this chapter.

REFERENCES

[1]   Dolk H, Loane M, Garne E. Congenital heart defects in Europe: prevalence and perinatal mortality,

2000 to 2005. Circulation 2011; 123(8): 841-9.
[http://dx.doi.org/10.1161/CIRCULATIONAHA.110.958405] [PMID: 21321151]

[2]   Hoffman JIe. The global burden of congenital heart disease. Cardiovasc J Afr 2013; 24(4): 141-5.
[http://dx.doi.org/10.5830/CVJA-2013-028] [PMID: 24217047]

[3]   Corno AF. "Functionally" univentricular hearts: impact of pre-natal diagnosis. Front Pediatr 2015; 3: 15.
[http://dx.doi.org/10.3389/fped.2015.00015] [PMID: 25774365]

[4]   Zhang YF, Zeng XL, Zhao EF, Lu HW. Diagnostic value of fetal echocardiography for congenital heart disease: a systematic review and meta-analysis. Medicine (Baltimore) 2015; 94(42): e1759.
[http://dx.doi.org/10.1097/MD.0000000000001759] [PMID: 26496297]

[5]   Hoffman JI, Kaplan S. The incidence of congenital heart disease. J Am Coll Cardiol 2002; 39(12): 1890-900.
[http://dx.doi.org/10.1016/S0735-1097(02)01886-7] [PMID: 12084585]

[6]   Vanpraagh R, Ongley PA, Swan HJ. Anatomic types of single or common ventricle in man: morphologic and geometric aspects of 60 necropsied cases. Am J Cardiol 1964; 13: 367-86.
[http://dx.doi.org/10.1016/0002-9149(64)90453-9] [PMID: 14128647]

[7]   Anderson RH, Becker AE, Wilkinson JL. Proceedings: Morphogenesis and nomenclature of univentricular hearts. Br Heart J 1975; 37(7): 781-2.
[PMID: 1156496]

[8]   Anderson RH, Cook AC. Morphology of the functionally univentricular heart. Cardiol Young 2004; 14 (Suppl. 1): 3-12.
[http://dx.doi.org/10.1017/S1047951104006237] [PMID: 15244133]

[9]   Wilkinson JL, Anderson RH. Anatomy of functionally single ventricle. World J Pediatr Congenit Heart Surg 2012; 3(2): 159-64.
[http://dx.doi.org/10.1177/2150135111421508] [PMID: 23804770]

[10]   Vanpraagh R, Vanpraagh S, Vlad P, Keith JD. Diagnosis of the anatomic types of single or common ventricle. Am J Cardiol 1965; 15: 345-66.
[http://dx.doi.org/10.1016/0002-9149(65)90329-2] [PMID: 14263032]

[11]   Tynan MJ, Becker AE, Macartney FJ, Jiménez MQ, Shinebourne EA, Anderson RH. Nomenclature and classification of congenital heart disease. Br Heart J 1979; 41(5): 544-53.
[http://dx.doi.org/10.1136/hrt.41.5.544] [PMID: 465224]

[12]   Anderson RH, Shinebourne EA, Gerlis LM. Criss-cross atrioventricular relationships producing paradoxical atrioventricular concordance or discordance. Their significance to nomenclature of congenital heart disease. Circulation 1974; 50(1): 176-80.
[http://dx.doi.org/10.1161/01.CIR.50.1.176] [PMID: 4835263]

[13]   Muñoz-Castellaños L, Espinola-Zavaleta N, Keirns C. Anatomoechocardiographic correlation double inlet left ventricle. J Am Soc Echocardiogr 2005; 18(3): 237-43.
[http://dx.doi.org/10.1016/j.echo.2004.11.009] [PMID: 15746713]

[14]   Dobell AR, Van Praagh R. The Holmes heart: historic associations and pathologic anatomy. Am Heart J 1996; 132(2 Pt 1): 437-45.
[http://dx.doi.org/10.1016/S0002-8703(96)90443-3] [PMID: 8701908]

[15]   Shiraishi H, Silverman NH. Echocardiographic spectrum of double inlet ventricle: evaluation of the interventricular communication. J Am Coll Cardiol 1990; 15(6): 1401-8.
[http://dx.doi.org/10.1016/S0735-1097(10)80031-2] [PMID: 2329242]

[16]   Anderson RH, Tynan M, Freedom RM, *et al.* Ventricular morphology in the univentricular heart. Herz 1979; 4(2): 184-97.
[PMID: 447181]

[17]   Rigby ML, Anderson RH, Gibson D, Jones OD, Joseph MC, Shinebourne EA. Two dimensional echocardiographic categorisation of the univentricular heart. Ventricular morphology, type, and mode of atrioventricular connection. Br Heart J 1981; 46(6): 603-12.
[http://dx.doi.org/10.1136/hrt.46.6.603] [PMID: 7317227]

[18]   Comstock CH. Normal fetal heart axis and position. Obstet Gynecol 1987; 70(2): 255-9.
[PMID: 3299186]

[19]   Tongsong T, Tongprasert F, Srisupundit K, Luewan S. The complete three-vessel view in prenatal detection of congenital heart defects. Prenat Diagn 2010; 30(1): 23-9.
[PMID: 19911415]

[20]   Yoo SJ, Lee YH, Kim ES, *et al.* Three-vessel view of the fetal upper mediastinum: an easy means of detecting abnormalities of the ventricular outflow tracts and great arteries during obstetric screening. Ultrasound Obstet Gynecol 1997; 9(3): 173-82.
[http://dx.doi.org/10.1046/j.1469-0705.1997.09030173.x] [PMID: 9165680]

[21]   Bravo-Valenzuela NJ, Peixoto AB, Araujo Júnior E. Prenatal diagnosis of congenital heart disease: A review of current knowledge. Indian Heart J 2018; 70(1): 150-64.
[http://dx.doi.org/10.1016/j.ihj.2017.12.005] [PMID: 29455772]

[22]   Schneider C, McCrindle BW, Carvalho JS, Hornberger LK, McCarthy KP, Daubeney PE. Development of Z-scores for fetal cardiac dimensions from echocardiography. Ultrasound Obstet Gynecol 2005; 26(6): 599-605.
[http://dx.doi.org/10.1002/uog.2597] [PMID: 16254878]

[23]   Pasquini L, Mellander M, Seale A, *et al.* Z-scores of the fetal aortic isthmus and duct: an aid to assessing arch hypoplasia. Ultrasound Obstet Gynecol 2007; 29(6): 628-33.
[http://dx.doi.org/10.1002/uog.4021] [PMID: 17476706]

[24]   Rizzo G, Capponi A, Cavicchioni O, Vendola M, Pietrolucci ME, Arduini D. Application of automated sonography on 4-dimensional volumes of fetuses with transposition of the great arteries. J Ultrasound Med 2008; 27(5): 771-6.
[http://dx.doi.org/10.7863/jum.2008.27.5.771] [PMID: 18424653]

[25]   Yeo L, Romero R. Color and power Doppler combined with Fetal Intelligent Navigation Echocardiography (FINE) to evaluate the fetal heart. Ultrasound Obstet Gynecol 2017; 50(4): 476-91.
[http://dx.doi.org/10.1002/uog.17522] [PMID: 28809063]

[26]   Allan LD, Huggon IC. Counselling following a diagnosis of congenital heart disease. Prenat Diagn 2004; 24(13): 1136-42.
[http://dx.doi.org/10.1002/pd.1071] [PMID: 15614846]

[27]   Donofrio MT, Levy RJ, Schuette JJ, *et al.* Specialized delivery room planning for fetuses with critical congenital heart disease. Am J Cardiol 2013; 111(5): 737-47.
[http://dx.doi.org/10.1016/j.amjcard.2012.11.029] [PMID: 23291087]

[28]   Słodki M, Respondek-Liberska M, Pruetz JD, Donofrio MT. Fetal cardiology: changing the definition of critical heart disease in the newborn. J Perinatol 2016; 36(8): 575-80.
[http://dx.doi.org/10.1038/jp.2016.20] [PMID: 26963427]

[29]   Khairy P, Poirier N, Mercier LA. Univentricular heart. Circulation 2007; 115(6): 800-12.
[http://dx.doi.org/10.1161/CIRCULATIONAHA.105.592378] [PMID: 17296869]

[30]   Anderson RH, Macartney FJ. Classification and Nomenclature of Congenital Heart Defects.Surgery for Congenital Heart Defects. 3rd ed. West Sussex: John Wiley & Sons 2006; pp. 3-11.
[http://dx.doi.org/10.1002/0470093188.ch1]

[31]   Edwards D, Maleszewski JJ. Classification and Terminology of Cardiovascular Anomalies.Moss & Adams's Heart Disease in Infants, Children and Adolescents. 28th ed. Baltimore, MD: Williams and Wilkins 2013; pp. 48-51.

[32]   Ngeh N, Api O, Iasci A, Ho SY, Carvalho JS. Criss-cross heart: report of three cases with double-inlet ventricles diagnosed *in utero*. Ultrasound Obstet Gynecol 2008; 31(4): 461-5.
[http://dx.doi.org/10.1002/uog.5300] [PMID: 18383472]

[33]   Fyler DC. Trends.Nadas' Pediatric Cardiology. 4th ed. Philadelphia, PA: Hanley & Belfus 1992; pp. 273-80.

[34]   Anderson RH, Shinebourne EA, Gerlis LM. Criss-cross atrioventricular relationships producing paradoxical atrioventricular concordance or discordance. Their significance to nomenclature of congenital heart disease. Circulation 1974; 50(1): 176-80.
[http://dx.doi.org/10.1161/01.CIR.50.1.176] [PMID: 4835263]

[35]   Marino B, Sanders SP, Pasquini L, Giannico S, Parness IA, Colan SD. Two-dimensional echocardiographic anatomy in crisscross heart. Am J Cardiol 1986; 58(3): 325-33.
[http://dx.doi.org/10.1016/0002-9149(86)90071-8] [PMID: 3739923]

[36]   Lev M, Rowlatt UF. The pathologic anatomy of mixed levocardia. A review of thirteen cases of atrial or ventricular inversion with or without corrected transposition. Am J Cardiol 1961; 8: 216-63.
[http://dx.doi.org/10.1016/0002-9149(61)90209-0] [PMID: 13761307]

[37]   Ya J, Erdtsieck-Ernste EB, de Boer PA, *et al.* Heart defects in connexin43-deficient mice. Circ Res 1998; 82(3): 360-6.
[http://dx.doi.org/10.1161/01.RES.82.3.360] [PMID: 9486664]

[38]   Anderson RH, Smith A, Wilkinson JL. Disharmony between atrioventricular connections and segmental combinations: unusual variants of "crisscross" hearts. J Am Coll Cardiol 1987; 10(6): 1274-7.
[http://dx.doi.org/10.1016/S0735-1097(87)80130-4] [PMID: 3680796]

[39]   Kim DY, Cho SR, Park SD, Chung HK. Double outlet of right in Criss-Cross heart: surgical experience of one case. Korean J Thorac Cardiovasc Surg 1997; 30: 1242-6.

[40]   Fontes VF, de Souza JA, Pontes Jùnior SC. Criss-cross heart with intact ventricular septum. Int J Cardiol 1990; 26(3): 382-5.
[http://dx.doi.org/10.1016/0167-5273(90)90102-B] [PMID: 2312210]

[41]   O'Leary PW, Hagler DJ. Cardiac Malpositions and Abnormalities of Atrial and Visceral Situs Anomalies.Moss & Adams's Heart Disease in Infants, Children and Adolescents. 28th ed. Baltimore, MD: Williams and Wilkins 2013; p. 201.

[42]   Ravi P, Fruitman D, Mills L, Colen T, Hornberger LK. Prenatal diagnosis of the criss-cross heart. Am J Cardiol 2017; 119(6): 916-22.
[http://dx.doi.org/10.1016/j.amjcard.2016.11.046] [PMID: 28215417]

[43]   Shirakawa A, Kaji T, Hayabuchi Y, Nakayama S, Maeda K, Irahara M. Prenatal three-dimensional color Doppler imaging showing crossover of the inflow streams of two ventricles in a case of criss-cross heart. J Echocardiogr 2017; 15(4): 191-3.
[http://dx.doi.org/10.1007/s12574-017-0339-3] [PMID: 28484959]

[44]   Tsukimori K, Kitadai Y, Kan N. Prenatal diagnosis of criss-cross heart using 4-dimensional color doppler rendering. Pediatr Cardiol 2019; 40(1): 237-9.
[http://dx.doi.org/10.1007/s00246-018-1990-9] [PMID: 30255311]

[45]   Oliveira ÍM, Aiello VD, Mindêllo MM, Martins YdeO, Pinto VC Jr. Criss-cross heart: report of two cases, anatomic and surgical description and literature review. Rev Bras Cir Cardiovasc 2013; 28(1): 93-102.
[http://dx.doi.org/10.5935/1678-9741.20130014] [PMID: 23739938]

CHAPTER 2

Fetal Myocardial and Pericardial Diseases

Ana B. Bianchi* and **Ihosvanny Gonzalez**

Maternal-Fetal Medicine Unit, Hospital Center "Pereira Rossell", Montevideo, Uruguay

Abstract: This chapter provides an overview of the most frequent pathologies of the myocardium and pericardium during fetal life. Considering that some of these pathologies constitute a group of uncommon conditions, they are of interest from the point of view of their prognostic and therapeutic value. Besides, they are also within the most striking pathologies found in the screening of the fetal heart, and the ones which cause greater anxiety in the family and professional environment. Progress has been made in different diagnostic techniques, outlining some therapeutic advancements, as well as in the importance of new technologies that allow to deepen our knowledge of the functional defects of the cardiac muscle during fetal life.

Keywords: Cardiomyopathies, Cardiac function, Cardiac tumors, Congenital heart defects, Ebstein disease, Fetus, Pericardial effusion, Strain, Speckle tracking, Ultrasound echocardiography, Ventricular dilatation, Ventricular diverticula, Ventricular hypertrophy.

INTRODUCTION

Congenital heart diseases (CHD) are the most frequent severe congenital malformations. They affect approximately 0.8-1% of the newborn population [1]. With the advances in technology, it is possible to visualize and examine the fetal heart from the onset of its formation in patients with a risk of developing some CHD. Knowledge of the anatomy of the cardiac structures and assessment of the images during fetal development allow an early diagnosis of certain congenital conditions with significant pathophysiological implications. It also allows to plan the moment of birth and work with a multidisciplinary team towards the best resolution and treatment of these newborns who, in spite of all the progress made in pediatric cardiac surgery, represent a global mortality of 15% and a substantial impact on the quality of life of the survivors and their families [1, 2].

*** Corresponding author Ana B Bianchi:** Maternal-Fetal Medicine Unit, Hospital Center "Pereira Rossell", Bulevar Artigas 1550, 11600, Montevideo, Uruguay; E-mail: anabbianchi@gmail.com

Edward Araujo Júnior, Nathalie Jeanne M. Bravo-Valenzuela and Alberto Borges Peixoto (Eds.)
All rights reserved-© 2020 Bentham Science Publishers

FETAL HEART SCREENING: STEPS TO FOLLOW

A complete and precise study of the fetal structural anatomy, cardiac function and blood vessels, as well as study of the physiology of the fetal cardiovascular system and heart rate, are necessary to detect malformation patterns and functional alterations. A complementary and essential part of the study is the assessment of the myocardial function, valvular insufficiencies and volume overloads, evaluating signs of heart failure that affect fetus development. On the other hand, the feto-placental circulation should also be observed to detect signs of inadequate oxygenation and lack of development and growth [3 - 9]. The presence of pericardial effusion should not be left aside (physiologic if less than 2 mm and if the atrioventricular level is not exceeded).

DEFINITION

Cardiomyopathies constitute a heterogeneous set of processes, which affect the cardiac muscle and cause a wide spectrum of cardiac dysfunctions. Fetal cardiomyopathy, whether primary or secondary in nature, represents up to 11% of the heart diseases diagnosed in the uterus [8 - 10]. The American Heart Association has proposed the following definition: "cardiomyopathies are a heterogeneous group of diseases of the myocardium associated with mechanical and/or electrical dysfunction which usually exhibit inappropriate ventricular hypertrophy or dilation, and are due to a variety of causes that frequently are genetic" [3]. The 1995 report from the World Health Organization (WHO) refers to cardiomyopathies as those "diseases of myocardium associated with cardiac dysfunction".

Cardiomyopathies are the main cause of global fetal cardiomegaly, and are classified according to the physiopathological model or by etiological/pathogenic factors. They are a disorder of the cardiac muscle, which may present as a primary disorder or may be associated with structural anomalies or pericardial disease. They constitute approximately 2% of the CHD in children born alive [10, 11].

Secondary fetal cardiomyopathy may be caused by a number of conditions, including fetal arrhythmias, structural heart disease, twin-to-twin transfusion syndrome, fetal anemia, fetal infection with myocarditis, and autoimmune maternal disorders. The *in utero* occurrence is reported to be between 8% and 11%. There are three different presentations in the fetus. The congestive or dilated form is the most common and presents with dilated, poorly contracting chambers, atrioventricular regurgitation and often, associated hydrops fetalis (pleural and pericardial effusions, ascites, and skin thickening) [1]. The second most common type of cardiomyopathy is the hypertrophic form. Hypertrophic cardiomyopathies are recognized by markedly thickened ventricular walls and septum. The third form, a restrictive cardiomyopathy, is unusual in the fetus, manifesting primarily as endocardial fibroelastosis [12]. Dilated cardiomyopathies can be divided into two categories. The first includes cardiomyopathies resulting from high-output failure caused by severe fetal anemias, or volume overload from massive arteriovenous shunting. The second one includes only cardiomyopathies.

ASSESSMENT OF CARDIOMEGALY

1- Cardiothoracic ratio. The diameter of the fetal heart should represent one-third of the thorax diameter,

2- Myocardial function. Measured by the systolic shortening fraction using the systolic shortening ratio that should reach values > 0.30,

3- Increase in atrial contractility identified in the ductus venosus flow with a zero or negative "a" wave in diastolic phase,

4- The presence of insufficiency of the tricuspid and mitral valves,

5- Pericardial effusion,

6- Hydrops fetalis.

GROWTH OF THE RIGHT AND LEFT ATRIUM

The growth of the right atrium may be due to different factors:

1- Tricuspid insufficiency,

2- Secondary to non-structural alterations, like tachycardia,

3- Extracardiac etiology, as in the case of arteriovenous malformations and constriction of the ductus arteriosus.

A rare extracardiac cause is the absence of ductus venosus when the umbilical vein is directly connected to the right atrium [9 - 15].

Intracardiac causes focus on two main possibilities: Ebstein's disease and tricuspid valve dysplasia. Ebstein's disease consists of a displacement of the septal and posterior tricuspid valve leaflets at the ventricular-atrial junction toward the right ventricle, with a reduction in the size of the functional ventricle caused by the atrialization of the inflow tract of that same ventricle and the thickened valves.

There is a rare pathology named idiopathic dilatation of the right atrium, where there is an excessive growth of the atrium of undefined cause, with a normal tricuspid ring and without regurgitation [16].

In the cases of growth of the left atrium, mitral regurgitation is a possible cause only if the flow through the foramen ovale is restricted. Other causes of mitral insufficiency are abnormalities intrinsic to the valve (infrequent) or secondary to severe obstructions of the aortic valve (stenosis or atresia).

VENTRICULAR DILATATIONS

The isolated dilatation of the right ventricle is observed in the agenesis of pulmonary valves, whereas the isolated dilatation of the left ventricle is observed in cases of severe aortic insufficiencies. When a segment of the heart is affected, as in the coarctation of the aorta, the interruption of the aortic arch and in total anomalous pulmonary vein drainage, the parts which affected are the right atrium and right ventricle. When faced with a total/partial cardiomegaly, it is important not only to look for cardiovascular causes, but also to consider its possible relation with extracardiac causes, and to make a comprehensive assessment of the fetus [17].

There are several etiologies and anatomical and functional features that lead to alterations in the heart function. Among them are viral and bacterial infections, congenital metabolic errors and maternal diabetes. Etiologies are also connected to viral diseases and infections, such as those caused by Parvovirus B19 and Coxsackie B, toxoplasmosis, syphilis, rubella, cytomegalovirus and herpes simplex (TORCH), being the most frequent causes [3, 4].

Severe fetal anemias result in high-output failure when the fetal heart increases the cardiac output, heart rate or ejection volume – or both – to solve the peripheral oxygen requirements. The arrhythmia-induced cardiomyopathy (tachycardia or bradycardia) is the most frequent cause of non-immune fetal hydrops [6, 7].

Fetal supraventricular tachycardia is the most frequent sustained fetal arrhythmia. It can present with congestive cardiomyopathy when the rapid heart rate results from a shortened diastole, so that myocardial perfusion (most of which occurs in diastole) is markedly decreased [18]. The identification of fetal arrhythmia is determined in the chronological relation between the contractions of the atria and ventricles. This identification can be done through Doppler techniques, like tissue imaging techniques, or more simply with the simultaneous registration of pulsed Doppler in the superior vena cava/ascending aorta or pulmonary artery/pulmonary vein. The superior vena cava/ascending aorta Doppler method provides a dynamic marker consisting of atrial (venous a 'wave') and ventricular contractions (aortic flow), which allows to perform a reliable analysis of the underlying mechanism of the arrhythmia [18, 19].

The direct damage to the myocardium, another cause of cardiomyopathy, includes fetal infection, tachycardia-induced cardiomyopathies and fetal anoxia. It is necessary to consider severe fetal hypoxias among the main causes of cardiomegaly due to decreased cardiac contractility.

OTHER CAUSES

• Inflammatory cardiomyopathy (myocarditis and cardiac dysfunction):

o Idiopathic,

o Autoimmune,

o Infectious (Chagas disease, human immunodeficiency virus, enterovirus, adenovirus, cytomegalovirus).

• Metabolic cardiomyopathy:

o Endocrine causes: thyrotoxicosis, hypothyroidism, adrenal insufficiency, pheochromocytoma, acromegaly, and diabetes mellitus;

o Storage and infiltrative diseases: hemochromatosis, glycogen storage disease, Hurler syndrome, Niemann-Pick disease, Fabry-Anderson disease, Hand-Schüller-Christian disease, Morquio-Ullrich disease;

o Deficiency diseases: alterations of potassium metabolism, magnesium deficiency, selenium deficiency, nutritional alterations, such as Kwashiorkor, anemia and beriberi;

o Primary and secondary amyloidosis. familial mediterranean fever.

• Cardiomyopathy due to systemic diseases:

o Connective tissue disease: systemic lupus erythematosus, polyarteritis nodosa, rheumatoid arthritis, scleroderma and dermatomyositis;

o Infiltrative and granulomatous diseases: sarcoidosis and leukemia.

• Cardiomyopathies due to muscular dystrophy:

o Duchenne, Myotonic dystrophy.

• Cardiomyopathy due to neuromuscular alterations:

o Friedreich's ataxia, Noonan syndrome.

• Cardiomyopathy due to toxic or sensitive reactions.

CARDIAC TUMORS

Cardiac tumors are rare in fetal life. In a series of more than 10,000 fetal explorations, 794 explorations detected a fetal cardiac disorder and 1.4% of these corresponded to fetal cardiac tumors [13]. Several retrospective studies of fetal echocardiography results revealed a prevalence of fetal cardiac tumors which ranged between 0.14% and 1.9%, and no metastatic heart tumors were found [14] Table **1**.

Table 1. Distribution of fetal cardiac tumors.

Rhabdomyoma 40–89%
Teratoma 15–19%
Fibroma 12–16%
Hemangioma 5%
Myxoma 2–4%
Angioma 5%
Lipoma very rare

Cardiac tumors are usually benign. They may be solitary or multiple, and arise from the left and right ventricles and the ventricular septum. Clinical manifestations of fetal heart tumors vary considerably from case to case. The affected fetus may be asymptomatic (especially when tumors are small) or present with ventricular/inflow obstruction, fetal hydrops, arrhythmias, congestive heart failure, or even sudden death.

Fetal pericardial teratomas are a significant etiology of pericardial effusion and fetal hydrops, and may lead to cardiac compression (affecting the right atrium, right ventricle, aorta, pulmonary artery, or superior vena cava), cardiac tamponade and fetal death [16]. A rapidly growing pericardial teratoma in a fetus can cause tamponade, which requires urgent fetal intervention; similar to a pericardial teratoma, a pericardial hemangioma can lead to congestive heart failure, pericardial effusion, thrombocytopenia, cardiac arrhythmias, tamponade and cardiac compression. Fetal tumors involving cardiac conduction systems are especially prone to cause cardiac block and severe arrhythmias [16, 17, 20 - 22].

Tuberous sclerosis was found in 76% of cases of fetal heart rhabdomyoma diagnosed prenatally or at autopsy; 21% of the complexes were familial and 79%

were sporadic [16]. The relationship between the tuberous complex and cardiac rhabdomyoma suggests that the cardiac tumor may be an early manifestation of the genetic disorder. Most cases of tuberous sclerosis can be attributed to a deletion mutation in the TSC2 and PKD1 genes [20].

Fibroids are less echogenic than rhabdomyomas, and unlike these, they present anechoic zones and have no genetic link. Hemangiomas present mixed echogenicity and are located predominantly in the base of the heart; on the other hand, teratomas protrude from ventricular walls and have heterogeneous aspect with solid cystic zones.

Tumors may evolve toward regression in the case of rhabdomyomas or hemangiomas, or toward a valvular obstruction with pericardial effusions, or lead to fetal hydrops and severe hemodynamic compromise in addition to fetal arrhythmias.

Fetal cardiac tumors are detectable between 20 and 30 weeks of gestation, without excluding the possibility of earlier diagnosis depending on the equipment and the expertise of the explorers [17]. The echocardiography plays an important role in the prenatal diagnosis of cardiac tumors (Fig. **1**) and may provide alternative findings related to tumors, such as cardiomegaly, pericardial effusions, arrhythmias, ventricular outflow tract obstruction, and hypokinesia. In addition, cardiac magnetic resonance imaging (MRI) may provide the necessary evidence for a differential diagnosis of benign and malignant tumors. However, fetal heart structure is not easily assessed by magnetic resonance imaging in a clinical setting, due to difficulties of synchronizing with the rapid heartbeat. Furthermore, infarcted and degenerative tissues within a pericardial hemangioma can cause misdiagnosis by computed tomography [1, 10]. Therefore, a definitive diagnosis will depend on the histological exams.

FETAL CARDIAC CIRCULATION

Thus, the right ventricle preferably maintains the thoracic and abdominal circulation by ductal arch while the left ventricle maintains the coronary and cerebral circulation by aortic arch. Therefore, both ventricles and arteries support the systemic pressure of the aorta [5]. Fetal circulation is completed by continuing with the abdominal aorta where the blood flow is distributed to the abdominal organs and iliac arteries and circulation of lower limbs. In this way, the fetal heart maintains a proportionate intrafetal circulation by transporting the O_2 saturated blood through its interauricular communication to the left heart, while the right heart uses the ductus arteriosus with the most desaturated blood to the descending aorta [15].

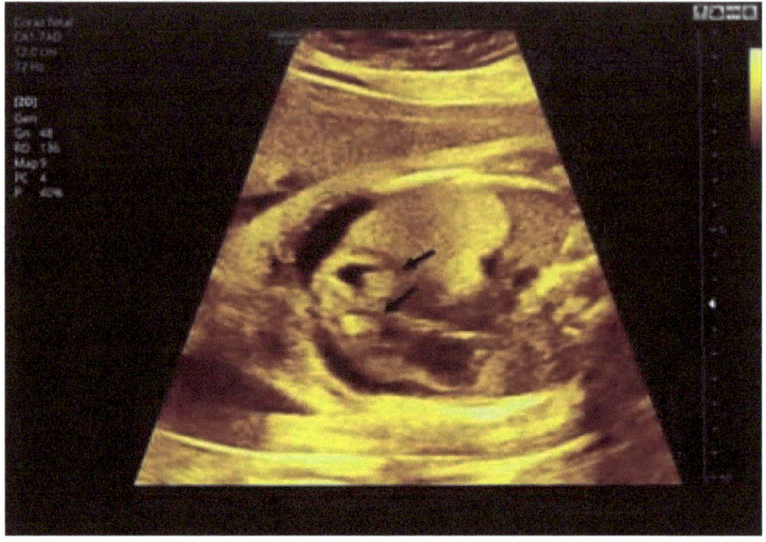

Fig. (1). Fetal cardiac tumors (arrows).

The inadequate contraction of the heart to maintain cardiac output and tissue perfusion causes fetal heart failure [23]. In this heart failure scenario, the fetus responds with peripheral vasoconstriction as a response to cardiovascular stress caused by an increase of catecholamines and natriuretic factor. The redistribution of the arterial flow and cardiac output is done to vital organs.

ULTRASOUND FINDINGS

Hypertrophic Cardiomyopathies

Hypertrophic cardiomyopathy presents with thickened ventricular walls arising from the enlargement of myocardial cells, resulting in decreased ventricular adaptability. This can lead to poor diastolic filling of the heart (diastolic dysfunction), which in turn leads to decreased cardiac output. Ventricular hypertrophy occurs in most recipient twins in twin-to-twin transfusion syndrome.

A familial history of cardiomyopathy, especially hypertrophic cases, can be the result of gene mutations whose inherited transmission is usually autosomal dominant (50% risk of transmission from a heterozygous parent). Prenatal identification of disorders, such as Marfan and Loeitz-Dietz syndromes causes dilation of the aortic root or valvular abnormalities that can lead to cardiomyopathy [12] (Fig. **2**).

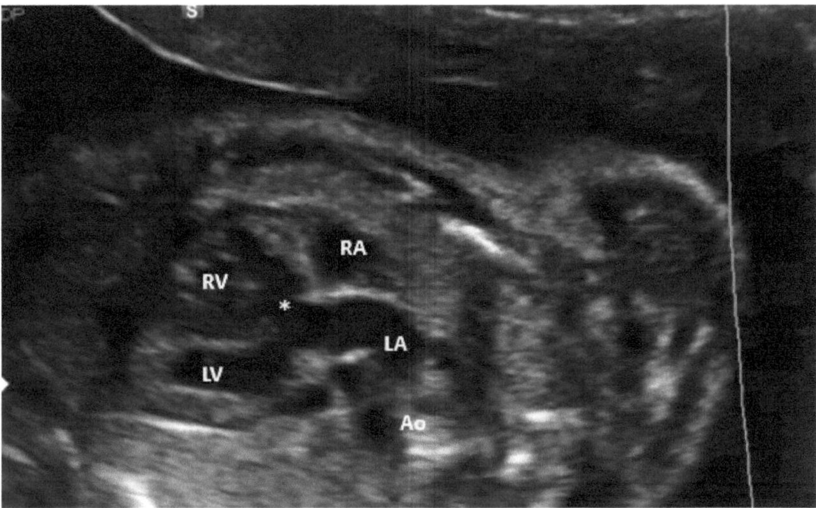

Fig. (2). Left outflow tract view of the heart with a ventricular septal defect (*). LA: left atrium; LV: left ventricle; RV: right ventricle; RA: right atrium; Ao: aorta.

The echocardiography is useful not only for detecting structural heart disease, but it is also critical in evaluating fetal well-being. The cardiothoracic ratio, the systolic myocardial shortening fraction determined with M-mode, as well as the diastolic filling pattern through the atrioventricular (AV) valves have been used in the functional assessment of the fetal heart with a variable reproducibility. More consistent information on right ventricular compliance is obtained with the study of the depth of the "a" wave through the ductus venosus on Doppler flow recordings [15].

The myocardial performance index (MPI) has also been applied in prenatal life for a more global functional cardiac evaluation; this index is based on time intervals during the cardiac cycles [9]. It has been shown that the pulsed Doppler of the aortic isthmus between the origin of the left subclavian artery and the aortic end of the ductus arteriosus provide reliable information on the peripheral fetal circulatory dynamics, as well as the relative systolic performance of each ventricle [24]. During the fetal life, the aortic isthmus occupies a unique position at the cross-road between the two parallel arterial systems. It represents the only shunt between the aortic and pulmonary arches as well as the supradiaphragmatic (directed to the brain) and infradiaphragmatic (directed to the placenta) circulations. Any change in individual ventricular performance or in peripheral vascular resistances are reflected in the isthmic Doppler flow pattern [2 - 4].

Two-dimensional (2D) and Doppler echocardiography have become an essential component in the assessment of anatomic anomalies of the heart, and an important tool in the assessment of fetal cardiac function. There are several techniques to assess fetal cardiovascular function, and they can be used to identify fetal cardiovascular involvement with a variety of cardiac and non-cardiac conditions [9].

With the advent of new ultrasound diagnostic technologies developed by the industry we have recently acquired powerful and promising tools to assess fetal cardiovascular function. With the ultrasound speckle tracking technique, longitudinal and circumferential strain are investigated, opening up new fields for the clinical monitoring of fetal heart diseases and hemodynamic alterations [25, 26]. In this context, 2D Strain acquires relevance and is ready to be a part of conversations in the years to come (Fig. **3**).

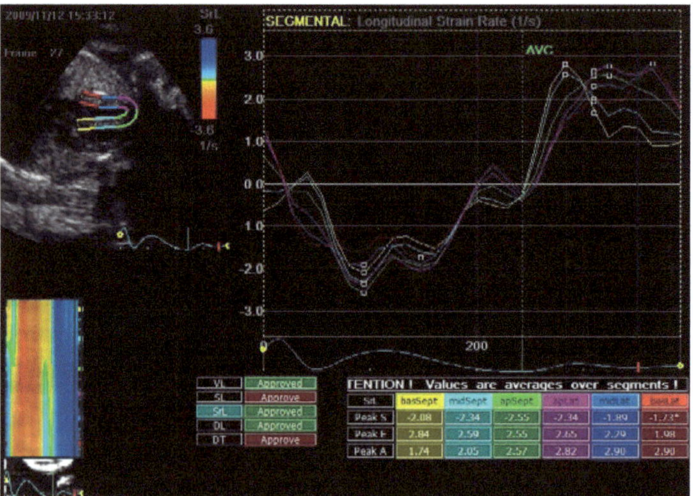

Fig. (3). Ventricle 2D strain.

DEFINITION OF STRAIN: DEFINITION OF STRAIN OR TENSION

Strain is one way of measuring the amount of local deformation of an object caused by an applied force (expressed in %). Strain is obtained by adding (integrating) the instantaneous strain rate values from a start point to an end point in a given amount of time. The 2D Strain is a technique derived from the technology of recognition and monitoring of the ultrasound Speckle. Basically, this equipment recognizes a certain wave pattern in the tissue and tracks it, obtaining an initial and final position [27]. To such an extent, that it is possible to use Speckle tracking to calculate all derivatives and equations that use these data to provide, as well as the tissue Doppler, precise information about tissue tracking (TT), wave rate (TDI), strain (ST) and strain rate (SR) [28] (Fig. **4**).

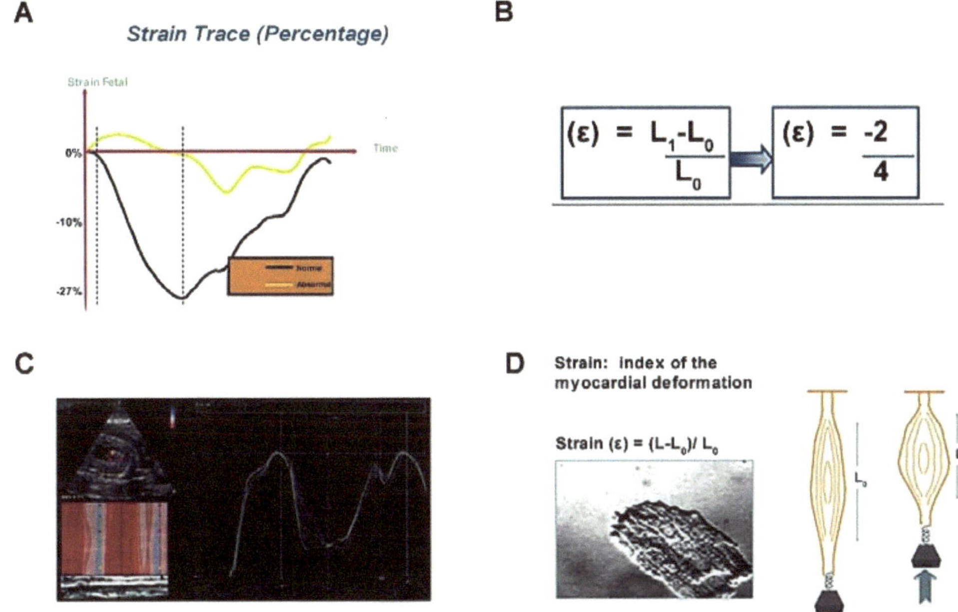

Fig. (4). Strain – Strain rate calculation and equations about tissue tracking.

VENTRICULAR WALL ANEURYSMS OR DIVERTICULA

Ventricular wall aneurysms or diverticula are protrusions of the ventricular walls that progress asymptomatically but can lead to hemodynamic complications and death [29]. They may result from a weakening of the ventricular wall during embryogenesis, infections or ischemia. Diverticula have a narrow connection with the ventricle, with myocardial fibers in the composition of their walls. They may affect the right or the left ventricle, and are more common in the apex. Complications include rupture, arrhythmia, pericardial effusion and hydrops. In the absence of hemodynamic impairment, pericardial effusion can have a favorable outcome. In the case of heart failure, a pericardiocentesis can be performed for good fetal lung development [30, 31].

Aneurysms are characterized by a unilobulated or multilobulated bulging of a ventricular wall segment, presenting a wide neck, fibrotic tissue and akinesia. They can be asymptomatic or lead to complications with pericardial effusion, embolism, rupture, and arrhythmia and heart failure. The differential diagnosis between aneurysm and diverticula is performed in the prenatal period, with a better prognosis for diverticula, with pericardial effusion being the most frequent complication. Color Doppler shows the connection between the ventricle and the diverticulum, showing an oscillating pattern between them, and retrograde flow from the diverticulum to the ventricle [29].

CONCLUSION

In the modern age, structural heart diseases and arrhythmias are expected to be diagnosed with precise details within the uterus. The aim of the fetal cardiologist has become to understand the fetus as a patient, knowing that fetal circulation differs from postnatal circulation, that coronary heart disease may progress in the uterus and that heart function and the stability of the cardiovascular system perform important functions in fetal well-being. In fetuses at risk for cardiovascular disease, collaboration among all caregivers is essential. This document has been created using what is currently known and practiced in the highly advanced and highly specialized field of fetal heart care. Additional studies are needed to determine more accurate indications for referral, better diagnostic protocols for CHD detection, and standardized treatment strategies to prevent cardiovascular involvement and progression of the disease. Given the rarity of many conditions, national and international multidisciplinary collaboration is essential as we assume our role as specialized caregivers for fetuses with cardiovascular disease.

CONSENT FOR PUBLICATION

Not applicable.

CONFLICT OF INTEREST

The authors confirm that the contents of this chapter have no conflict of interest.

ACKNOWLEDGEMENTS

Declare none.

REFERENCES

[1]   Donofrio MT, Moon-Grady AJ, Hornberger LK, *et al.* Diagnosis and treatment of fetal cardiac disease: a scientific statement from the American Heart Association. Circulation 2014; 129(21): 2183-242.
[http://dx.doi.org/10.1161/01.cir.0000437597.44550.5d] [PMID: 24763516]

[2]   McAuliffe FM, Trines J, Nield LE, Chitayat D, Jaeggi E, Hornberger LK. Early fetal echocardiography-a reliable prenatal diagnosis tool. Am J Obstet Gynecol 2005; 193(3 Pt 2): 1253-9.
[http://dx.doi.org/10.1016/j.ajog.2005.05.086] [PMID: 16157147]

[3]   Bishop KC, Kuller JA, Boyd BK, Rhee EH, Miller S, Barker P. Ultrasound examination of the fetal heart. Obstet Gynecol Surv 2017; 72(1): 54-61.
[http://dx.doi.org/10.1097/OGX.0000000000000394] [PMID: 28134395]

[4]   Díaz Góngora G, Sandoval Reyes N, Vélez Moreno J, Carrillo Ángel G. Cardiología Pediátrica.

Bogotá: McGraw-Hill 2003; pp. 281-95.

[5]   Buyens A, Gyselaers W, Coumans A, *et al.* Difficult prenatal diagnosis: fetal coarctation. Facts Views Vis ObGyn 2012; 4(4): 230-6.
[PMID: 24753914]

[6]   Kleinman CS, Nehgme RA. Cardiac arrhythmias in the human fetus. Pediatr Cardiol 2004; 25(3): 234-51.
[http://dx.doi.org/10.1007/s00246-003-0589-x] [PMID: 15360116]

[7]   Hornberger LK, Sahn DJ. Rhythm abnormalities of the fetus. Heart 2007; 93(10): 1294-300.
[http://dx.doi.org/10.1136/hrt.2005.069369] [PMID: 17890709]

[8]   Carvalho JS, Allan LD, Chaoui R, *et al.* ISUOG Practice Guidelines (updated): sonographic screening examination of the fetal heart. Ultrasound Obstet Gynecol 2013; 41(3): 348-59.
[http://dx.doi.org/10.1002/uog.12403] [PMID: 23460196]

[9]   Michelfelder E, Allen C, Urbinelli L. Evaluation and management of fetal cardiac function and heart failure. Curr Treat Options Cardiovasc Med 2016; 18(9): 55.
[http://dx.doi.org/10.1007/s11936-016-0477-3] [PMID: 27423668]

[10]   Cardiac screening examination of the fetus: guidelines for performing the 'basic' and 'extended basic' cardiac scan. Ultrasound Obstet Gynecol 2006; 27(1): 107-13.
[PMID: 16374757]

[11]   Lee W, Allan L, Carvalho JS, *et al.* ISUOG consensus statement: what constitutes a fetal echocardiogram? Ultrasound Obstet Gynecol 2008; 32(2): 239-42.
[http://dx.doi.org/10.1002/uog.6115] [PMID: 18663769]

[12]   Groves AM, Fagg NL, Cook AC, Allan LD. Cardiac tumours in intrauterine life. Arch Dis Child 1992; 67(10 Spec No): 1189-92.
[http://dx.doi.org/10.1136/adc.67.10_Spec_No.1189] [PMID: 1444556]

[13]   Yuan SM. Fetal cardiac tumors: clinical features, management and prognosis. J Perinat Med 2018; 46(2): 115-21.
[http://dx.doi.org/10.1515/jpm-2016-0311] [PMID: 28343178]

[14]   Nii M, Hamilton RM, Fenwick L, Kingdom JC, Roman KS, Jaeggi ET. Assessment of fetal atrioventricular time intervals by tissue Doppler and pulse Doppler echocardiography: normal values and correlation with fetal electrocardiography. Heart 2006; 92(12): 1831-7.
[http://dx.doi.org/10.1136/hrt.2006.093070] [PMID: 16775085]

[15]   Carvalho JS, Prefumo F, Ciardelli V, Sairam S, Bhide A, Shinebourne EA. Evaluation of fetal arrhythmias from simultaneous pulsed wave Doppler in pulmonary artery and vein. Heart 2007; 93(11): 1448-53.
[http://dx.doi.org/10.1136/hrt.2006.101659] [PMID: 17164485]

[16]   Fouron JC, Fournier A, Proulx F, *et al.* Management of fetal tachyarrhythmia based on superior vena cava/aorta Doppler flow recordings. Heart 2003; 89(10): 1211-6.
[http://dx.doi.org/10.1136/heart.89.10.1211] [PMID: 12975422]

[17]   Raboisson MJ, Fouron JC, Sonesson SE, Nyman M, Proulx F, Gamache S. Fetal Doppler echocardiographic diagnosis and successful steroid therapy of Luciani-Wenckebach phenomenon and endocardial fibroelastosis related to maternal anti-Ro and anti-La antibodies. J Am Soc Echocardiogr 2005; 18(4): 375-80.
[http://dx.doi.org/10.1016/j.echo.2004.10.023] [PMID: 15846168]

[18]   Jaeggi ET, Fouron JC, Silverman ED, Ryan G, Smallhorn J, Hornberger LK. Transplacental fetal treatment improves the outcome of prenatally diagnosed complete atrioventricular block without structural heart disease. Circulation 2004; 110(12): 1542-8.
[http://dx.doi.org/10.1161/01.CIR.0000142046.58632.3A] [PMID: 15353508]

[19]   Horigome H, Nagashima M, Sumitomo N, *et al.* Clinical characteristics and genetic background of

congenital long-QT syndrome diagnosed in fetal, neonatal, and infantile life: a nationwide questionnaire survey in Japan. Circ Arrhythm Electrophysiol 2010; 3(1): 10-7.
[http://dx.doi.org/10.1161/CIRCEP.109.882159] [PMID: 19996378]

[20]   Milanesi R, Baruscotti M, Gnecchi-Ruscone T, DiFrancesco D. Familial sinus bradycardia associated with a mutation in the cardiac pacemaker channel. N Engl J Med 2006; 354(2): 151-7.
[http://dx.doi.org/10.1056/NEJMoa052475] [PMID: 16407510]

[21]   Friedman D, Buyon J, Kim M, Glickstein JS. Fetal cardiac function assessed by Doppler myocardial performance index (Tei Index). Ultrasound Obstet Gynecol 2003; 21(1): 33-6.
[http://dx.doi.org/10.1002/uog.11] [PMID: 12528158]

[22]   Huhta JC, Paul JJ. Doppler in fetal heart failure. Clin Obstet Gynecol 2010; 53(4): 915-29.
[http://dx.doi.org/10.1097/GRF.0b013e3181fdffd9] [PMID: 21048458]

[23]   Fouron JC. The unrecognized physiological and clinical significance of the fetal aortic isthmus. Ultrasound Obstet Gynecol 2003; 22(5): 441-7.
[http://dx.doi.org/10.1002/uog.911] [PMID: 14618654]

[24]   Fouron JC, Gosselin J, Raboisson MJ, *et al.* The relationship between an aortic isthmus blood flow velocity index and the postnatal neurodevelopmental status of fetuses with placental circulatory insufficiency. Am J Obstet Gynecol 2005; 192(2): 497-503.
[http://dx.doi.org/10.1016/j.ajog.2004.08.026] [PMID: 15695993]

[25]   Matsuura Y, Daimon M, Notomi Y, Miyasaka N, Yamaguchi Y, Doi S. Feasibility and reproducibility of fetal left ventricular twist using two-dimensional speckle-tracking analysis in a japanese population. Int Heart J 2019; 60(3): 671-8.
[http://dx.doi.org/10.1536/ihj.18-480] [PMID: 31105153]

[26]   Cotran RS, Kumar V, Collins T. Robbins Patología estructural y funcional. 6th ed. Madrid: McGraw-Hill Interamericana 2000; p. 162.

[27]   Lowe JB, Williams JC, Robb D, Cole D. Congenital diverticulum of the left ventricle. Br Heart J 1959; 21(1): 101-6.
[http://dx.doi.org/10.1136/hrt.21.1.101] [PMID: 13618466]

[28]   Deng J, Rodeck CH. Current applications of fetal cardiac imaging technology. Curr Opin Obstet Gynecol 2006; 18(2): 177-84.
[http://dx.doi.org/10.1097/01.gco.0000192987.99847.a4] [PMID: 16601479]

[29]   Di Salvo G, Russo MG, Paladini D, *et al.* Two-dimensional strain to assess regional left and right ventricular longitudinal function in 100 normal foetuses. Eur J Echocardiogr 2008; 9(6): 754-6.
[http://dx.doi.org/10.1093/ejechocard/jen134] [PMID: 18490298]

[30]   Willruth AM, Geipel AK, Fimmers R, Gembruch UG. Assessment of right ventricular global and regional longitudinal peak systolic strain, strain rate and velocity in healthy fetuses and impact of gestational age using a novel speckle/feature-tracking based algorithm. Ultrasound Obstet Gynecol 2011; 37(2): 143-9.
[http://dx.doi.org/10.1002/uog.7719] [PMID: 20549769]

[31]   Kapusta L, Mainzer G, Weiner Z, *et al.* Second trimester ultrasound: reference values for two-dimensional speckle tracking-derived longitudinal strain, strain rate and time to peak deformation of the fetal heart. J Am Soc Echocardiogr 2012; 25(12): 1333-41.
[http://dx.doi.org/10.1016/j.echo.2012.09.011] [PMID: 23200418]

CHAPTER 3

Fetal Cardiac Tumors

Maria Respondek-Liberska[1,2,*]

[1] *Fetal Malformations and Prevention Department, Medical University of Lodz, Poland*

[2] *Cardiology Department Research Institute Polish Mother's Memorial Hospital, Lodz, Poland*

Abstract: Fetal cardiac tumors (FCT) are rare anomalies (about 1% among prenatal cardiac problems). There are more frequent multiple FCT and less frequent single FCT. The FCT occur in the population of healthy young mothers and risk factors are not easily detectable, but environmental factors (benzapirin?) could play a role. Basic ultrasound (US) anatomy in the 1st and 2nd trimester usually is normal and FCT are usually detected in the second half of pregnancy. In the majority of cases the fetus's growth is normal. In each case, targeted fetal echocardiography should be performed in a fetal cardiology center. The very first problem is to discriminate between normal heart anatomy and congenital heart defect. The second goal of fetal echocardiography in FCT is to make an assessment of the hemodynamic status of the fetus. Extracardiac and additional anomalies coexisting in cases of FTC can be divided into two types *i.e.*, frequent and rare. An experienced fetal cardiologist can not only make a proper diagnosis but also should counsel parents about the short-term prognosis for the fetus (about his future during prenatal life) as well as long term prognosis (after birth and later on). In cases of maternal decision to continue the pregnancy, fetal echocardiography monitoring should be offered to evaluate possible hemodynamic changes, to prepare both fetus and pregnant woman for optimal time for delivery and perinatal care. The main goal would be to avoid prematurity and to confirm fetal well-being, despite the cardiac abnormality. Details of echocardiography and postnatal outcome are presented in rhabdomyoma, teratoma, fibroma, myxoma and hemangioma. The way of delivery in surgical resection of cardiac tumors in newborns is discussed. In differential diagnosis, "bright spot" is discussed. Suggested management – algorithm of perinatal care in cases of FCT is presented with emphasis on cooperation of a perinatal team. FCT can be diagnosed at 20 weeks of pregnancy, which allows to start echocardiographic monitoring, taking into consideration the potential risk of hemodynamic progression. FCT (both multiple and single) can be the first sign of tuberous sclerosis complex in later prenatal or postnatal life. Single FCT other than rhabdomyoma can be asymptomatic in newborns, but may require an early surgical resection, therefore delivery in tertiary centers is recommended. FCT are a good example of the practical value of prenatal cardiology development.

---

[*] **Corresponding author Maria Respondek-Liberska:** Fetal Malformations and Prevention Department, Medical University of Lodz, Poland; Tel: +48 602 45 19 09; E-mail: majkares@uni.lodz.p

Keywords: Differential diagnosis, Fibroma, Myxoma and Hemangioma, Perinatal management, Rhabdomyoma, Teratoma, Type of delivery.

Fetal cardiac tumors are rare anomalies. These are intracardiac masses located within a lumen or walls of cardiac chambers, in their septa or pericardium, of different sizes (from a few millimeters up to few centimeters). The prenatal diagnosis by ultrasound has been known since the eighties of the last century [1]. The Polish National Prenatal Cardiac Pathology Registry (www.ORPKP.pl) shows the prevalence of intracardiac tumors to be 1.05% [2]. In the years 2004-2016, amongst 8112 fetuses in Poland, (Europe), there were 85 fetuses with cardiac tumors, including 52 cases of multiple cardiac tumors (0.64%) and 33 single anomalies (0.4%) (Figs. **1** and **2**).

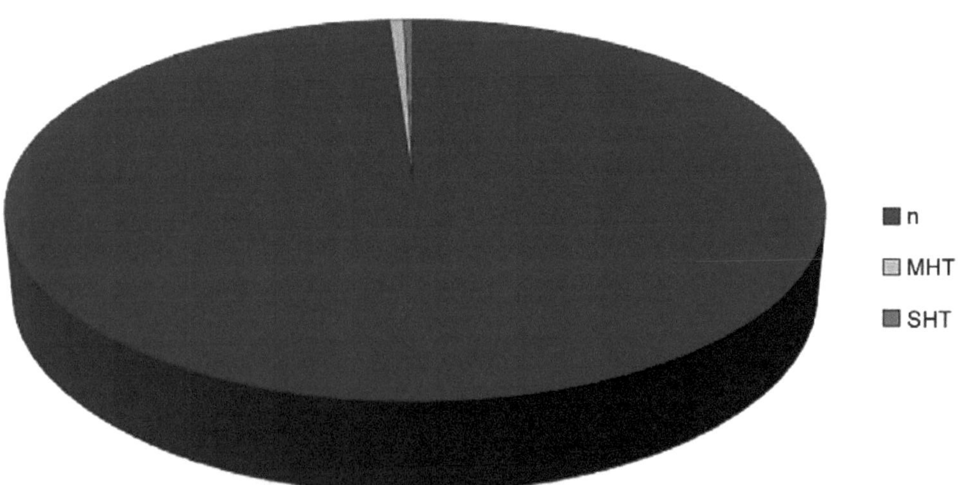

Fig. (1). Data from National Registry of Fetal Cardiac Anomalies in Poland (www.ORPKP.pl) in years 2004-2016 amongst 8112 fetuses with cardiac problems, 85 fetuses were diagnosed with cardiac tumors, including 52 cases of multiple cardiac tumors and 33 cases of single cardiac tumors (1.05% of total).

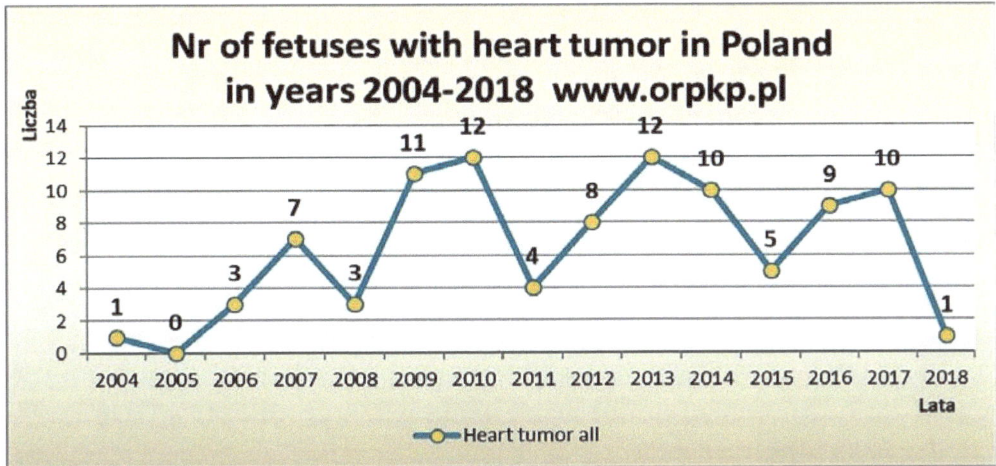

Fig. (2). Number of fetuses with heart tumor per year in Poland in years 2004-2018 www.orpkp.

Fetal cardiac tumors occur in the population of healthy young mothers, usually expecting their first child. Risk factors are not easily detectable. In the analysis by our Department, a hypothesis was put forward suggesting the relationship between maternal place of residency and ecological situation of that region [3]. A high concentration of polycyclic aromatic hydrocarbons (including benzapirin) was found in certain areas of Poland, so benzene can be a suspected factor, however this needs further work-up.

In the majority of cases, the first trimester scan is normal, with nuchal translucency as well as nasal bone assessment. Moreover, biochemical tests and basic ultrasound anatomy scan in the 1st and 2nd trimester are normal. Heart tumors are usually detected later on, so usually this is the problem that occurs in the second half of pregnancy (since 20 weeks of gestation until term at 39 weeks of gestation) [3]. In the majority of cases, presence of fetal cardiac tumor had no influence on the fetuses growth.

Usually heart tumors are easy to detect *in utero* by two-dimensional (2D) ultrasound during screening obstetrical ultrasound. Real time 2D visualization allows to pin-point an exact location of the tumor or tumors. After detecting the problem, fetal echocardiography should be performed, optimally in a fetal cardiology center. There are at least two important reasons for such a rule. First, that tertiary center has greater experience than primary care obstetricians or ultrasonographers who may have dealt only once with such a problem during their practice. The second reason is also crucial; in rare conditions such as heart tumors tertiary centers, there is a chance to collect series of such cases for epidemiological analysis and perhaps future prevention.

In tertiary centers, the very first problem is to discriminate between normal heart anatomy and congenital heart defect. Congenital heart defect and fetal heart tumor are rare [3]. In our center, we have seen coexistance of heart tumor with tetralogy of Fallot (with good outcome), hypoplastic left heart syndrome (bad outcome), complete atrioventricular canal (bad outcome) and aortic stenosis (50% bad outcome). In the literature, there is a case report on single ventricle repair in heart tumor [4].

The second goal of fetal echocardiography in heart tumor is to make an initial assessment of the hemodynamic status of the fetus, and its intracardiac and peripheral flows (umbilical artery and middle cerebral artery), to rule out any extracardiac anomalies (Table **1**).

Table 1. Extracardiac anomalies in fetuses with heart tumors.

Extracardiac anomalies:
• Polyhydramnios
• Oligohydramnios
• Small for gestational age
• Central nervous system tumor
• Hydrothorax or ascites
• Kidney tumor
• Pyelectasis
• Situs inversus
• Hydrops testis

Additional anomalies coexisting in cases of fetal heart tumors can be divided into frequent and rare (Table **2**). The frequent anomalies include cardiomegaly, pericardial effusion, tricuspid regurgitation and myocardial hypertrophy. Other functional echocardiographic anomalies such as aortic valve stenosis, foramen ovale restriction, right atrium enlargement, arrhythmia (premature atrial contractions), mitral valve stenosis and pulmonary insufficiency are seen sporadically.

An experienced fetal cardiologist can not only make a proper diagnosis, but also should counsel parents about the short-term prognosis for that particular fetus (about his future during prenatal life) as well as long-term prognosis (after birth and later on). In the event in which the pregnant woman decides to continue the pregnancy, fetal echocardiography monitoring should be offered to evaluate possible hemodynamic changes, to prepare both fetus and pregnant woman for optimal time for delivery and perinatal care. The second counseling for family should be provided. The main goal would be to avoid prematurity and to confirm fetal well-being, despite the cardiac abnormality.

Table 2. Fetal echocardiography additional anomalies in fetal heart with tumor.

	Frequent	Rare
Normal heart anatomy	+	
Congenital heart defects		+
Normal heart anatomy since embryogenesis but tumor mass may change intracardiac flows mimicking heart defect		+
Cardiomegaly	+	
Pericardial effusion	+	
Tricuspid valve regurgitation	+	
Myocardial hypertrophy (SEP > 4 mm)	+	
Aortic valve stenosis (increased maximum velocity across aorta valve)		+
Mitral valve stenosis		+
Pulmonary regurgitation		+
Foramen ovale restriction		+
Right atrium enlargement		+
Akinesis of the wall of the fetal heart		+
Fetal heart arrhythmia (premature atrial contractions or supraventricular tachycardia)		+

SEP: interventricular septum.

In case of polyhydramnios, amnioreduction can be offered; in case of arrhythmias, anti-arrhythmic transplacental treatment should be given, while in case of lung development delay, steroids could be considered. In case of rapid growth of the tumor, an experimental surgery, for instance in Children's Hospital of Philadelphia [5] or in The Fetal Treatment Center - University of California, San Francisco, California [6], could be considered if that is the maternal wish. In majority of cases regarding fetal cardiac tumors, surgery is postponed for postnatal life [3, 7].

During the postnatal life, in neonates or children, the prognosis of the tumor is established based on histopathological evaluation, while before birth, it is usually not possible. So, proper fetal echocardiography by an experienced fetal cardiologist in fetal cardiac center is so far the main source of information. Maybe, in the near future, new ultrasound techniques such as tissue harmonic imaging would be added, or any newer ultrasound modalities [8]. Today, practical counseling in fetal cardiology in case of intracardiac tumors is much more difficult compared to clinical situations in pediatric cardiology. Other diagnostic methods which are used at referral center is fetal magnetic resonance imaging (MRI), specially to look for additional nodules in central nervous systems or to rule out their presence [9, 10]. In countries where legal termination of pregnancy is possible, the woman has to make her final decision before the histopathological evaluation [11, 12].

The most common type of fetal cardiac tumor is rhabdomyoma (76-83%). It is usually multiple (but can also be single), is homogenous, well-circumscribed mass, variable in size and location (Fig. **3**). It may appear in right and left ventricle, in the interventricular septum or at the level of interatrial septum. In case of "good localization", for instance close to apex, usually the intracardiac flows, despite the presence of multiple tumors, are laminar (Figs. **4** and **5**). Their size is variable from 3-4 mm to 10-15 mm. In the majority of cases, they do not compromise cardiac function, but some of them may create an obstructive lesion for the fetal valve and then mimic, for instance, pulmonary or aortic stenosis. Rhabdomyomas can be a cause of fetal arrhythmias.

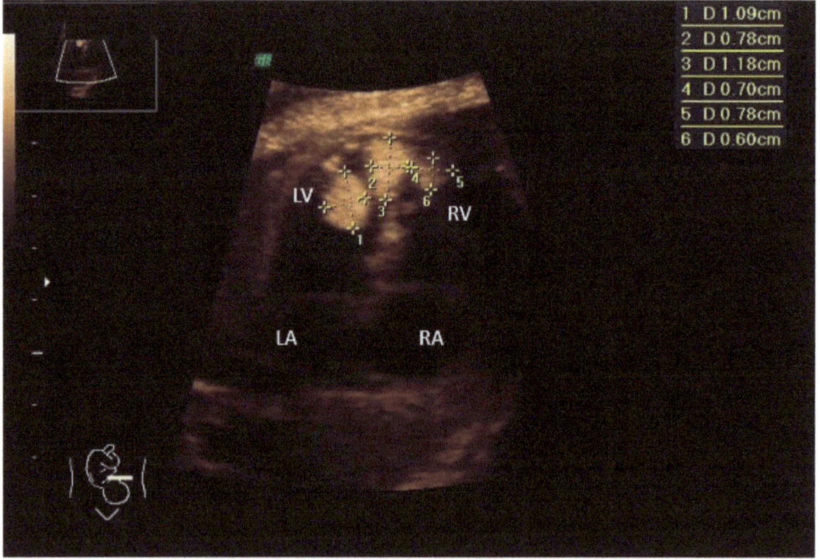

Fig. (3). Fetus at 33rd week of gestation with multiple rhabdomyoma close to apex, both in left and right ventricle. LA: left atrium; LV: left ventricle; RA: right atrium; R: right ventricle.

These tumors usually appear not sooner than at the 20th week of gestation. Predominantly, they increase in size in the 3rd trimester and before term. In the event of coexisting fetal hydrops and arrhythmia resistant to treatment, cardiomegaly in about 12% of cases and intrauterine or neonatal death has been observed. However, in the majority of cases (about 80%), patients with rhabdomyoma are alive and usually during infancy tumors disappear, partially or completely; however, their medical history is continued as other tumor masses may appear in the central nervous system or in the kidneys [13]. This clinical manifestation is known as tuberous sclerosis or Bourneville–Pringle disease (Figs. **6** to **8**). Genetic background was established in these cases: mutation in the Hamartin (TSC-1) and Tuberin (TSC-2) genes, located on 9q34 and 16p13 chromosomes. Hamartin and tuberin are responsible for tumor suppression. In Bourneville-Pringle disease, nodules, especially hamartomas may be present in the skin, brain, kidneys and visceral organs. Cardiac tumors are usually rhabdomyomas. The spectrum of the disease is very wide: ranging from asymptomatic to severe epilepsy and mental delay.

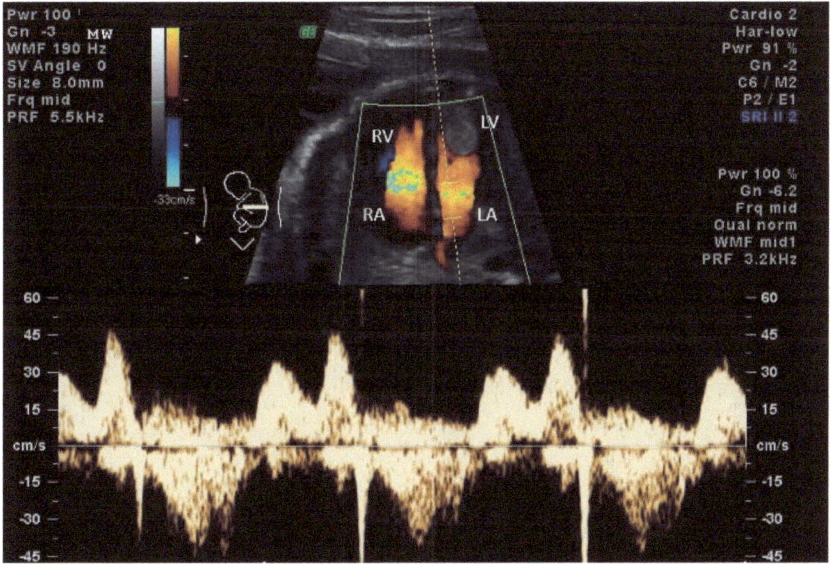

Fig. (4). The same fetus from (Fig. **3**) - intracardiac blood flows in color Doppler at the level of mitral valve - normal inflow (above the zero line) and outflow (below the zero line). LA: left atrium; LV: left ventricle; RA: right atrium; RV: right ventricle.

The early prenatal diagnosis might also be confirmed by cordocentesis and molecular testing, especially by the family history of epilepsy, chronic headaches, skin lesions (nodules or café – au lait spots).

In neonates with prenatally confirmed disease, early neurological counseling is offered and anti-epileptic treatment is introduced as early as possible through the 1st and 2nd year of postnatal life to avoid future epilepsy and deterioration in child's development. In Europe, a multicenter program Epi-Stop was developed and coordinated by prof. Jozwik from Warsaw-Poland [14].

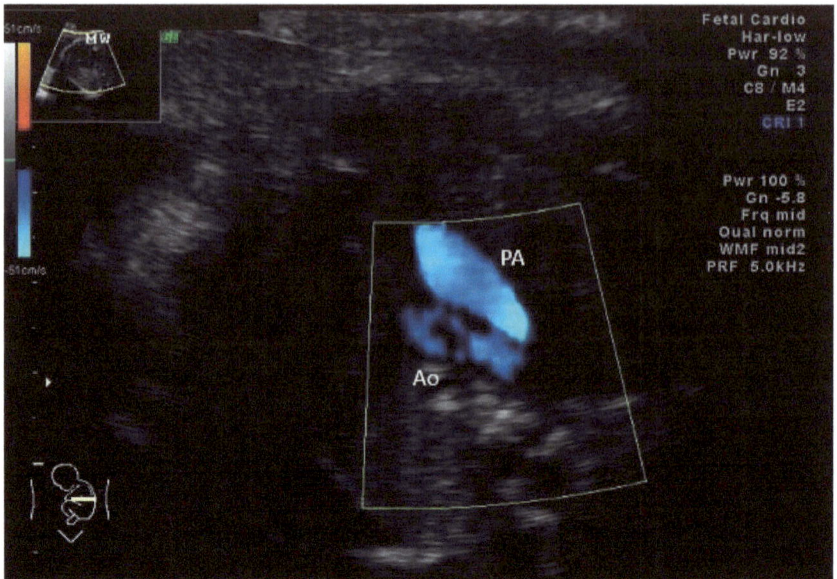

Fig. (5). The same fetus from Figs. (**3** and **4**) -the same direction of blood flow in pulmonary artery (PA) and aorta (Ao) at the level of mediastinum

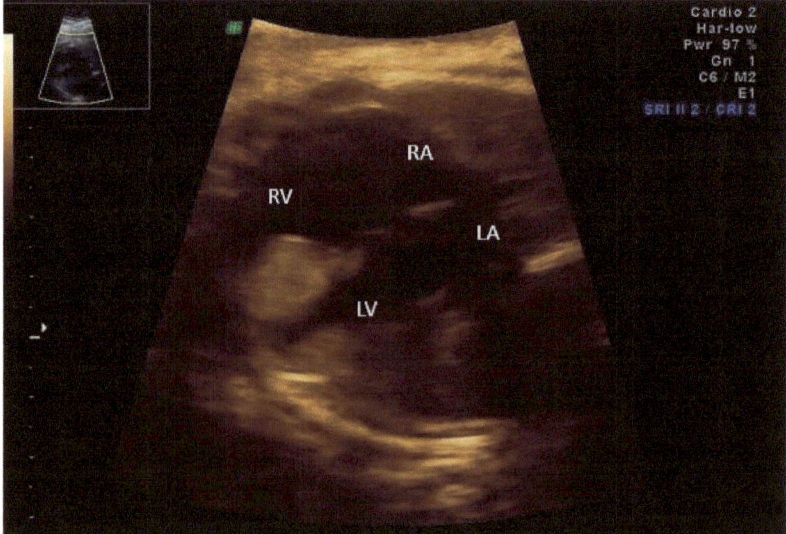

Fig. (6). Postnatal magnetic resonance imaging (MRI) of the same patient from Figs. (**4** and **5**) as a newborn - two tumors in frontal lobes (arrows) – Bourneville syndrome. LA: left atrium; LV: left ventricle; RA: right atrium; RV: right ventricle.

Single cardiac tumor in the lower part of the interventricular septum at 33rd week of gestation with multiple cardiac rhabdomyomas everolimus [15], a mammalian target of rapamycin inhibitor has been reported to be an effective drug to cause tumor remission. Neonatal cardiac surgery for the resection of primary cardiac tumors found by fetal echocardiography has been reported sporadically [13, 17].

The importance of the diagnosis of tuberous sclerosis is exemplified by the neurodevelopmental complications, with four-fifths of the patients showing epilepsy, and two-thirds having delayed development. The presence of multiple cardiac tumors suggested a higher risk of being affected by tuberous sclerosis. The tumors generally regress after birth, and cardiac-related problems are rare after the perinatal period. Tuberous sclerosis and the associated neurodevelopmental complications dominate the clinical picture, and should form an important aspect of the prenatal counselling of parents [18]. So, in long-term prognosis, rhabdomyoma tumors shrink and become clinically less important over time, however, other health problems could be more important [19].

The other fetal cardiac tumor might be teratoma. It is a cystic pericardiac tumor, usually in size of more than 10-15 mm. In comparison, teratoma does not occur in the heart, but with close contact with aorta or pulmonary artery or mediastinum. Usually it is a single tumor, nonhomogeneous, with irregular shape and echogenicity (Fig. **9**). Usually, there is moderate pericardial effusion. Large teratoma may cause heart compression, fetal hydrops and intrauterine death. A multidisciplinary team approach is recommended to choose the best time for delivery: not too early and not too late [11].

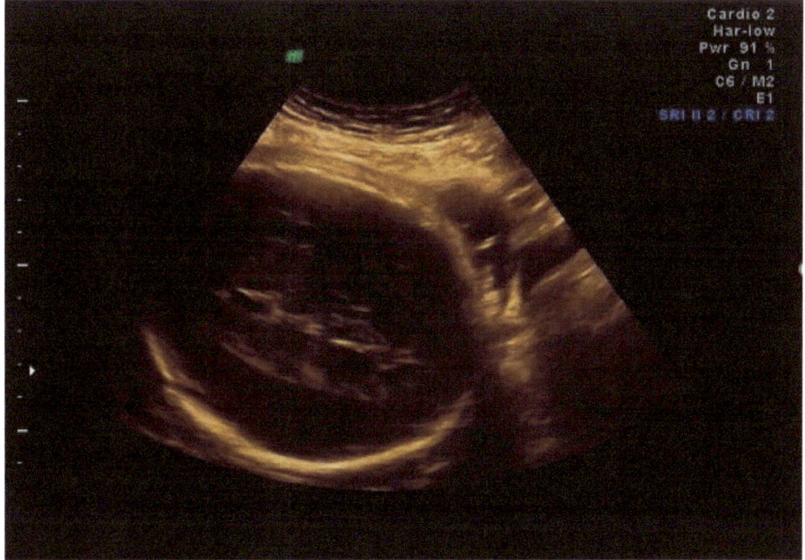

Fig. (7). The same fetus from Fig. (**6**) - ultrasound of his head - no evidence of lesions in central nervous system

Fetuses with teratoma demonstrate several clinical symptoms, from asymptomatic to mild pericadial effusion up to hydrops fetalis. Yinon *et al.* [11] reported about 40 cases of fetuses with different intracardiac tumors, including 3 with teratomas and none of them survived.

In case of significant pericardial effusion and imminent secondary tamponade, pericardiocentesis might be considered in tertiary center. Such a procedure implemented by Sklansky *et al.* [20] in one of the twins allowed continuation of the pregnancy until the 35th week of gestation and resection was performed after birth. One year later, both the twins were alive and well and had no evidence of tumor recurrence.

In the case presented in Fig. (**9**), the time of delivery was planned in advance by obstetricians together with fetal cardiologist and cardiac surgeon. The complete excision of the tumor was performed on the 4th day of postnatal life and neonate was discharged home 3 weeks later. At the age of 6 months and 12 months, he was asymptomatic with no abnormalities on echocardiography and ultrasound examination (abdomen and transfontanelle scans).

In the differential diagnosis of fetal heart tumor, one should also keep in mind fibroma. It is usually a single mass: 15-30 mm, may have a cystic form, but usually is homogeneous, rounded and may be a cause of pericardial effusion (Figs. **10** and **11**). Such a tumor detected prenatally can be in selected cases successfully surgically removed in neonates [21].

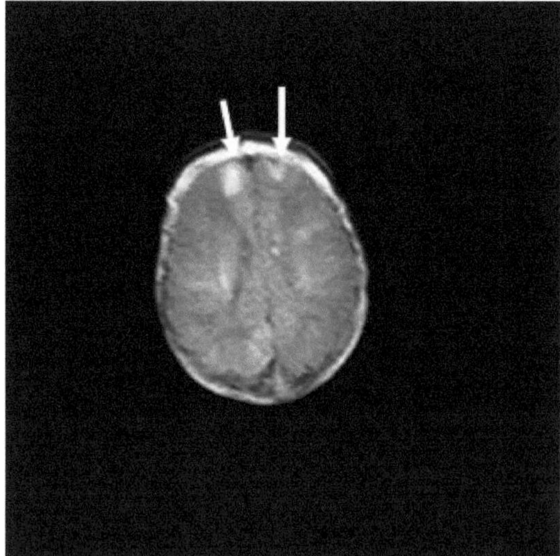

Fig. (8). Postnatal magnetic resonance imaging (MRI) of the same patient from Figs. (**6** and **7**) Two tumors in frontal lobes - Bourneville syndrome in newborn.

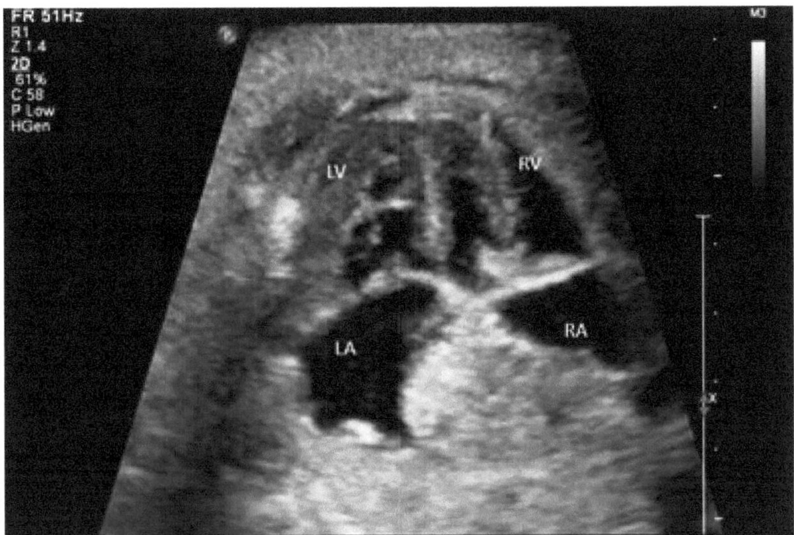

Fig. (9). The same fetus as on (Fig. **8**) – showing the tumor at the level of fetal abdomen with small pericardial Huge tumor at the level of the right atrium (RA): nonhomogenous, not regular, without compressing mitral or tricuspid valve. Elective cesarean section and successful cardiac surgery on day 4th on postnatal life. By histopathology evaluation - teratoma . Neonate was live born, however died before cardiac surgery. LA: left atrium; LV: left ventricle; RV: right ventricle.

Myxoma is another single cardiac tumor. Paladini *et al.* [22] reported one such case that presented as a right atrial mass, at 23 weeks' gestation and moving across foramen ovale to left atrium later on. It was followed until delivery and myxoma removed at the 20th day of postnatal life. Another case of fetal cardiac myxoma was reported by Rios *et al.* [23] where surgery was successfully performed on the 8th day of postnatal life.

A very rare form of prenatal heart tumor is hemangioma. After prenatal diagnosis, the newborns were successfully operated, during the first and second week of postnatal life [24, 25].

The prognosis cannot be made only on the basis of the size of the tumor or location, number of the tumors or even histopathology. The cardiovascular condition of the fetus assessed longitudinally by echocardiography is the best method to choose the optimal time of delivery. Before the final interpretation of fetal echocardiography, other data about the fetus condition should be taken into consideration, including amniotic fluid index, Doppler blood flow in umbilical and middle cerebral arteries, his biometry (normal? too small for gestational age? too large lung's for gestational age?), other extracardiac anomalies (hydrothorax? hydronephrosis?), lung's maturation.

The type of delivery in majority of cases of fetal heart tumors in our center as well as in the literature were cesarean sections, but vaginal delivery is also recommended [26]. In the majority of cases, newborns were born at term (in our center with an average of birth weight 2989 g ranging 2000-3950 g, with 10 or 9 Apgar score at 1st min) [7].

In cases of prenatal surgery, the delivery was elective cesarean section at 38 weeks of gestation [5]. Majority of newborns in our center were discharged home after 10-15 days of observation, in general good condition, without clinical symptoms, for further ambulatory care, without the need for cardiac surgery.

Surgical resection of the cardiac tumors was performed on 4 newborns in our center with teratomas or fibromas at the 2nd, 4th, 8th and 16th day of life (average 7.5 day) [7]. Time of hospitalization of these newborns was from 10 to 53 days (without one-day hospitalization of the newborn that passed away in his first day of postnatal life). There were 4 deaths in cases of single heart tumor (31%) on the 1st, 2nd and 11th day (before the resection of the tumor) and in one case, on the 28th day after the operation.

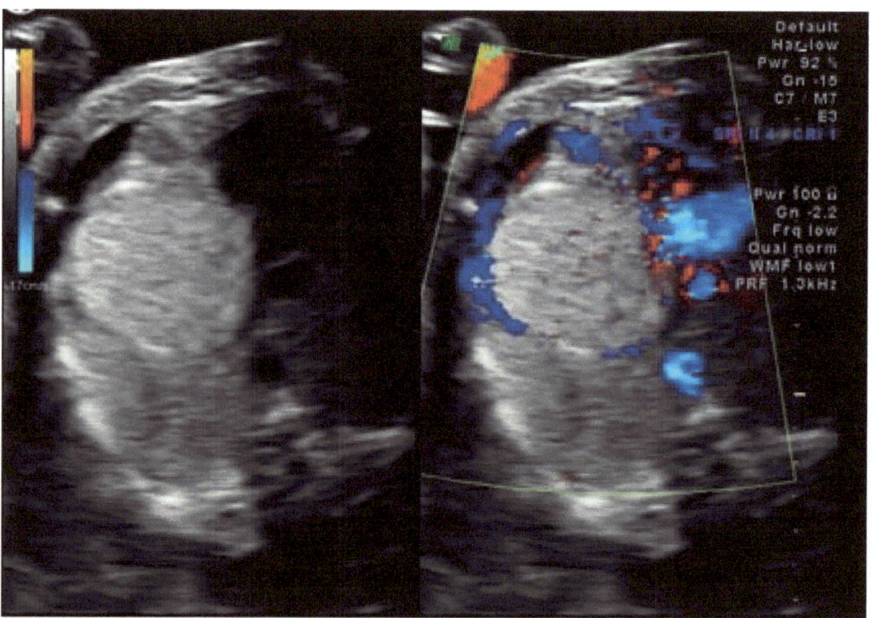

Fig. (10). 36 mm tumor at the level of mediastinum in a fetus at 24th week of gestation: regular and homogenous.

In differential diagnosis, hyperechogenic spots in heart chambers, known as "bright spots" can be misinterpreted as small cardiac tumors, therefore they should also be taken into consideration. By ultrasound examination, these appears as homogenous, hyperechogenic nodules with benign contours and oval shape, known in the literature also as "golf ball sign". Because of the possibility of progression, it may be initially labeled as "bright spot" is initially known as "bright spot" and is finally diagnosed as a cardiac tumor. More intense observation in selected cases is justified. Sokolowski and Respondek-Liberska concerning echogenic intracardiac focus in patients with prenatally diagnosed hyperechogenic spot in heart cavity, pointed out the possible role of the infectious factor, which can also be the cause of low birth weight in these cases [27].

Suggested management – algorithm of perinatal care in cases of fetal heart tumor is presented with emphasis on perinatal team in our most recent publication [28].

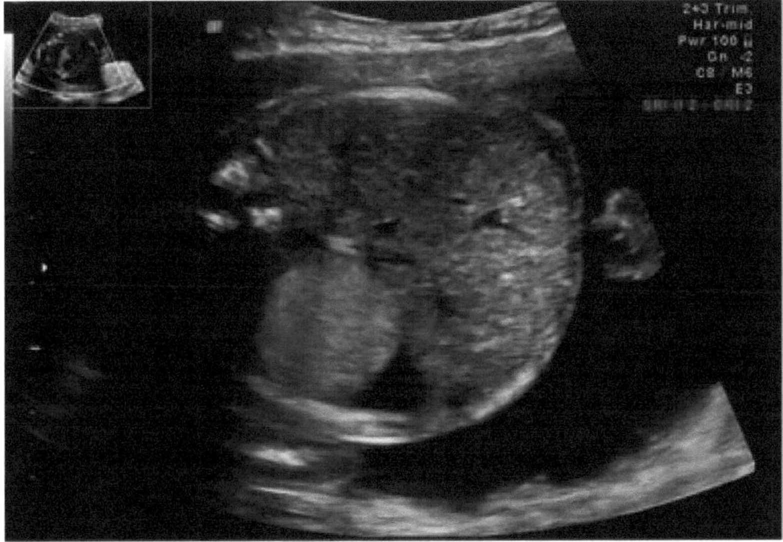

Fig. (11). The same fetus from (Fig. **10**) - small pericardial effusion (arrow). Neonate was live born, however died before cardiac surgery (it was fibroma).

CONCLUSION

1. Fetal cardiac tumors can be diagnosed at 20 weeks of pregnancy, which allows to start echocardiographic monitoring, taking into consideration the potential risk of hemodynamic progression.
2. Fetal cardiac tumors (both multiple and single) can be the first sign of tuberous sclerosis complex in later prenatal or postnatal life.
3. Single cardiac tumor other than rhabdomyoma can be asymptomatic in newborn, but may require an early surgical resection, therefore delivery in tertiary centers is recommended.
4. Fetal cardiac tumors are a good example of the practical value of prenatal cardiology development.

CONSENT FOR PUBLICATION

Not applicable.

CONFLICT OF INTEREST

The authors confirm that the contents of this chapter have no conflict of interest.

ACKNOWLEDGEMENTS

Declare none.

REFERENCES

[1]　DeVore GR, Hakim S, Kleinman CS, Hobbins JC. The *in utero* diagnosis of an interventricular septal cardiac rhabdomyoma by means of real-time-directed, M-mode echocardiography. Am J Obstet Gynecol 1982; 143(8): 967-9.
[http://dx.doi.org/10.1016/0002-9378(82)90484-7] [PMID: 7102774]

[2]　Kordjalik P, Tobota Z, Respondek-Liberska M. Selected data from the Polish National Prenatal Cardiac Pathology Registry from the year 2016. Prenat Cardiol 2017; 7: 7-11.
[http://dx.doi.org/10.1515/pcard-2017-0002]

[3]　Więckowska K, Piątek K, Respondek-Liberska M. Heart tumors in 33 fetuses – review of twenty two years of the single center experience. Pren Cardiol 2016; 6(1): 22-30.

[4]　Mir A, Ikemba CM, Veeram Reddy SR. Hypoplastic left heart syndrome secondary to intrauterine rhabdomyoma necessitating single ventricle palliation. Ann Pediatr Cardiol 2014; 7(3): 207-9.
[http://dx.doi.org/10.4103/0974-2069.140851] [PMID: 25298697]

[5]　Rychik J, Khalek N, Gaynor JW, *et al.* Fetal intrapericardial teratoma: natural history and management including successful *in utero* surgery. Am J Obstet Gynecol 2016; 215(6): 780.e1-7.
[http://dx.doi.org/10.1016/j.ajog.2016.08.010] [PMID: 27530489]

[6]　Sydorak RM, Kelly T, Feldstein VA, *et al.* Prenatal resection of a fetal pericardial teratoma. Fetal Diagn Ther 2002; 17(5): 281-5.
[http://dx.doi.org/10.1159/000063180] [PMID: 12169812]

[7]　Żalińska A, Korabiewska S, Krekora M, *et al.* Single fetal cardiac tumors and follow-up based on 13 cases from the Fetal Cardiac Referral Center in 1993-2017. Prenat Cardiol 2017; 7: 43-9.
[http://dx.doi.org/10.1515/pcard-2017-0007]

[8]　Hosono T, Chiba Y, Kanai H, Kanagawa T. Initial experiences of tissue harmonic imaging in the diagnosis of fetal cardiac tumors. Ultrasound Obstet Gynecol 2002; 19(4): 400-2.
[http://dx.doi.org/10.1046/j.1469-0705.2002.00664.x] [PMID: 11952972]

[9]　Kivelitz DE, Mühler M, Rake A, Scheer I, Chaoui R. MRI of cardiac rhabdomyoma in the fetus. Eur Radiol 2004; 14(8): 1513-6.
[http://dx.doi.org/10.1007/s00330-003-2062-x] [PMID: 14551725]

[10]　Mühler MR, Rake A, Schwabe M, *et al.* Value of fetal cerebral MRI in sonographically proven cardiac rhabdomyoma. Pediatr Radiol 2007; 37(5): 467-74.
[http://dx.doi.org/10.1007/s00247-007-0436-y] [PMID: 17357805]

[11]　Yinon Y, Chitayat D, Blaser S, *et al.* Fetal cardiac tumors: a single-center experience of 40 cases. Prenat Diagn 2010; 30(10): 941-9.
[http://dx.doi.org/10.1002/pd.2590] [PMID: 20721876]

[12]　Yu Q, Zeng W, Zhou A, Zhu W, Liu J. Clinical value of prenatal echocardiographic examination in

the diagnosis of fetal cardiac tumors. Oncol Lett 2016; 11(2): 1555-9.
[http://dx.doi.org/10.3892/ol.2015.4061] [PMID: 26893779]

[13]   Schlaegel F, Takacs Z, Solomayer EF, Abdul-Kaliq H, Meyberg-Solomayer G. Prenatal diagnosis of giant cardiac rhabdomyoma with fetal hydrops in tuberous sclerosis. J Prenat Med 2013; 7(3): 39-41.
[PMID: 24175016]

[14]   Słowińska M, Jóźwiak S, Peron A, *et al.* Early diagnosis of tuberous sclerosis complex: a race against time. How to make the diagnosis before seizures? Orphanet J Rare Dis 2018; 13(1): 25.
[http://dx.doi.org/10.1186/s13023-018-0764-z] [PMID: 29378663]

[15]   Mlczoch E, Hanslik A, Luckner D, Kitzmüller E, Prayer D, Michel-Behnke I. Prenatal diagnosis of giant cardiac rhabdomyoma in tuberous sclerosis complex: a new therapeutic option with everolimus. Ultrasound Obstet Gynecol 2015; 45(5): 618-21.
[http://dx.doi.org/10.1002/uog.13434] [PMID: 24913039]

[16]   Niewiadomska-Jarosik K, Stanczyk J, Janiak K, *et al.* Prenatal diagnosis and follow-up of 23 cases of cardiac tumors. Pediatr Cardiol 2004; 25: 252-73.

[17]   Yuan SM. Fetal primary cardiac tumors during perinatal period. Pediatr Neonatol 2017; 58(3): 205-10.
[http://dx.doi.org/10.1016/j.pedneo.2016.07.004] [PMID: 28043830]

[18]   Degueldre SC, Chockalingam P, Mivelaz Y, *et al.* Considerations for prenatal counselling of patients with cardiac rhabdomyomas based on their cardiac and neurologic outcomes. Cardiol Young 2010; 20(1): 18-24.
[http://dx.doi.org/10.1017/S1047951109992046] [PMID: 20092673]

[19]   Lacey SR, Donofrio MT. Fetal cardiac tumors: prenatal diagnosis and outcome. Pediatr Cardiol 2007; 28(1): 61-7.
[http://dx.doi.org/10.1007/s00246-005-0876-9] [PMID: 17308946]

[20]   Sklansky M, Greenberg M, Lucas V, Gruslin-Giroux A. Intrapericardial teratoma in a twin fetus: diagnosis and management. Obstet Gynecol 1997; 89(5 Pt 2): 807-9.
[http://dx.doi.org/10.1016/S0029-7844(97)00031-8] [PMID: 9166328]

[21]   Atallah J, Robertson M, Rebeyka IM, Dyck J, Noga ML. Antenatal diagnosis and successful surgical removal of a large right ventricular fibroma. Pediatr Cardiol 2006; 27(4): 493-6.
[http://dx.doi.org/10.1007/s00246-006-1260-0] [PMID: 16835803]

[22]   Paladini D, Tartaglione A, Vassallo M, Martinelli P. Prenatal ultrasonographic findings of a cardiac myxoma. Obstet Gynecol 2003; 102(5 Pt 2): 1174-6.
[PMID: 14607047]

[23]   Ríos JC, Chávarri F, Morales G, *et al.* Cardiac myxoma with prenatal diagnosis. World J Pediatr Congenit Heart Surg 2013; 4(2): 210-2.
[http://dx.doi.org/10.1177/2150135112472210] [PMID: 23799738]

[24]   Sharma J, Hirata Y, Mosca RS. Surgical repair in neonatal life of cardiac haemangiomas diagnosed prenatally. Cardiol Young 2009; 19(4): 403-6.
[http://dx.doi.org/10.1017/S1047951109004168] [PMID: 19442320]

[25]   Eckstein FS, Heinemann MK, Mielke GJ, Greschniok A, Bader P, Ziemer G. Resection of a large right atrial hemangioma in a neonate after prenatal diagnosis. Ann Thorac Surg 1999; 68(3): 1074-5.
[http://dx.doi.org/10.1016/S0003-4975(99)00659-1] [PMID: 10510016]

[26]   Paladini D, Palmieri S, Russo MG, Pacileo G. Cardiac multiple rhabdomyomatosis: prenatal diagnosis and natural history. Ultrasound Obstet Gynecol 1996; 7(1): 84-5.
[http://dx.doi.org/10.1046/j.1469-0705.1996.07010084.x] [PMID: 8932639]

[27]   Sokolowski L, Respondek-Liberska M. The follow up of 114 fetuses and newborns (without chromosomal aberrations) with echogenic intracardiac focus detected in prenatal US. Prenat Cardiol 2014; 4: 6-10.

[28]   Strzelecka I, Sylwestrzak O, Krekora M, Przysło Ł, Gach A, Respondek-Liberska M. Fetal cardiac tumours in a referral prenatal cardiology centre – series of 37 cases with neonatal follow-up. Prenat Cardiol 2019.
[http://dx.doi.org/10.5114/pcard.2019.92399]

CHAPTER 4

Premature Closure of the Foramen Ovale and the Ductus Arteriosus

Eliane Lucas[1,2,3], **Carla Verona Barreto Farias**[4,5] and **Nathalie Jeanne Magioli Bravo-Valenzuela**[5,6,*]

[1] *Department of Pediatrics, Bonsucesso Federal Hospital (HFB-MS), Rio de Janeiro-RJ, Brazil*

[2] *Department of Pediatrics, University Center Organ Mountains (UNIFESO), Teresópolis-RJ, Brazil*

[3] *Department of Pediatrics, Central Hospital of the Army (HCE), Rio de Janeiro-RJ, Brazil*

[4] *Department of Pediatrics, Fernandes Figueira Institute, Oswaldo Cruz Foundation (IFF-FIOCRUZ), Rio de Janeiro-RJ, Brazil*

[5] *Discipline of Pediatrics (Pediatric Cardiology), Department of Medicine, Federal University of Rio de Janeiro (UFRJ), Rio de Janeiro-RJ, Brazil*

[6] *Discipline of Fetal Medicine, Department of Obstetrics, Paulista School of Medicine, Federal University of São Paulo (EPM-UNIFESP), São Paulo-SP, Brazil*

Abstract: The foramen ovale and the ductus arteriosus are fetal circulation shunt sites, and the appropriate flow profile in these shunts allows the maintenance of fetal hemodynamic stability. The presence of restrictive or closed foramen ovale and/or ductus arteriosus may lead to poor fetal outcomes, such as right ventricular failure, neonatal pulmonary hypertension, or even death. Fetal echocardiography is the main tool for the diagnosis and assessment of premature closure of the foramen ovale and/or ductus arteriosus, and its intrauterine and/or postnatal management. In some cases, fetal intervention or soon after birth may be required in the presence of fetal hemodynamic instability.

Keywords: Abnormal cardiac position, Ductus arteriosus, Echocardiography, Foramen ovale, Premature constriction of fetal ductus arteriosus, Restrictive or closed foramen ovale.

* **Corresponding author Nathalie J. M. Bravo-Valenzuela:** Discipline of Fetal Medicine, Department of Obstetrics, Paulista School of Medicine, Federal University of São Paulo (EPM-UNIFESP), R. Napoleão de Barros, 871/875, 04024-002, São Paulo-SP, Brazil; Tel/Fax: +55 11 5571-0761; E-mail: njmbravo@cardiol.br

RESTRICTED OR CLOSED FORAMEN OVALE

The foramen ovale (FO) is a channel at the interatrial septum level that is of great importance during fetal life. It provides the only pathway for oxygenated maternal blood to enter the left heart and upper body of the fetus. It is estimated that 65% of the blood flow from the inferior vena cava (IVC) runs through the FO into the left atrium (LA) and left ventricle (LV), promoting LV development and directing oxygenated blood to the coronary and cerebral arteries [1].

The formation of the atrial septum (AS) begins in the 4th week of gestation with the cranial dorsal migration of the septum primum towards the endocardial cushion. During the 5th and 6th weeks of intrauterine life, the development of the septum secundum begins. In this developing septum secundum, a channel is formed, the FO. And the free border of the septum primum is screened in the ultrasound as the FO membrane (Figs. **1** and **2**).

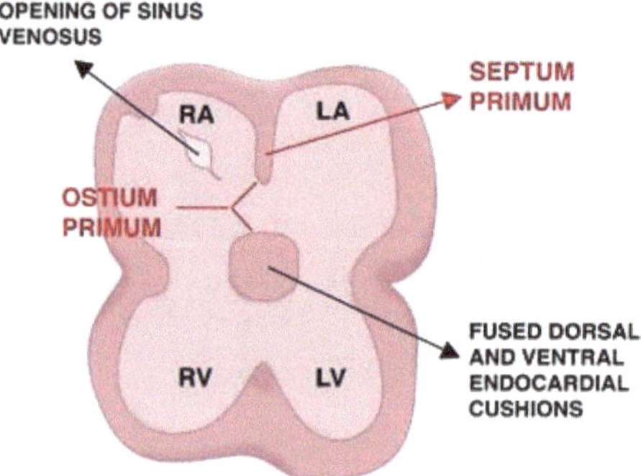

Fig. (1). Embryological septation of the atria. RA: right atrium; LA: left atrium; RV: right ventricle; LV: left ventricle.

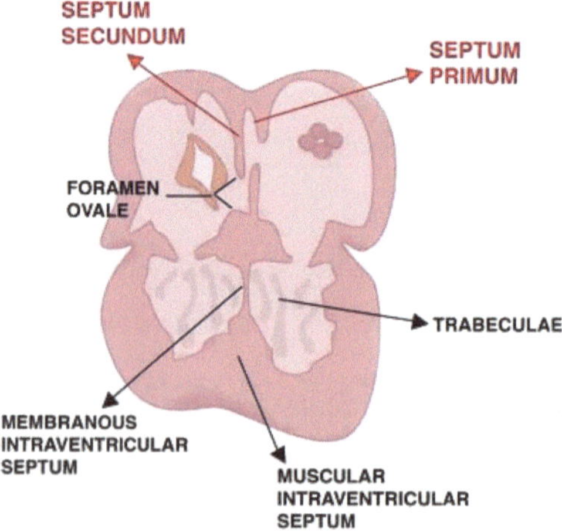

Fig. (2). Free border of the septum primum (foramen ovale membrane).

In the fetus, ventricular development is stimulated by the preload blood volume. However, for the left side of the heart, the FO is an important limiting factor, particularly in cases of a restrictive foramen ovale (rFO) or premature closure. In normal fetal physiology, it is not the oval hole of the septum that constitutes the area restricting the flow to the LA, but rather the horizontal area between the FO valve and the atrial septum above the FO (Fig. **3**) [2].

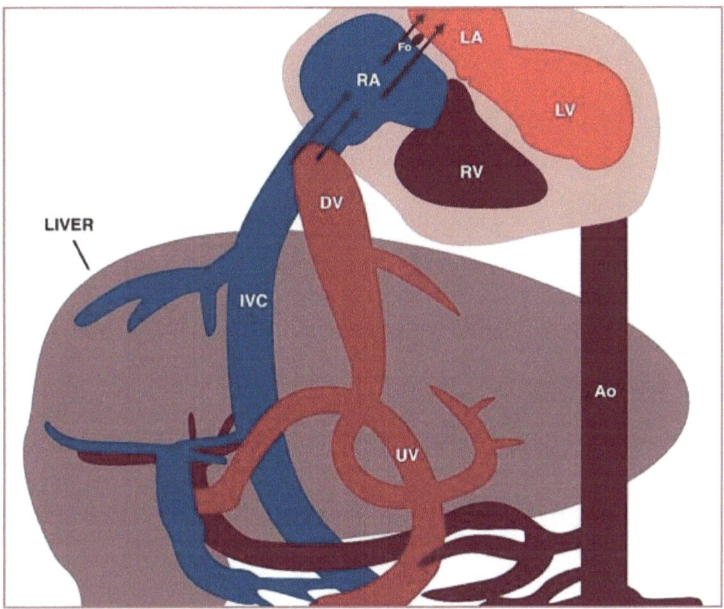

Fig. (3). Flow profile at the Fo; red: flow to the left atrium; blue: flow to the right atrium (RA). IVC: inferior vena cava; UV: umbilical vein; DV: ductus venosus; RA: right atrium; Fo: foramen ovale; LA: left atrium; RV: right ventricle; LV: left ventricle; Ao: aorta.

The first description of a closed foramen ovale (cFO) appeared in 1981 in a paper by Redel and Hansmann using the Doppler, who described two cases. In 1989, Fraser reported factors linked to the redundancy of the FO, thus leading to its greater migration to the upper and lower portions associated with lesser mobility of the septum primum [3, 4].

Subsequently, Chobot *et al.* demonstrated an increase in flow speed through an rFO on the echocardiogram [5]. Restricted or closed foramen ovale (rFO/cFO) are more frequently found in fetuses with congenital heart defects, especially in cases requiring a left-right atrial level shunts (hypoplasia of the left chambers), right-left shunts (right heart hypoplasia), or with heart diseases in which the left atrial pressure rises (mitral / aortic atresia and transposition of the great arteries [6, 7].

Important hemodynamic changes occur in the presence of rFO/cFO, depending mainly on gestational age and the degree of flow restriction. When the event occurs at the onset of gestation, severe left ventricular hypoplasia is frequently associated, in contrast, at later phases it may develop with few repercussions in the LV, although right heart failure and atrial septum aneurysm may be present [8].

Restricted or Closed Foramen Ovale with Structurally Normal Heart

The presence of rFO or cFO in a fetus with no congenital heart disease (CHD) is a very rare condition, although it is one of the causes of right chamber dilatation in a fetus (Table **1**). In cases where there is interatrial septum aneurysm, there may be difficulties in the accuracy of FO diameter, or it may also be confused with cortriatriatum [6].

Table 1. Differential diagnosis of causes for right-ventricular enlargement and redundant atrial septum.

Right-ventricular enlargement	Premature constriction of the ductus arteriosus Arteriovenosus malformations Aneurysm of the Galen vein Absent ductus venosus Coarctation of the aorta Intrauterine growth restriction
Redundant atrial septum	Cortriatriatum

Uzun *et al.* found 1.4% fetuses with rFO or cFO in the presence of increased RA and right ventricle (RV) in hearts without other structural defects [9]. The dilated dimensions of the right cavities, hypermobility or redundancy of the interatrial septum primum, increased right/left flow, and accentuation of the posterior angle of the ductus arteriosus were the most constant findings (Fig. **4**). The diagnosis of rFO by fetal echocardiography may be made according to the following published echocardiographic criteria: FO ≤ 2.5mm (obtained at four-chamber view), FO Doppler ≥ 40 cm/s, FO/right atrium ratio<0.3, and FO/diameter of ascending aorta ratio<0.52 (Table **2**) [9]. The complete closure of the FO was considered as being the absence of an FO aperture and flow, in a Doppler color study.

Table 2. Echocardiographic findings in restrictive foramen ovale.

Cardiac Structure	Measurements
Foramen ovale FO diameter	≤ 2.5 mm
FO Doppler	≥ 40 cm/s
Redundant atrial septum	Yes

(Table 2) cont.....

Cardiac Structure	Measurements
FO/RA ratio	<0.3
FO/aorta ratio	<0.52
FO/atrial septum length ratio	<0.33
Right ventricle Dilated right ventricle	>+2 (Z score)
Right/left ventricle size ratio	>1.2
Moderate tricuspid regurgitation	Yes
Cardiac output Right/ combined ventricular output ratio	>0.65
Right/left ventricular output ratio	>1.42
Pulmonary artery Pulmonary/aorta	>1.2
Ductus arteriosus and Aortic isthmus Posterior angulated ductus	Yes
Nonrestrictive anterior ductus Aortic isthmus-to-ductus ratio	Yes <0.74

FO: foramen ovale; RA: right atrium.

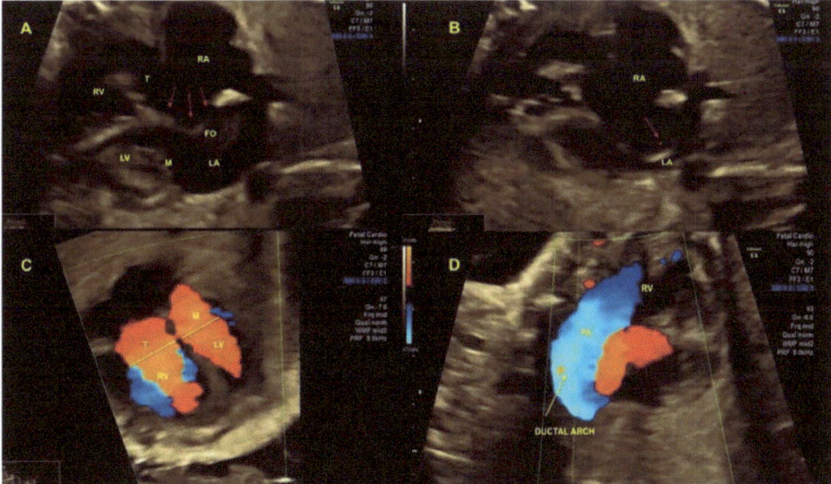

Fig. (4). Fetal echocardiogram of a 32 weeks fetus rFO and no other cardiac defects: note the redundant atrial septum (red arrows) (**A** and **B**), the enlargement of the right RA (**B**) and RV with RV/LV ratio > 1.5 (**C**) and the posterior angulated ductus arteriosus with no restrictive flow (**D**). RA: right atrium; LA: left atrium; RV: right ventricle; LV: left ventricle; FO: forame ovale; rFO: restricted forame ovale; M: mitral valve; T: tricuspid valve; PA: pulmonary artery.

The studies show the importance of performing a study of fetal ventricular function in situations of hemodynamic changes such as rFO and cFO. The blood that returns though the IVC, the size of FO and RV filling are important factors in the assessment of the function of LV. This occurs in the same way at RV function. In these cases, the calculation of the RV function is thus necessary. The assessment of global contractility is applied to the ejection fraction or shortening fraction, using M-mode altered only at a late stage of ventricular dysfunction. Other diastolic (E/A) or combined (systolic and diastolic) function parameters such as the myocardial performance index (MPI) or the Tei index, tricuspid annular plane systolic excursion (TAPSE) (Fig. **5**), pulmonary vein, FO pulsatility, and lateral tissue Doppler of the right ventricle (Fig. **6**) are also indicators used to improve the accuracy of the assessment [10].

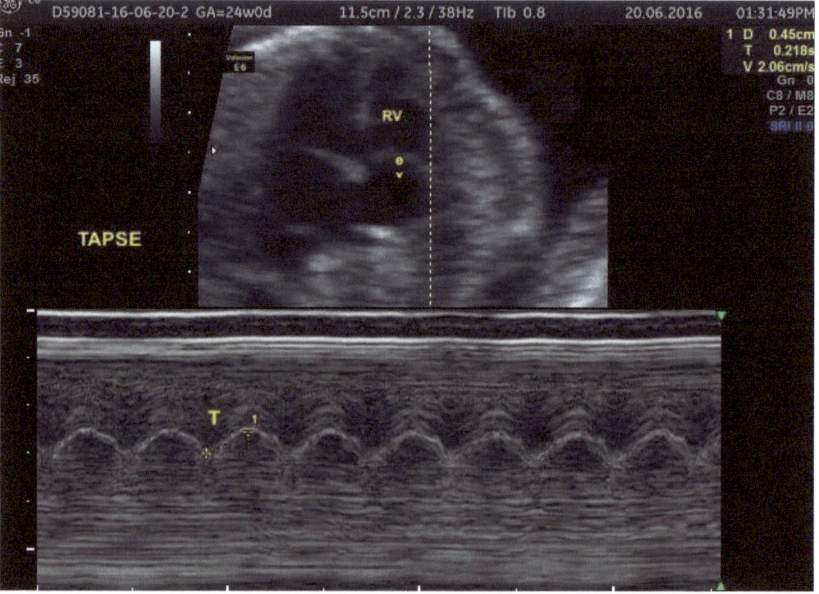

Fig. (5). The maximum systolic excursion of tricuspid valve (TAPSE) assessment in the apical four-chamber view of the fetal hear, by M-mode. T: TAPSE = 4.5 mm. RV: right ventricle.

More recently, Gu *et al.* evaluated a robust cohort with 9,704 fetuses, observing only 0.89% with rFO and 0.07% cFO in the group without CHD [11]. These groups were also identified as having major alterations: dilation of the right atrium and ventricle, tricuspid regurgitation, and pericardial effusion. No fetal deaths were noted during follow-up, but neonatal mortality was very significant (40%) in the cFO group. The literature shows that rFO/cFO without CHD is considered a benign presentation; however, some cases may manifest in the neonatal period associated with pulmonary hypertension [9].

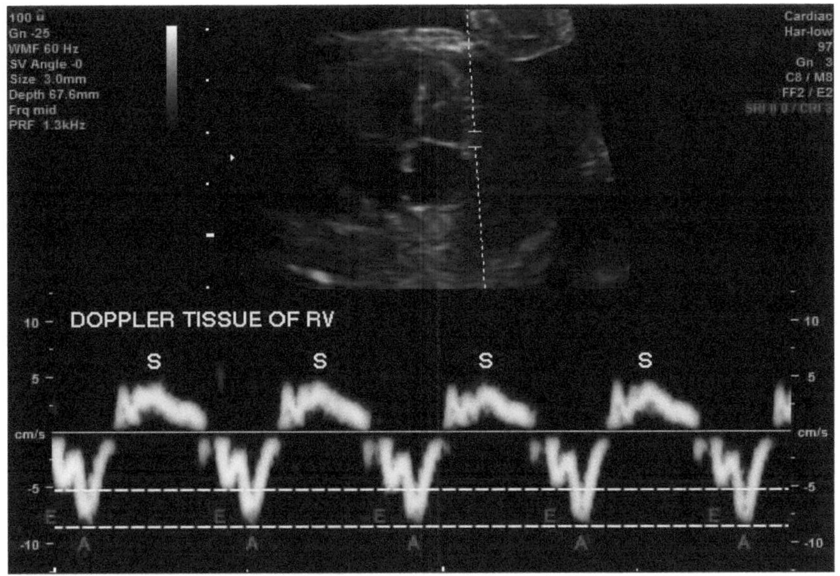

Fig. (6). Lateral tissue Doppler of the right ventricle. RV: right ventricle; E: e wave (rapid filling of RV); A: a wave (slow filling of RV); S: s wave (RV systolic wave).

Restrictive or Closed Foramen Ovale with Congenital Heart Disease

The patency of the FO is important for maintaining normal fetal cardiac flow [5]. Foramen ovale restriction or closure has a greater incidence in fetuses with CHDs and required atrial shunting and/or left atrial hypertension [6].

Foramen ovale restriction or closure in fetuses with CHD may lead to hemodynamic damage *in utero* or after birth. Some studies suggest performing serial ultrasound assessment for at-risk fetuses with CHD in order to preserve fetal well-being, program the timing and mode of delivery, and develop management protocols for *in utero* and postnatal care, such as the maintenance of a fetal FO shunt in these cases [6, 12].

Hypoplastic left heart syndrome (HLHS) and dextro-transposition of the great arteries (d-TGA) may be at greater risk of immediate neonatal distress if echocardiographic features of the restriction of the FO are found during serial evaluations [13]. According to Donofrio *et al.*, a fetus with HLHS or d-TGA with restrictive or closed FO has a stratified postnatal level of care (LOC) of 3 or 4, where a cardiac instability and the need for urgent intervention may occur soon after birth [14].

Balloon atrial septostomy (BAS) is a procedure that enlarges atrial communication and is the accepted standard for improving cyanosis by allowing atrial level shunting [15]. These fetuses with LOC 3 or 4 must generally be assisted and/or delivered at or near centers able to perform a BAS procedure *In utero* in some cases of HLHS or immediately after birth. Respondek-Liberska *et al.* in a retrospective analysis of 16 cases concluded that for a fetus with CHD that relies on atrial shunting, assessment of the FO is extremely important during the prenatal stage [16]. Prenatal echocardiography data restriction of the FO as FO diameter of 4 mm or less, shunt across the FO with a peak velocity greater than 70 cm/s and reversal flow in pulmonary veins must be taken into account as valuable information suggesting high priority for a fetal procedure or early postnatal cardiac procedure.

Dextro – Transposition of the Great Arteries

In a fetus with dextro – transposition of the great arteries (d-TGA), FO restriction is secondary to the outcome of hemodynamic alterations, in that the physiopathology of highly oxygenated blood in the left ventricle is pumped directly to the pulmonary artery. When researching fetal lambs, Konduri *et al.* [17] found that a 13% increase in oxygen saturation was associated with a three-fold increase in pulmonary blood flow. This blood then returns to the fetal heart through the pulmonary veins and may cause the oxygen saturation in the left ventricle to be even higher than that in the normal heart, with the left atrial pressure increasing from 4 to 8 mmHg [18].

In critical d-TGA, described as requiring a BAS procedure within the first 24 hours after delivery, a prenatal diagnostic criteria for post-delivery FO restriction is important, because even a short delay in performing the procedure (*e.g.* that interval during transfer to a tertiary cardiac center) can lead to cyanosis, acidosis, multiorgan failure, and death, owing to the failure to restore proper hemodynamic conditions before undergoing cardiac surgery [18].

In recent publications, echocardiographic criteria have been proposed for a diagnosis of restriction or closure of the foramen ovale in d-TGA [12, 14, 15, 19, 20]:

1) Hypermobile septum, defined as a septum primum flap that oscillates between both atria [15],

2) Angle of septum primum < 30°, the angle between the septum primum and the rest of the atrial septum [21],

3) Lack of swinging motion of septum or "tethered" septum,

4) Bowing of atrial septum > 50%, the aneurysmal septum primum bulged 50% of the way across to the left atrial free wall [21],

5) Intact atrial septum.

Punn *et al.* also included as a feature of restrictive FO the restrictive atrial septum: small orifice with color Doppler flow aliasing across the atrial septum [15]. Słodki *et al.* in a recent retrospective study of 51 patients with singleton pregnancies diagnosed prenatally with fetal d-TGA, prenatal sonographic features like increased pulmonary venous blood flow (at the entrance into the left atrium) with a cut-off value of 41 cm/s provided maximum specificity (100%) and positive predictive value (100%) for prenatally predict the need for BAS procedure early before delivery [18]. In this study, a flattened FO valve was also a statistically significant variable observed in 52% of patients who required a BAS in the first 24 hours after birth [18].

Hypoplastic Left Heart Syndrome with Restrictive or Intact Atrial Septum

The hearts of fetuses diagnosed with HLHS have an elevated left atrial pressure, because this pressure may increase as the disease progresses, with the flow across the FO becoming bidirectional and eventually left to right [22]. This physiopathology leads to a stop on left ventricle growth, and while the FO is becoming restrictive, or even closed, the pulmonary venous return in the fetal heart will be impaired, so associated severe fetal pulmonary vascular disease may occur with a poor prognostic soon after birth.

Assessment of the FO flow is recommended every four to six weeks by serial ultrasound evaluation with Doppler evaluation of the flow pattern in pulmonary veins. Finding a ratio of forward pulmonary vein flow to reverse flow of less than 3 (the pulmonary flow is expressed as a velocity-time integral) is an indirect feature of restrictive FO, meaning that there is a high probability of needing intervention to open the atrial septum *in utero* or early after birth [23, 24]. Some authors also proposed echocardiographic criteria for the diagnosis of restriction or closure of the foramen ovale in HLHS. The ratio of forward pulmonary vein (PV) flow to reversed flow of less than three (where the pulmonary vein flow is expressed as a velocity-time integral) denotes a severe obstruction in FO, and for diagnostic of moderate obstruction of the foramen ovale in HLHs, the echocardiographic find is a ratio of forward/reverse (f/r) pulmonary vein flow < 5 and >3 [12, 14, 19, 20] (Fig. **7**). In a review publication of fetal interventions for structural heart disease, the echocardiographic features for consideration of fetal intervention for HLHS and rFo/cFO are: intact atrial septum (IAS) or ≤ 1 mm atrial septum defect, and PV r/s < 3 [24, 25].

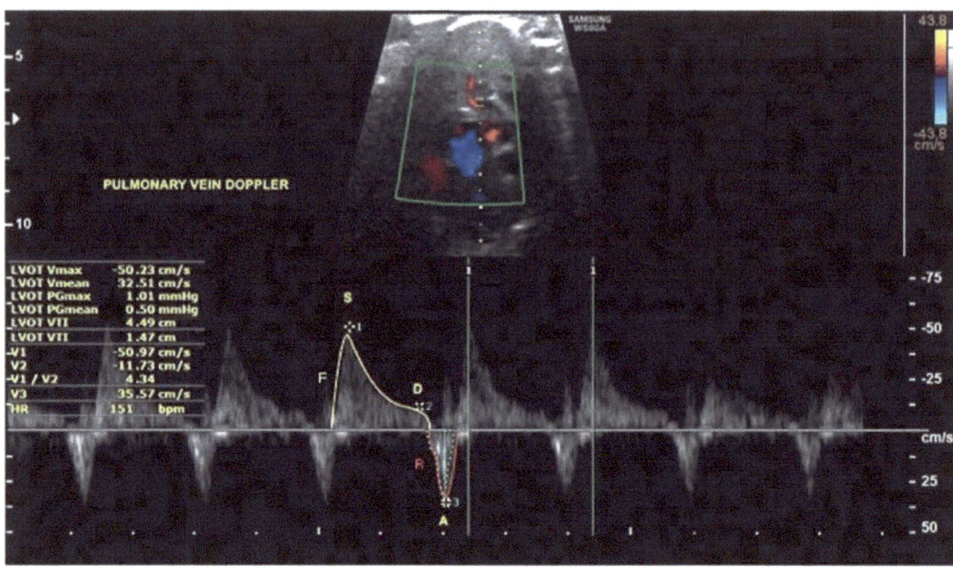

Fig. (7). Pulmonary vein Doppler in a case of a 27 week's fetus with hypoplastic left heart syndrome (HLHS) and restrictive foramen ovale. Ratio of velocity-time integral of forward (4.4 cm) to reverse PV flow (1.4 cm) = 3.1PV: pulmonary vein; F: forward PV flow (S+D waves); S: systolic wave of PV; R: reverse PV flow.

Echocardiographic criteria for the diagnosis of rFo/cFO in d-TGA and HLHS are summarized in Table **3**.

Table 3. Echocardiographic features of restrictive / closed foramen in congenital heart diseases.

CHD	Echocardiographic features
d-TGA	- Hypermobile septum - Angle of septum primum < 30° - Lack of swinging motion of septum or "tethered" septum - Bowing of atrial septum > 50% - Intact atrial septum (IAS) - PV blood flow > 41cm/s *
HLHS	- PV Doppler: forward to reversed (f/r) VTI ratio: moderate obstruction f/r < 5 and > 3 severe obstruction f/r < 3 - IAS or atrial septum ≤ 1 mm *

CDH: congenital heart disease; d-TGA: dextro-transposition of the great arteries; HLHS: hypoplastic left heart syndrome; PV: pulmonary vein; VTI: velocity-time integral

2-PREMATURE CLOSURE OF THE DUCTUS ARTERIOSUS

Introduction

Premature constriction of the ductus arteriosus (DA) is not a structural cardiac malformation, but it is a functional abnormality that we must rule out during the diagnostic investigation of fetuses with right chambers enlargement, signs of heart failure and hydrops. Depending upon the degree and duration of the ductal constriction, it may be related to severe conditions with fetal heart failure, fetal hydrops, and even fetal or neonatal death.

Ductus Arteriosus- Embryology and Anatomy

The DA derives from the distal portion of the sixth aortic arch. Around the 29th day of fetal development, after the division of the truncus arteriosus by the aorticopulmonary septum, the ventral aorta and pulmonary artery are created. Thus, the sixth aortic arch becomes the pulmonary arch. On the right side, it becomes the proximal segment of the right pulmonary artery and on the left, it remains during fetal life as the DA. After birth, the functional closure of the DA occurs and it continues to function as an arterial ligament [26 - 28].

The DA is a vessel that connects the trunk of the pulmonary artery to the descending thoracic aorta, distally to the left subclavian artery. When the aortic arch is positioned to the right instead of in the normal topography (to the left), the DA may be positioned to the right, joining the right pulmonary artery to the right aortic arch below the right subclavian artery. The DA is rarely bilateral. During fetal life, the DA is a large vessel with a relatively uniform diameter, and its post-natal closure begins at the pulmonary extremity. Histologically, the media of the DA is predominantly composed of layers of smooth muscle arranged in a spiral, while the middle layers of the aorta and pulmonary artery mainly comprise elastic fibers [29, 30].

Mechanisms of Ductal Constriction and Hemodynamic Fetal Repercussions

Around the 6th week of gestation, the DA is sufficiently developed to handle most of the cardiac output (CO) of the right ventricle and in the third trimester approximately 40% of the combined CO is directed to this vessel. Thus, the DA allows directing the flow of pulmonary circulation that has high vascular resistance to the descending aorta and to placental circulation, being the latter a low resistance circulation [2, 31].

As already described, the media of the DA wall is predominantly muscular and increasingly so from the second to the third trimester of gestation, which makes this vessel more sensitive to vasoconstrictor factors [30 - 32]. Several studies have shown the vasodilator effect of prostaglandins on the DA (prostaglandin E2 in particular) [33]. In the production of prostaglandins, the enzymes cyclooxygenase-1 and 2 (COX-1 and COX-2) convert arachidonic acid to prostacyclins, thromboxane A2, and prostaglandins through oxygenation. COX-1 is expressed endogenously (*e.g.*, in platelets) and COX-2 is expressed by cells involved in inflammation, being induced by cytokines and other mediators at sites of inflammation [34, 35].

After the second trimester, it is well known that the administration of anti-inflammatory medications in pregnant women can cause constriction of the DA by interfering with the prostaglandin pathway. Thus, nonsteroidal anti-inflammatory drugs, such as indomethacin, nimesulide, diclofenac, ibuprofen, aspirin, and even paracetamol are examples of cyclooxygenase (COX) inhibiting medications and therefore have the potential to cause ductal constriction in fetuses [30, 36 - 40]. Among the anti-inflammatory drugs listed above, researchers extensively studied indomethacin and ductal restriction reportedly occurs several hours after maternal ingestion. It has been observed that ductal sensitivity can increase with gestational age, from the second to the third trimester, ranging from 5%–10% before 27 weeks up to 100% after 34 weeks [30, 31, 41]. Corticosteroids (nonsteroidal anti-inflammatory drugs) may also cause intrauterine ductal constriction. This effect is dose related and can be potentiated when associated with nonsteroidal anti-inflammatory drugs (synergism) [42]. Several studies demonstrated that other substances, such as retinoic acid, prostanoid EP4 receptors, and L-arginine analogs (L-name: nitric oxide synthesis inhibitors), can also induce ductal constriction [43 - 45].

Although some cases of ductal constriction have been described as idiopathic, an increasing number of authors reported an association between intrauterine ductal constriction and maternal consumption of a polyphenol-rich diet during the third trimester of pregnancy [46 - 48]. Polyphenols are substances characterized by having one or more hydroxyl groups bonded to one or more aromatic rings. There are the flavonoid and non-flavonoid polyphenols. Flavonoids are present in many foods and beverages consumed in the human diet and are known for their health benefits for a large part of the population. They have anti-inflammatory and antioxidant actions. However, studies have shown that, in the third trimester of pregnancy, the consumption of polyphenol-rich foods for a period of two weeks or more can interfere with DA flow with a risk of ductal constriction [49 - 53]. The mechanism proposed for the action of polyphenols on the flow of the DA is by COX and prostaglandin inhibition, mainly PGE2 [53, 54]. The main foods and beverages with a high concentration of polyphenols (> 30 mg per 100 mg or 100 mL) are: herbal teas, mate tea, dark chocolate, natural fruits and juices (oranges, red and purple grapes, strawberries and other berries), some vegetables (*e.g.*, red onions, tomatoes, and green herbs), oils (olive and soy), and red wine [55, 56]. Consequently, several studies suggest that pregnant women (class II, level A) should be warned to avoid excess consumption of polyphenol-rich foods in the third trimester of gestation to prevent DA constriction [57 - 59]. Therefore, the consumption of low-nutrition foods or beverages with high concentrations of polyphenols (herbal teas, mate tea, and dark chocolate) should be avoided in the 3rd trimester of gestation. Nutritional polyphenol-rich foods can be consumed in moderation, including the following: lettuce (10 leaves per day); red apple (without peel); orange (fruit or juice, 1 unit or 200 mL per day); red, pink, or white grapes (fruit or juice, 10 units per week); olive oil (up to 1 teaspoon per day); and herbs (12 teaspoons per day). Foods with a polyphenol concentration of less than 30 mg per 100 g can be freely consumed [58].

Fetal premature closure of DA evolves with hemodynamic repercussion for the fetus. The increase in resistance due to the duct flow obstruction will results in enlargement of the right chambers and pulmonary arteries, right ventricular (RV) hypertrophy, tricuspid and/or pulmonary insufficiency, and lastly RV systolic dysfunction. Increased pressure in the RV, especially in cases in which tricuspid insufficiency is more pronounced, contributes to increase FO shunting (from the RV to the LV), thereby overloading the LV. Although the rapid enlargement of the aortic isthmus enables fetal peripheral perfusion to be maintained for several days, ductal flow restriction can lead to failure of the RV with compromise to the LV, fetal cardiac failure, hydrops, and even fetal or neonatal death [60].

Ductal Constriction - Prenatal Diagnosis

The image of the DA in the sagittal plane (ductal arch) is crucial for the evaluation of ductal flow (Figs. **8** and **9**). The increased pressure in the pulmonary artery in cases of ductal constriction causes an increase in systolic and diastolic peaks of the ductal Doppler with a consequent reduction in the ductal pulsatility index (PI). The ductal PI [systolic peak velocity minus diastolic velocity / time averaged velocity] can be calculated by the equipment after manual tracing of the ductal flow waveform. For this evaluation, the Doppler sample should be positioned on the descending aorta at the end of the DA, assisted by color Doppler aligned as parallel as possible, at an angle < 30° (without using angle correction) (Fig. **10**). Thus, the echocardiographic diagnosis of ductal constriction in the presence of turbulent duct flow on color Doppler is confirmed when the pulse-wave Doppler parameters are as follows: a peak systolic velocity > 140 cm/s, ductal peak diastolic velocity > 30 cm/s, and PI < 2.2 (Fig. **11**) [61 - 63].

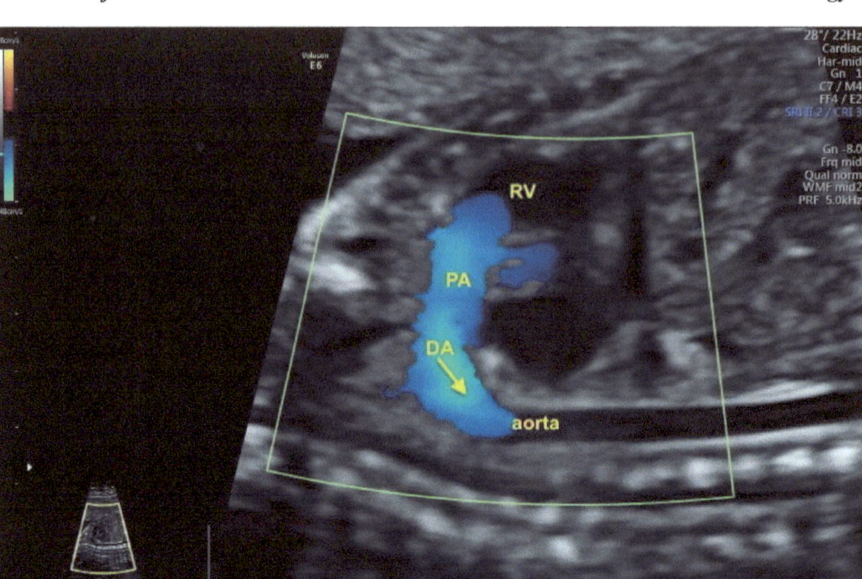

Fig. (8). Color Doppler of ductal arch: ductus arteriosus with normal flow. RV: right ventricle; PA: pulmonary artery; DA: ductus arteriosus.

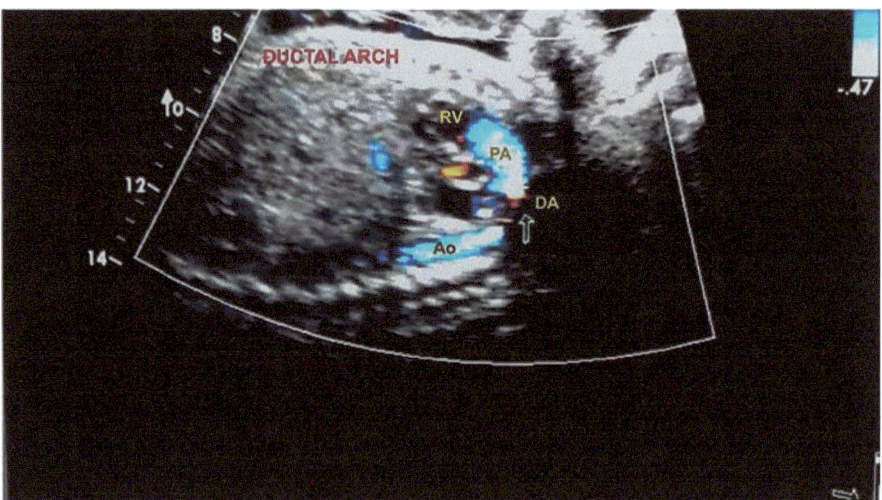

Fig. (9). Color Doppler of ductal arch: ductal flow obstruction in a case of ductus arteriosus constriction after administration of anti-inflammatory medication. Note the presence of turbulent flow (arrow). RV; right ventricle; PA: pulmonary artery; DA: ductus arteriosus; Ao: aorta.

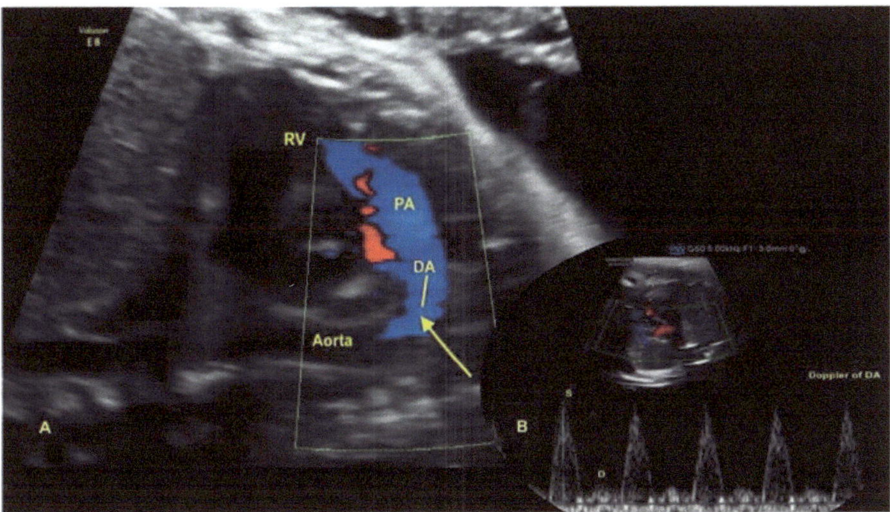

Fig. (10). Color Doppler of ductus arteriosus in the sagittal plane of the ductal arch (A). The pulsed-Doppler sample should be positioned on the descending aorta at the end of the DA (arrow) (B). DA: ductus arteriosus; S: systolic wave of DA flow; D: diastolic wave of DA flow; RV: right ventricle; PA: pulmonary artery.

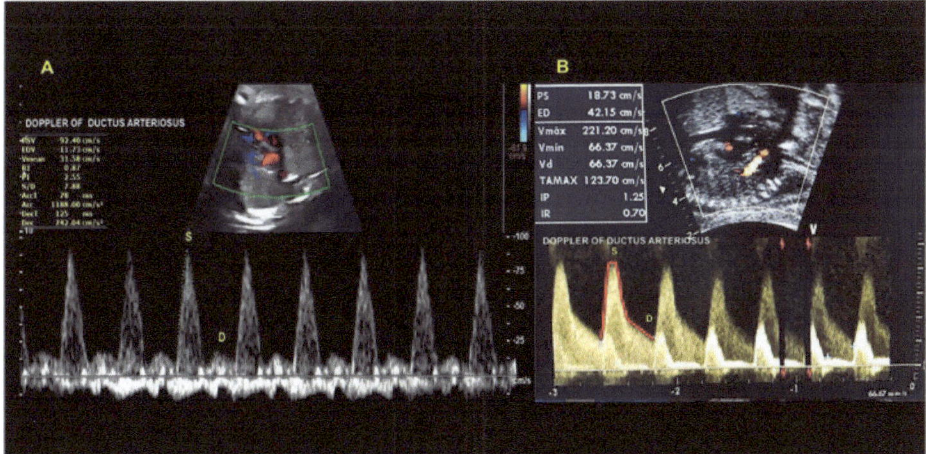

Fig. (11). **(A)** Ductus arteriosus (DA) without blood flow restriction with normal pulsatility index (PI= 2.55). **(B)** DA with blood flow restriction (pulsed Doppler sonography). Note the decreased pulsatility index (PI =1.25) and the systolic (221 cm/s) and diastolic (42.15 cm/s) peak velocities in case B. S: systolic wave of DA flow; D: diastolic wave of DA flow.

Cases of ductal constriction with any sign of hemodynamic compromise plus PI< 1.0 or cases of total ductal occlusion are considered as severe. Regarding the severity of the fetal hemodynamic compromise, it is considered as mild when the heart chambers are normal and tricuspid and/or pulmonary insufficiency is mild or absent, being moderate when there is RV dilatation without contractile dysfunction. The hemodynamic compromise is severe when there are RV dilatation and ventricular hypertrophy associated with significant tricuspid and/or pulmonary insufficiency. Complete closure of the DA is rare in fetal life and its diagnosis is confirmed by the absence of transductal flow on color Doppler. The use of advanced technology such as with high resolution Doppler (HD-flow) and realistic color Doppler with 3D and 4D spatiotemporal image correlation (STIC) may greatly assist in this evaluation (Fig. **12**).

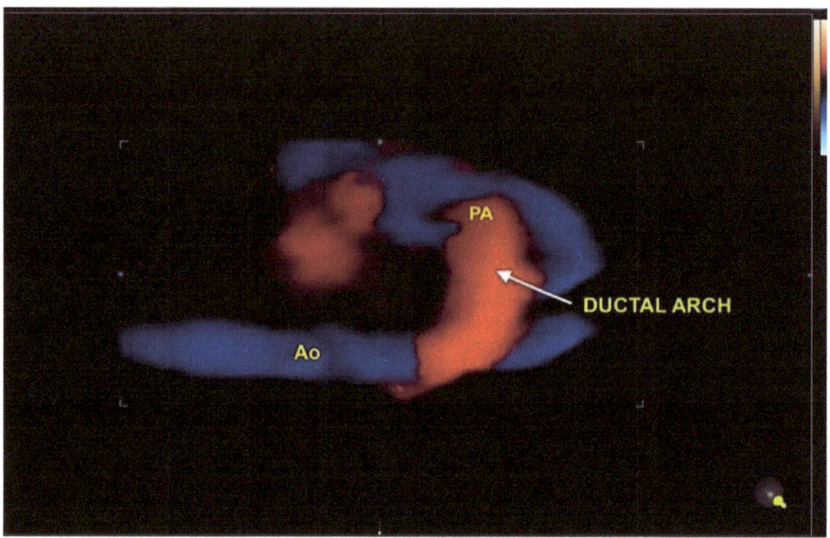

Fig. (12). Ductus arteriosus with normal blood flow in a 27-week fetus viewed in the ductal arch acquired with 4D spatiotemporal image correlation (STIC) and realistic color Doppler. Ao: aorta; PA: pulmonary artery.

The four-chamber view may reveal ventricular asymmetry with the signs of RV overload (RV dilatation, hypertrophy, and dysfunction) (Fig. **13**). The RV outflow tract and three vessels views enable the assessment of the pulmonary artery which can be enlarged in cases of ductal restriction (Fig. **14**). Several functional cardiac parameters, such as the fractional shortening of the RV, MPI or Tei index and the annular plane systolic excursion (TAPSE), should be combined to analyze RV function (Fig. **15**) [64, 65]. Finally, the cardiovascular profile score or 10-point score should be used to assess fetal heart failure (Fig. **16**). This score can help predict the prognosis of these fetuses in terms of the risk of progression to hydrops [66].

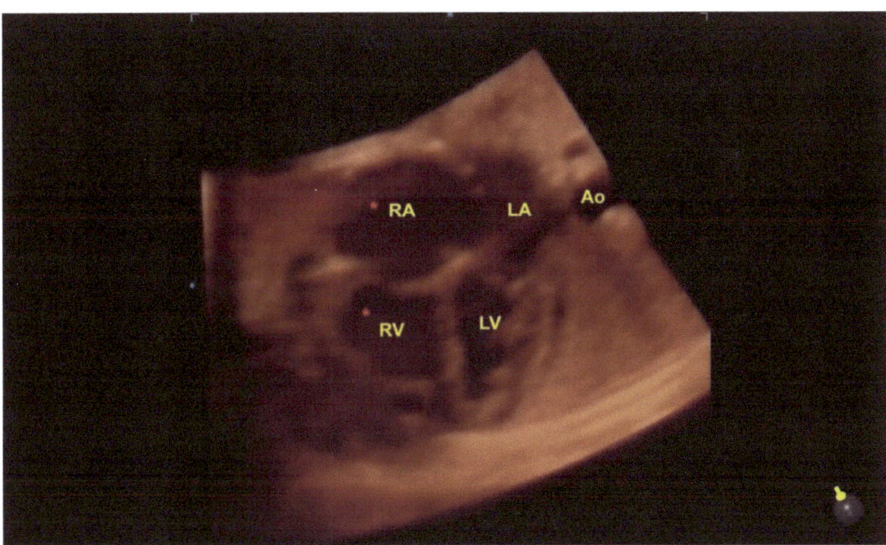

Fig. (13). 3D/4D fetal echocardiogram (4-chamber view with Cristal Vue™) showing an enlargement of the right chambers (*) in a case of ductus arteriosus constriction in a 32-week fetus. LA: left atrium; RA: right atrium; RV: right ventricle; LV: left ventricle; Ao: aorta.

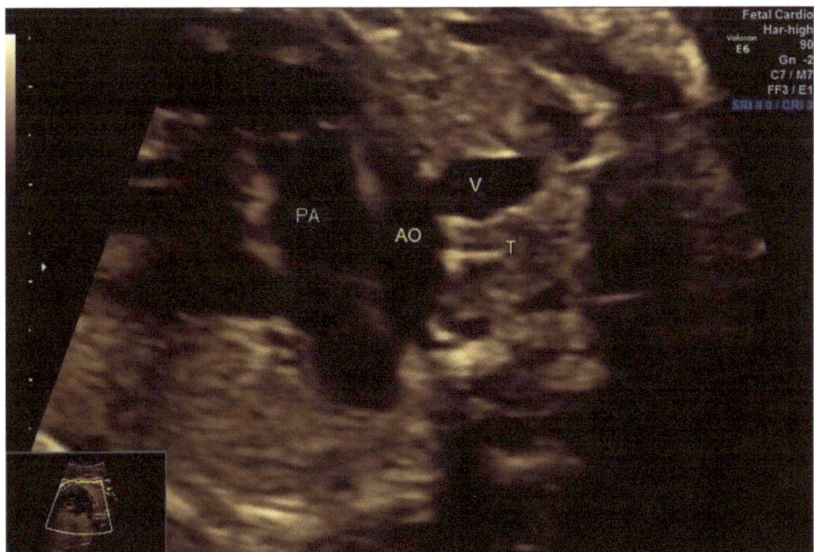

Fig. (14). Three-vessel view of the trachea showing an enlargement of the pulmonary artery trunk in a case of premature constriction of the ductus arteriosus due to consumption of polyphenol-rich foods. PA: pulmonary artery; AO: aorta; T: trachea; V: superior vena cava.

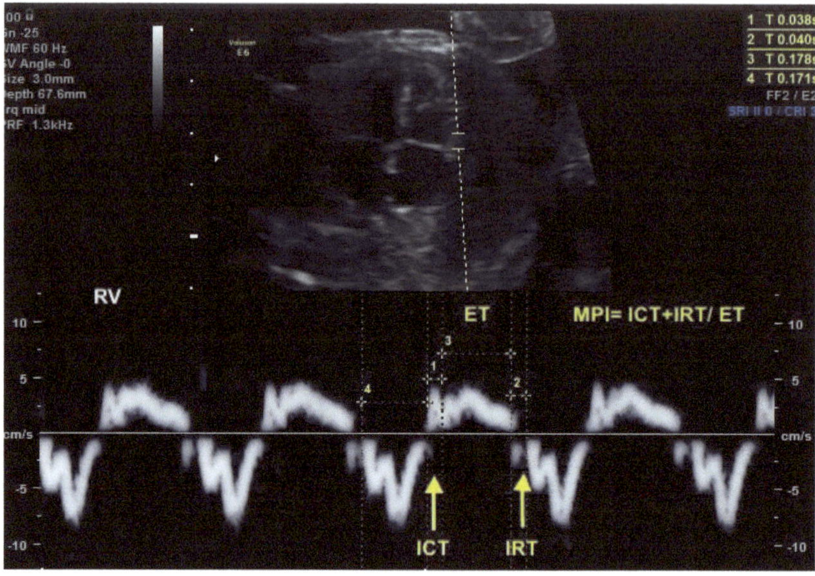

Fig. (15). Myocardial performance index (MPI) or Tei index of the right ventricle (RV) determined by tissue Doppler using the inflow and outflow values of the RV. MPI = IVCT + IVRT/ET. MPI: myocardial performance index; ICT: isovolumetric contraction time; IVRT: isovolumetric relaxation time; ET: ejection time.

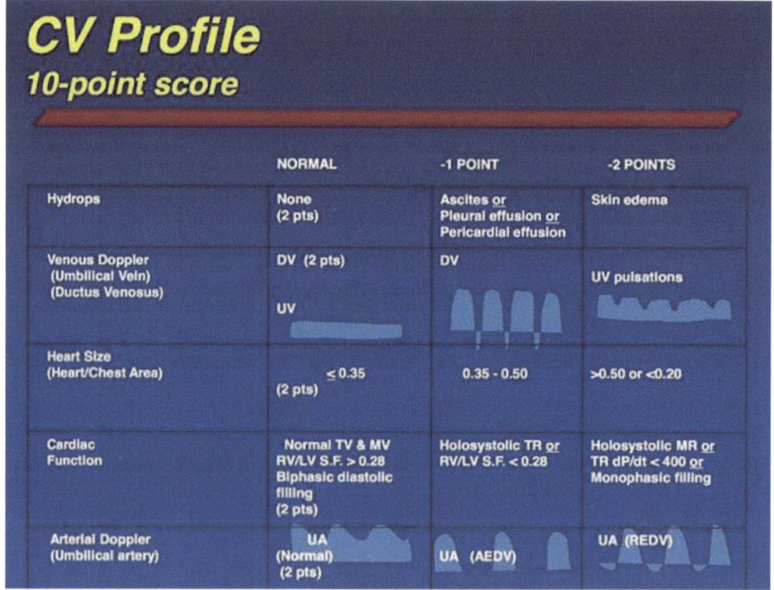

	NORMAL	-1 POINT	-2 POINTS
Hydrops	None (2 pts)	Ascites or Pleural effusion or Pericardial effusion	Skin edema
Venous Doppler (Umbilical Vein) (Ductus Venosus)	DV (2 pts) UV	DV	UV pulsations
Heart Size (Heart/Chest Area)	≤ 0.35 (2 pts)	0.35 - 0.50	>0.50 or <0.20
Cardiac Function	Normal TV & MV RV/LV S.F. > 0.28 Biphasic diastolic filling (2 pts)	Holosystolic TR or RV/LV S.F. < 0.28	Holosystolic MR or TR dP/dt < 400 or Monophasic filling
Arterial Doppler (Umbilical artery)	UA (Normal) (2 pts)	UA (AEDV)	UA (REDV)

Fig. (16). Parameters used in the cardiovascular (CV) profile to evaluate fetal heart failure. Normal score, 10; high risk, <7. UA: umbilical artery; DV: ductus venosus; SF: shortening fraction; MI: mitral insufficiency; MR: mitral valve regurgitation; TI: tricuspid insufficiency; TR: tricuspid valve regurgitation; UA: umbilical artery; UV: umbilical vein; AEDV: absent end-diastolic velocity; REDV: reversed end-diastolic velocity (Cortesy of Prof. James C. Huhta).

Differential diagnoses are the following: coarctation of aorta, tricuspid insufficiency due to congenital anomalies, and isolated dilatation of the right cavities. In coarctation of the aorta, the diameter of the aortic isthmus is reduced (Z score < −2.0) (Fig. **17**), in dysplasia of the tricuspid valve the leaflets are thickened, in the Ebstein anomaly there is apical displacement of the posterior and septal leaflets; and in the isolated dilatation of the right cavities, as the name indicates, there are no associated alterations and the flow of the DA is normal.

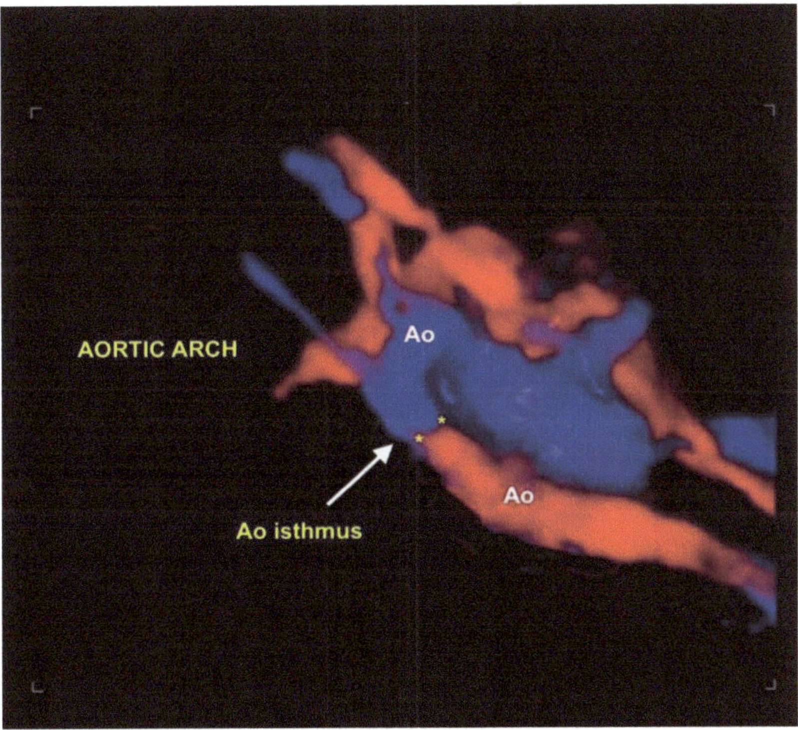

Fig. (17). 3D/4D spatiotemporal image correlation (STIC) acquisition combined with realistic view (color Doppler) of the aortic arch in a case of coarctation of the aorta. Aortic isthmus with Z score < −2.0. Ao: aorta.

Ductal Constriction- Progression and Prenatal Management

Initially, it is very important to identify an agent that may cause the ductal constriction through a detailed investigation about the intake of medications, foods, and beverages (rich in polyphenols) that may have caused this closure. If such intake is identified it should be halted immediately. Subsequent management will depend on hemodynamic compromise. In clinical practice, ductal flow generally returns to normal in mild and moderate cases, with subsequent normalization of the hemodynamic changes after suspending administration or intake of the causal agent. In general, in clinical practice the delivery is recommended if the hemodynamic repercussions are severe. The risk of death is high in cases of endocardial ischemia, systolic dysfunction of the RV, and hydrops. If no etiological agent for the ductal constriction is identified, delivery may be recommended depending on gestational age and the hemodynamic status of the fetus.

Monitoring of DA flow and of fetal hemodynamic repercussions by fetal echocardiography is indicated every 24–48 h until ductal flow is re-established or delivery occurs. Following birth, many findings that signaled RV overload may take 3 weeks or longer to disappear. Several studies associated prenatal constriction of the DA with neonatal pulmonary hypertension [32, 37, 57].

Ductal constriction may be associated with heart disease, such as d-TGA, which makes the condition even more serious, and ultimately lethal if associated with a restrictive FO [20]. In contrast, in cases of Ebstein anomaly or severe tricuspid dysplasia with circular shunt physiology, researchers suggest that ductal constriction may be beneficial [50].

CONCLUSION

• The restrictive FO in fetuses without associated CHD has a good prognosis in most cases.

• The rFO or cFO has a higher incidence in fetuses with CHD.

• In congenital heart defects such as d-TGA or HLHS, the FO profile can predict fetal or newborn outcomes, and serial echocardiographic assessments of FO regarding restriction and/or closure features may direct the appropriate management of the fetus and/or the newborn, with the main objective of maintaining the hemodynamic stability of the patient.

• In fetuses with CHD, rFo/cFO is more frequent during the third trimester of gestation as pulmonary blood flow increases.

• A healthcare team must be very well trained, in order to deal with patients with diagnosed fetal CHD and rFo/cFO, being able to perform pre or postnatal atrial septostomy promptly, thus reducing morbidity and mortality before or after cardiac surgery.

• Premature closure of the DA is a functional anomaly that should always be ruled out during diagnostic investigation of fetuses with heart failure and hydrops.

• Initially, it is essential to conduct a detailed investigation about the intake of medications, foods, and beverages (rich in polyphenols) that might cause ductal closure and suspend their administration or consumption when identified.

• The presence of turbulent duct flow on color Doppler with ductal peak systolic velocity > 140 cm/s, ductal peak diastolic velocity > 30 cm/s, and pulsatility index < 2.2 confirm the echocardiographic diagnosis of prenatal ductal constriction.

CONSENT FOR PUBLICATION

Not applicable.

CONFLICT OF INTEREST

The authors confirm that the contents of this chapter have no conflict of interest.

ACKNOWLEDGEMENTS

The authors acknowledge Liana Bravo-Valenzuela e Silva graphic designer at Pedicor Pediatric Cardiology center in Brazil for editing figures to this chapter.

REFERENCES

[1]   Rudolph AM. Circulation in the normal fetus and cardio-vascular adaptations to birth.Fetal Cardiology: Embryology, Genetics, Physiology, Echocardiographic Evaluation, Diagnosis and Perinatal Management of Cardiac Diseases. 2nd ed. New York, NY: Informa Heathcare 2009; pp. 131-51.

[2]   Kiserud T. Physiology of the fetal circulation. Semin Fetal Neonatal Med 2005; 10(6): 493-503.
        [http://dx.doi.org/10.1016/j.siny.2005.08.007] [PMID: 16236564]

[3]   Redel DA, Hansmann M. Fetal obstruction of the foramen ovale detected by two-dimensional Doppler echocardiograhy.Echocardiology. Developments in Cardiovascular MedicineDordrecht: Springer 1981; pp. 425-9.
        [http://dx.doi.org/10.1007/978-94-009-8299-4_47]

[4]   Kiserud T, Rasmussen S. Ultrasound assessment of the fetal foramen ovale. Ultrasound Obstet Gynecol 2001; 17(2): 119-24.
        [http://dx.doi.org/10.1046/j.1469-0705.2001.00331.x] [PMID: 11251919]

[5]   Chobot V, Hornberger LK, Hagen-Ansert S, Sahn DJ. Prenatal detection of restrictive foramen ovale. J Am Soc Echocardiogr 1990; 3(1): 15-9.
        [http://dx.doi.org/10.1016/S0894-7317(14)80294-0] [PMID: 2310587]

[6]   Donofrio MT, Bremer YA, Moskowitz WB, Moskowitz WB. Diagnosis and management of restricted or closed foramen ovale in fetuses with congenital heart disease. Am J Cardiol 2004; 94(10): 1348-51.
        [http://dx.doi.org/10.1016/j.amjcard.2004.07.133] [PMID: 15541266]

[7]   Tseng SY, Alsaied T, Barnard K, Hahn E, Divanovic AA, Cnota JF. Tricuspid atresia with restrictive foramen ovale: A rare combination with implications on fetal growth. Echocardiography 2019; 36(4): 800-2.
        [http://dx.doi.org/10.1111/echo.14267] [PMID: 30693549]

[8]   Chrysostomou C, Romaguera RL, Rodriguez MM. Giant aneurysm of the atrial septum associated with premature closure of foramen ovale. Cardiovasc Ultrasound 2005; 3: 20.
        [http://dx.doi.org/10.1186/1476-7120-3-20] [PMID: 16098228]

[9]   Uzun O, Babaoglu K, Ayhan YI, *et al.* Diagnostic ultrasound features and outcome of restrictive foramen ovale in fetuses with structurally normal hearts. Pediatr Cardiol 2014; 35(6): 943-52.
        [http://dx.doi.org/10.1007/s00246-014-0879-5] [PMID: 24585219]

[10]   Bravo-Valenzuela NJ, Peixoto AB, Nardozza LM, Souza AS, Araujo Júnior E. Applicability and technical aspects of two-dimensional ultrasonography for assessment of fetal heart function. Med Ultrason 2017; 19(1): 94-101.
[http://dx.doi.org/10.11152/mu-934] [PMID: 28180202]

[11]   Gu X, Zhang Y, Han J, Liu X, Ge S, He Y. Isolated premature restriction or closure of foramen ovale in fetuses: Echocardiographic characteristics and outcome. Echocardiography 2018; 35(8): 1189-95.
[http://dx.doi.org/10.1111/echo.14009] [PMID: 29756643]

[12]   Sanapo L, Pruetz JD, Słodki M, Goens MB, Moon-Grady AJ, Donofrio MT. Fetal echocardiography for planning perinatal and delivery room care of neonates with congenital heart disease. Echocardiography 2017; 34(12): 1804-21.
[http://dx.doi.org/10.1111/echo.13672] [PMID: 29287132]

[13]   Bensemlali M, Bajolle F, Laux D, *et al.* Neonatal management and outcomes of prenatally diagnosed CHDs. Cardiol Young 2017; 27(2): 344-53.
[http://dx.doi.org/10.1017/S1047951116000639] [PMID: 27225605]

[14]   Donofrio MT, Skurow-Todd K, Berger JT, *et al.* Risk-stratified postnatal care of newborns with congenital heart disease determined by fetal echocardiography. J Am Soc Echocardiogr 2015; 28(11): 1339-49.
[http://dx.doi.org/10.1016/j.echo.2015.07.005] [PMID: 26298099]

[15]   Punn R, Silverman NH. Fetal predictors of urgent balloon atrial septostomy in neonates with complete transposition. J Am Soc Echocardiogr 2011; 24(4): 425-30.
[http://dx.doi.org/10.1016/j.echo.2010.12.020] [PMID: 21324642]

[16]   Respondek-Liberska M, Płużańska J, Słodki M, *et al.* Early neonatal surgery for heart defects after prenatal diagnosis of restricted foramen ovale as the priority procedure? Prenat Cardiol 2015; 5: 24-9.

[17]   Konduri GG, Gervasio CT, Theodorou AA. Role of adenosine triphosphate and adenosine in oxygen-induced pulmonary vasodilation in fetal lambs. Pediatr Res 1993; 33(5): 533-9.
[http://dx.doi.org/10.1203/00006450-199305000-00022] [PMID: 8511029]

[18]   Słodki M, Axt-Fliedner R, Zych-Krekora K, *et al.* New method to predict need for Rashkind procedure in fetuses with dextro-transposition of the great arteries. Ultrasound Obstet Gynecol 2018; 51(4): 531-6.
[http://dx.doi.org/10.1002/uog.17469] [PMID: 28295809]

[19]   Donofrio MT, Moon-Grady AJ, Hornberger LK, *et al.* Diagnosis and treatment of fetal cardiac disease: a scientific statement from the American Heart Association. Circulation 2014; 129(21): 2183-242.
[http://dx.doi.org/10.1161/01.cir.0000437597.44550.5d] [PMID: 24763516]

[20]   Sanapo L, Moon-Grady AJ, Donofrio MT. Perinatal and delivery management of infants with congenital heart disease. Clin Perinatol 2016; 43(1): 55-71.
[http://dx.doi.org/10.1016/j.clp.2015.11.004] [PMID: 26876121]

[21]   Jouannic JM, Gavard L, Fermont L, *et al.* Sensitivity and specificity of prenatal features of physiological shunts to predict neonatal clinical status in transposition of the great arteries. Circulation 2004; 110(13): 1743-6.
[http://dx.doi.org/10.1161/01.CIR.0000144141.18560.CF] [PMID: 15364811]

[22]   Frommelt MA. Challenges and controversies in fetal diagnosis and treatment: hypoplastic left heart syndrome. Clin Perinatol 2014; 41(4): 787-98.
[http://dx.doi.org/10.1016/j.clp.2014.08.004] [PMID: 25459774]

[23]   Abuhamad A, Chaoui R. A practical guide to fetal echocardiography normal and abnormal hearts. 3rd ed. Philadelphia, PA: Wolters /Kluwer 2016; pp. 329-53.

[24]   Schidlow DN, Freud L, Friedman K, Tworetzky W. Fetal interventions for structural heart disease. Echocardiography 2017; 34(12): 1834-41.

[http://dx.doi.org/10.1111/echo.13667] [PMID: 29287139]

[25]   Pedra SR, Peralta CF, Crema L, Jatene IB, da Costa RN, Pedra CA. Fetal interventions for congenital heart disease in Brazil. Pediatr Cardiol 2014; 35(3): 399-405.
[http://dx.doi.org/10.1007/s00246-013-0792-3] [PMID: 24030590]

[26]   Elumalai G, Ebami TU. patent ductus arteriosus" embryological basis and its clinical significance. Elixir Embryology 2016; 100: 43433-8.

[27]   Sadler T, Langman J. Langman's Medical Embryology. 12th ed. Philadelphia, PA: Lippincott: Williams & Wilkins 2012; pp. 185-9.

[28]   Ho SY, Anderson RH. Anatomical closure of the ductus arteriosus: a study in 35 specimens. J Anat 1979; 128(Pt 4): 829-36.
[PMID: 489470]

[29]   Huhta JC, Moise KJ, Fisher DJ, Sharif DS, Wasserstrum N, Martin C. Detection and quantitation of constriction of the fetal ductus arteriosus by Doppler echocardiography. Circulation 1987; 75(2): 406-12.
[http://dx.doi.org/10.1161/01.CIR.75.2.406] [PMID: 3802445]

[30]   Moise KJ Jr, Huhta JC, Sharif DS, et al. Indomethacin in the treatment of premature labor. Effects on the fetal ductus arteriosus. N Engl J Med 1988; 319(6): 327-31.
[http://dx.doi.org/10.1056/NEJM198808113190602] [PMID: 3393194]

[31]   Kiserud T, Acharya G. The fetal circulation. Prenat Diagn 2004; 24(13): 1049-59.
[http://dx.doi.org/10.1002/pd.1062] [PMID: 15614842]

[32]   Tarcan A, Gürakan B, Yildirim S, Ozkiraz S, Bilezikçi B. Persistent pulmonary hypertension in a premature newborn after 16 hours of antenatal indomethacin exposure. J Perinat Med 2004; 32(1): 98-9.
[http://dx.doi.org/10.1515/JPM.2004.019] [PMID: 15008397]

[33]   Backes CH, Smith CV. Patent ductus arteriosus - a complex problem in need of a solid conceptual foundation. Circ J 2016; 80(3): 601-2.
[http://dx.doi.org/10.1253/circj.CJ-16-0057] [PMID: 26831254]

[34]   Majed BH, Khalil RA. Molecular mechanisms regulating the vascular prostacyclin pathways and their adaptation during pregnancy and in the newborn. Pharmacol Rev 2012; 64(3): 540-82.
[http://dx.doi.org/10.1124/pr.111.004770] [PMID: 22679221]

[35]   Fries S, Grosser T. The cardiovascular pharmacology of COX-2 inhibition. Hematology (Am Soc Hematol Educ Program) 2005; - 445-51.
[http://dx.doi.org/10.1182/asheducation-2005.1.445] [PMID: 16304418]

[36]   Prefumo F, Marasini M, De Biasio P, Venturini PL. Acute premature constriction of the ductus arteriosus after maternal self-medication with nimesulide. Fetal Diagn Ther 2008; 24(1): 35-8.
[http://dx.doi.org/10.1159/000132403] [PMID: 18504378]

[37]   Luchese S, Mânica JL, Zielinsky P. Intrauterine ductus arteriosus constriction: analysis of a historic cohort of 20 cases. Arq Bras Cardiol 2003; 81(4): 405-410, 399-404.
[http://dx.doi.org/10.1590/S0066-782X2003001200007] [PMID: 14666282]

[38]   Schiessl B, Schneider KT, Zimmermann A, Kainer F, Friese K, Oberhoffer R. Prenatal constriction of the fetal ductus arteriosus--related to maternal pain medication? Z Geburtshilfe Neonatol 2005; 209(2): 65-8.
[http://dx.doi.org/10.1055/s-2005-864116] [PMID: 15852232]

[39]   Lopes LM, Carrilho MC, Francisco RP, Lopes MA, Krebs VL, Zugaib M. Fetal ductus arteriosus constriction and closure: analysis of the causes and perinatal outcome related to 45 consecutive cases. J Matern Fetal Neonatal Med 2016; 29(4): 638-45.
[http://dx.doi.org/10.3109/14767058.2015.1015413] [PMID: 25708490]

[40]   Peña DP, Sara AB, Martínez-Peñuela CR, *et al.* Restricción del ductus arterioso fetal en gestante del tercer trimestre por consumo de paracetamol. Rev Cuba Obstet Ginecol 2016; 42: 493-501.

[41]   Dudley DK, Hardie MJ. Fetal and neonatal effects of indomethacin used as a tocolytic agent. Am J Obstet Gynecol 1985; 151(2): 181-4.
       [http://dx.doi.org/10.1016/0002-9378(85)90008-0] [PMID: 3970083]

[42]   Levy R, Matitiau A, Ben Arie A, Milman D, Or Y, Hagay Z. Indomethacin and corticosteroids: an additive constrictive effect on the fetal ductus arteriosus. Am J Perinatol 1999; 16(8): 379-83.
       [http://dx.doi.org/10.1055/s-1999-6814] [PMID: 10772195]

[43]   Shaul PW. Maternal vitamin A administration and the fetal ductus arteriosus. Pediatr Res 2001; 49(6): 744-6.
       [http://dx.doi.org/10.1203/00006450-200106000-00005] [PMID: 11385132]

[44]   Momma K, Nakanishi T, Imamura S. Inhibition of *in vivo* constriction of fetal ductus arteriosus by endothelin receptor blockade in rats. Pediatr Res 2003; 53(3): 479-85.
       [http://dx.doi.org/10.1203/01.PDR.0000049516.70216.2E] [PMID: 12595598]

[45]   Reese J, Veldman A, Shah L, Vucovich M, Cotton RB. Inadvertent relaxation of the ductus arteriosus by pharmacologic agents that are commonly used in the neonatal period. Semin Perinatol 2010; 34(3): 222-30.
       [http://dx.doi.org/10.1053/j.semperi.2010.02.007] [PMID: 20494739]

[46]   Enzensberger C, Wienhard J, Weichert J, *et al.* Idiopathic constriction of the fetal ductus arteriosus: three cases and review of the literature. J Ultrasound Med 2012; 31(8): 1285-91.
       [http://dx.doi.org/10.7863/jum.2012.31.8.1285] [PMID: 22837295]

[47]   Trevett TN Jr, Cotton J. Idiopathic constriction of the fetal ductus arteriosus. Ultrasound Obstet Gynecol 2004; 23(5): 517-9.
       [http://dx.doi.org/10.1002/uog.980] [PMID: 15133807]

[48]   Zielinsky P, Busato S. Prenatal effects of maternal consumption of polyphenol-rich foods in late pregnancy upon fetal ductus arteriosus. Birth Defects Res C Embryo Today 2013; 99(4): 256-74.
       [http://dx.doi.org/10.1002/bdrc.21051] [PMID: 24339037]

[49]   Rakha S. Excessive maternal orange intake - a reversible etiology of fetal premature ductus arteriosus constriction: a case report. Fetal Diagn Ther 2017; 42(2): 158-60.
       [http://dx.doi.org/10.1159/000453063] [PMID: 28746929]

[50]   Khoi LM. Premature constriction of fetal ductus arteriosus: role of maternal intake of non-steroidal anti- inflammatory drugs (NSAIDS) and polyphenol-rich foods. Int. J Drug Res Tech 2017; 8: 101-10.

[51]   Sridharan S, Archer N, Manning N. Premature constriction of the fetal ductus arteriosus following the maternal consumption of camomile herbal tea. Ultrasound Obstet Gynecol 2009; 34(3): 358-9.
       [http://dx.doi.org/10.1002/uog.6453] [PMID: 19705407]

[52]   Tanaka M, Miyakoshi K, Yamada M, Kadohira I, Minegishi K, Yoshimura Y. Functional foods for the fetus? Acta Obstet Gynecol Scand 2011; 90(10): 1172-3.
       [http://dx.doi.org/10.1111/j.1600-0412.2011.01167.x] [PMID: 21535430]

[53]   Zielinsky P, Piccoli AL Jr, Manica JL, *et al.* Maternal consumption of polyphenol-rich foods in late pregnancy and fetal ductus arteriosus flow dynamics. J Perinatol 2010; 30(1): 17-21.
       [http://dx.doi.org/10.1038/jp.2009.101] [PMID: 19641513]

[54]   Vian I, Zielinsky P, Zílio AM, *et al.* Increase of prostaglandin E2 in the reversal of fetal ductal constriction after polyphenol restriction. Ultrasound Obstet Gynecol 2018; 52(5): 617-22.
       [http://dx.doi.org/10.1002/uog.18974] [PMID: 29205592]

[55]   USDA   Database   for   the   Flavonoid   Content   of   Selected   Foods   Release 2019.https://www.ars.usda.gov/ARSUserFiles/80400525/Data/Flav/Flav_R03.pdf

[56]   Neveu V, Perez-Jiménez J, Vos F, *et al.* Phenol-Explorer: an online comprehensive database on

polyphenol contents in foods. Database (Oxford) 2010; 2010bap024
[http://dx.doi.org/10.1093/database/bap024] [PMID: 20428313]

[57]   Weichert J, Hartge DR, Axt-Fliedner R. The fetal ductus arteriosus and its abnormalities--a review. Congenit Heart Dis 2010; 5(5): 398-408.
[http://dx.doi.org/10.1111/j.1747-0803.2010.00424.x] [PMID: 21087423]

[58]   Vian I, Zielinsky P, Zílio AM, *et al.* Development and validation of a food frequency questionnaire for consumption of polyphenol-rich foods in pregnant women. Matern Child Nutr 2015; 11(4): 511-24.
[http://dx.doi.org/10.1111/mcn.12025] [PMID: 23316751]

[59]   Hahn M, Baierle M, Charão MF, *et al.* Polyphenol-rich food general and on pregnancy effects: a review. Drug Chem Toxicol 2017; 40(3): 368-74.
[http://dx.doi.org/10.1080/01480545.2016.1212365] [PMID: 27498715]

[60]   Gardiner HM. Response of the fetal heart to changes in load: from hyperplasia to heart failure. Heart 2005; 91(7): 871-3.
[http://dx.doi.org/10.1136/hrt.2004.047399] [PMID: 15958350]

[61]   Mielke G, Benda N. Reference ranges for two-dimensional echocardiographic examination of the fetal ductus arteriosus. Ultrasound Obstet Gynecol 2000; 15(3): 219-25.
[http://dx.doi.org/10.1046/j.1469-0705.2000.00078.x] [PMID: 10846778]

[62]   Zielinsky P, Manica JL, Piccoli AL Jr, *et al.* Fetal ductal constriction caused by maternal ingestion of green tea in late pregnancy: an experimental study. Prenat Diagn 2012; 32(10): 921-6.
[http://dx.doi.org/10.1002/pd.3933] [PMID: 22821626]

[63]   Zielinsky P, Piccoli AL Jr, Manica JL, *et al.* Reversal of fetal ductal constriction after maternal restriction of polyphenol-rich foods: an open clinical trial. J Perinatol 2012; 32(8): 574-9.
[http://dx.doi.org/10.1038/jp.2011.153] [PMID: 22052330]

[64]   Tongsong T, Wanapirak C, Piyamongkol W, *et al.* Fetal ventricular shortening fraction in hydrops fetalis. Obstet Gynecol 2011; 117(1): 84-91.
[http://dx.doi.org/10.1097/AOG.0b013e3181fc3887] [PMID: 21173648]

[65]   Van Mieghem T, Gucciardo L, Lewi P, *et al.* Validation of the fetal myocardial performance index in the second and third trimesters of gestation. Ultrasound Obstet Gynecol 2009; 33(1): 58-63.
[http://dx.doi.org/10.1002/uog.6238] [PMID: 18973212]

[66]   Huhta JC. Fetal congestive heart failure. Semin Fetal Neonatal Med 2005; 10(6): 542-52.
[http://dx.doi.org/10.1016/j.siny.2005.08.005] [PMID: 16199214]

CHAPTER 5

Fetal Cardiac Dysfunction Related to Extra-cardiac Conditions

Filomena Sileo[1], Emma Bertucci[1] and Francesco D'Antonio[2,3,*]

[1] Prenatal Medicine Unit, Obstetrics and Gynaecology Unit, Department of Medical and Surgical Sciences for Mother, Child, and Adult, University of Modena and Reggio Emilia, Modena, Italy

[2] Department of Clinical Medicine, Faculty of Health Sciences, UiT - The Arctic University of Norway, Tromsø, Norway

[3] Department of Obstetrics and Gynaecology, University Hospital of Northern Norway, Tromsø, Norway

Abstract: The main function of the heart is to provide an adequate perfusion to the different organs. This function is achieved through an adequate filling of the ventricles from the atria (diastole) and the subsequent contraction of the muscular walls in order to generate a sufficient pressure to eject blood from the ventricles into the aorta and pulmonary artery (systole). The inability of the heart to provide sufficient perfusion the body tissues is defined as "heart failure". In the fetus, heart failure is usually a late event characterized by cardiomegaly, atrioventricular regurgitation and fetal hydrops that occur after a subclinical period of cardiac dysfunction when the heart tries to adapt to the initial stages of an insult through cardiac remodelling. Different cardiac and extra-cardiac conditions can lead to fetal cardiac dysfunction and cardiac failure *in utero*. Intrinsic cardiac conditions potentially leading to heart failures include cardiomyopathies, structural abnormalities and persistent arrhythmias, while extrinsic causes comprise extra-cardiac lesions that contribute to heart failure through high output states, increased afterload, or cardiac compression resulting in low cardiac output and increased central venous pressures. The aim of this chapter is to provide an up-to-date on the causes, physiopathology, prenatal diagnosis and clinical implications of the most common extra-cardiac conditions potentially leading to fetal heart dysfunction.

Keywords: Congenital anomalies, Diagnosis/methods, Echocardiography, Fetus, Heart failure, Treatment outcome.

PRE AND POST-NATAL CIRCULATION

Understanding the differences between pre- and post-natal circulation is crucial to understand the pathophysiology of fetal heart dysfunction. In the postnatal life,

* **Corresponding author Francesco D'Antonio:** Department of Clinical Medicine, Faculty of Health Sciences, UiT-The Arctic University of Norway,Hansine Hansens veg 18, 9019 Tromsø, Norway; E-mail: dantoniofra@gmail.com

Edward Araujo Júnior, Nathalie Jeanne M. Bravo-Valenzuela and Alberto Borges Peixoto (Eds.)

the left (LV) and right (RV) ventricles work in series and pumps a similar amount of blood during each cardiac cycle. The desaturated blood from the body enters the right atrium through the inferior and superior vena cava, goes into the right ventricle and then reaches the lungs through the pulmonary artery and its branches. The blood is oxygenated in the lungs and reaches the left atrium through the pulmonary veins from which, through the mitral valve, goes into the left ventricle and then to rest of the body through the aorta. The two circulations are well separated in and the dysfunction of one ventricle may result in the heart failure.

In utero, the function of the lungs is achieved by the placenta and the two circulations work in parallel in view of the presence of three different communications systems (called "shunts): the foramen ovale (between the atria), the ductus arteriosus (between the pulmonary artery and aorta) and the ductus venosus (DV) (connecting the umbilical vein to the inferior vena cava at its inlet to the right atrium). The blood is oxygenated in the placenta and goes back to the fetus through the umbilical vein and reaches the right atrium through the DV bypassing the liver. The large majority of oxygenated blood is deviated from the DV into the left circulation and through the patent foramen ovale into the aorta. The remaining blood reaches the right ventricles through the inferior vena cava and is diverged towards the pulmonary artery and the lungs. However, because the high pressures in the pulmonary circulation due to collapsed lungs, the large majority of the blood entering in the pulmonary artery is deviated towards the aorta through the ductus arteriosum, providing perfusion preferentially to the lower body and the placenta.

In adults, the heart is able to adapt to both an increase in the preload (which reflects the volume of blood entering in the atria) and an increase in afterload (which reflects the pressure against which the heart has to contract in systole) according to the Frank-Starling mechanism [1 - 8]. This is partially true during fetal life because the fetal myocardium is less contractile and less compliant compared to post-natal life due to immaturity of both myocardial fibres and autonomic nervous system. Furthermore, the fetal heart already exerts its function at the top of its curve. The heart filling capacity is limited by the positive pressure exerted by the collapsed lungs. Moreover, the fast heart rate in fetal life prevents the possibility of increasing the cardiac output by increasing its rate [9]. Nevertheless, the fetal heart is still remarkably flexible and capable of adapting to functional or anatomical anomalies.

ULTRASOUND ASSESSMENT IN FETUSES WITH SUSPECTED HEART FAILURE

Assessment of fetuses at risk of heart failure requires a comprehensive assessment of fetal heart structure and function in order to detect the presence of dysfunction, quantify its severity and estimate the short- and long-term risk of cardiovascular morbidity.

The most common ultrasound parameters which should be assessed in fetuses with suspected heart failure are:

- ***Heart Size:*** Heart size is usually one third of the thorax and has to be routinely evaluated also in screening evaluation of the heart. The Cardio/Thoracic (C/T) area or circumference ratio is an index used to assess the dimension of the heart which is relatively stable through gestation with a mean value of 0.45 at 17 weeks and 0.50 at term (circumference ratio). Fetal cardiomegaly is one of the most commonly detected ultrasound signs in fetuses affected by heart failure and is defined as a C/T greater than two standard deviations (SD).
- ***Myocardial Function and Valve Regurgitation:*** Myocardial function is indirectly assessed by the global shortening and thickening of the walls of the ventricles and by the function of the atrioventricular and semi-lunar valves. The shortening fraction of a ventricle, which should be calculated by taking the difference between the diastolic and systolic dimensions and dividing by the diastolic dimension of each ventricle, should be more than 0.28 in fetuses with normal heart function. A myocardial compromise or an increase in the foetal ventricular workload can cause an abnormal shortening fraction; likewise, an increase in diastolic function usually reflects a reduced shortening fraction requiring a more intensive monitoring.

In normal conditions, both atrioventricular (AV) and semilunar valves are competent with no signs of regurgitation during the entire cardiac cycle. The presence of regurgitation may be a sign of altered cardiac physiology, although it can be occasionally detected in fetuses with normal heart function. Mild regurgitation, especially when detected in the right AV valve, is a relatively common finding with no haemodynamic significance. Conversely, holosystolic (involving the entire systole) tricuspid regurgitation with right atrial enlargement should be considered a sign of abnormal cardiac function and prompt further investigation, is usually abnormal and indicates the need for further investigation. While tricuspid regurgitation can be a reversible sign of heart failure, the progression to the mitral valve regurgitation is a sign of a significant increase in left ventricle wall stress and diastolic dysfunction. Regurgitation of all valves, including the semilunar valves, is usually a sign of more advanced congestive heart failure associated with acidosis in a very compromised fetus. Pulsed-Wave Doppler assessment of the atrioventricular valve can also add useful information on the diastolic function of the heart: in normal conditions, there is a constant proportion of atrial filling during the atrial contraction throughout gestation, while, in case of compromised diastolic function and fetal heart failure, there is a monophasic filling of the ventricles [3, 7].

- ***Left and Right Outflow Tracts:*** The aortic and pulmonary outflow tracts provide valuable information on the velocity and volume of blood ejected by either ventricle and allows afterload estimation of the cardiac function. Through velocity measurements and valve area, the right, left and combined cardiac output can be estimated; in normal fetuses, the cardiac combined output shows a continuous increment throughout gestation with predominance of the right ventricle.
- ***Venous Doppler:*** Assessment of venous Doppler, including the DV, inferior vena cava and umbilical vein, is also a fundamental part in the evaluation of fetuses with suspected heart failure. Presence of negative or reverse a wave in the DV, increased atrial reversal a wave in the inferior vena cava or pulsations in the umbilical wave can indicate increased inter-atrial pressure due to impaired heart function and increase the risk of heart failure.
- ***Myocardial Performance Index:*** The global ventricular function can be assessed through a non-geometrical index introduced by Tei *et al.* [10] called myocardial performance index (MPI) which incorporates systolic and diastolic intervals and becomes prolonged in case of ventricular dysfunction. MPI is calculated as the ratio between the sum of isovolumetric relaxation time and isovolumetric contraction time with the ejection time. Normally, MPI is relatively stable during gestation with a mean MPI value of 0.36 (range 0.28-0.44). It is considered a marker of global cardiac function and is affected by ventricular loading, cardiac contractility and relaxation abnormalities. Abnormal MPI is likely to reflect initial stages of cardiac adaptation to different perinatal insults and it has shown to be altered in intrauterine growth restriction (IUGR), maternal diabetes and twin-to-twin transfusion syndrome (TTTS) [11, 12].

EXTRA-CARDIAC ANOMALIES POTENTIALLY LEADING TO HEART FAILURE IN THE FETUS

Extra-cardiac anomalies may potentially lead to impaired cardiac dysfunction through three main mechanisms high output states, increased afterload, or cardiac compression resulting in low cardiac output and increased central venous pressures.

Fetal Anemia

Fetal anemia is a condition characterised by diminished oxygen carrying capacity to the developing tissue [13]. It is usually defined as a haemoglobin (Hb) concentration more than 2 SD below the mean for gestational age or a haematocrit (Hct) of less than 30%. Currently, the peak velocity in middle cerebral artery (MCA-PSV) Doppler is usually used as a non-invasive screening tool for fetal anemia, with MCA-PSV more than 1.5 MoM per gestational age identifying fetuses at high risk of severe anemia [14, 15].

The most common causes of fetal anemia are [15]:

- abnormal destruction of red blood cells, including red cell alloimmunization, Rh disease or antibodies towards atypical agents;

- abnormal production, including parvovirus B19 infection or rarely other infections which can cause a transient bone marrow suppression;

- inherited diseases, including case of alpha-thalassemia, erythrocyte enzymopathies or genetic diseases such as Fanconi anemia that can cause fetal anemia;

- other conditions as twin-polycythemia-anemia-sequence as complication in monochorionic-diamniotic pregnancy (usually after a selective fetoscopic laser photocoagulation in case of TTTS).

Cardiovascular Changes in Fetal Anemia

On ultrasound, fetuses affected by severe anemia presents with signs of hyperdynamic circulation. There is an increase in cardiac output with a decreased afterload and increased in myocardial stretching and filling pressure, thus resulting in cardiomegaly. The increasing demands of fetal myocardium are supplied by an increase in coronary perfusion reducing coronary resistance and increasing coronary pressure [16]. Unless the anemia is severe enough to cause myocardial ischemia, diminished function and consequent development of dilated cardiomyopathy [13]. When the adaptive mechanisms fail to compensate, fetal hydrops occurs potentially leading to intra-uterine death.

Treatment of Fetal Anemia

Intra-uterine transfusion represents the gold standard for managing fetuses affected by severe anemia close to terms. According to the cause and the gestational age at onset there might be the need for more than one transfusion. Conversely, iatrogenic preterm delivery may represent a reasonable option for cases affected by mild disease or presenting with anemia close to term.

Vein of Galen Malformations

Cerebral arterio-venous malformations may be responsible of heart failure in the fetus due to volume overload; the most frequent is the vein of Galen aneurysmal malformation (VGAM), which represents 1% of all paediatric congenital malformations. VGAM develops due to an error in early vasculogenesis in the first trimester; normally, the choroid plexus is responsible for fluid circulation within the neural tube between 6 and 10 weeks of gestation while the median prosencephalic vein (MProsV) of Markowski becomes responsible for venous drainage [17]. Later, between 10 and 11 weeks of gestation, the choroidal arteries progressively lose their role while the arterial network of the cortex matures; similarly, paired cerebral veins develop and drain into the MProsV of Markowski which at that point begins to involute and its caudal remnants join the internal cerebral veins to form the vein of Galen. A disruption in this mechanism may occur when there is the formation of a shunt between the choroid arterial network and the MProsV of Markowski. The bypass of the capillary bed promotes its enlargement as an aneurysm and prevents the normal development of the vein of Galen [18].

Cardiovascular Changes in Vein of Galen Aneurysmal Malformation

The presence of a VGAM causes a volume overload and may result in a congestive heart failure due to the high output status. VGAM determines an increase volume load to the cerebral venous system and to the heart due to preferential flow towards low resistance district. Consequently, almost 80% of the cardiac output can be diverged towards the brain, causing a marked dilatation of the sagittal and straight venous sinuses and cerebral venous system carrying this blood back to the heart [19]. Furthermore, the persistent venous congestion can cause a mass effect into the brain resulting in abnormal brain development and brain hypoplasia; cerebral haemorrhage and/or thrombosis into the veins can also occur [13, 20].

Associated cardiac findings in fetuses affected by VGAM include: dilatation of the superior vena cava due to increased venous return with subsequent dilatation of the right heart. The dilatation of the right ventricle can stretch the tricuspid anulus and consequently cause tricuspid regurgitation with dilatation of the right atrium. The cerebral steal may also result in reversed diastolic flow in the aortic isthmus, which can cause a reduced perfusion of peripheral organs, mainly and, the liver and kidneys [21, 22]. More importantly, the cerebral steal may also cause coarctation of the aorta as the blood flow in the aortic arch and descending aorta is decreased, resulting in an impaired growth of the aorta [13]. The high output status can also result in diastolic dysfunction of the heart, cardiomegaly, and pericardial effusion and, at a late stage, fetal hydrops.

Treatment of Fetal Vein of Galen Aneurysmal Malformation

There are no treatments available for this condition prenatally; a recently published series showed that VCGAM malformation is associated with only 36.7% of survival [22]. After birth, the VCGAM may undergo endovascular treatment with embolization of the lesion; this, in conjunction with a specialized management in intensive perinatal care centres, may lead to an improved perinatal outcome [23, 24].

Placental Chorioangioma

Chorioangioma is the most common non-trophoblastic vascular tumor of the placenta, with an estimated incidence of 1%. Although its precise etiology has not been completely elucidated, it is thought to be the results of an abnormal proliferation of vessels in various stages of differentiation – endotheliomatous, capillary, cavernous – in fibrous stroma arising from chorionic tissue [25 - 27]. Chorioangioma can vary in size from a few millimeters to several centimeters in diameter and may present as a single or, more rarely, as multiple masses [26].

The importance of prenatal diagnosis of chorioangioma relies in its potential association with adverse perinatal outcome. The pathophysiology behind the chorioangioma related fetal damage is likely to be secondary to the sustained alterations in fetal hemodynamic response which can lead to high-output cardiac failure and the development of hydrops. The size of the mass, presence of hydrops and gestational age at occurrence of cardiac failure have been reported to be the main determinants of perinatal outcome in pregnancies complicated by chorioangioma.

Placental chorioangioma can be detected prenatally with ultrasound; it usually appears as a hypo or hyperechoic mass within the placenta but well-circumscribed and distinct from the rest of the placenta (Fig. **1**). Sometimes it can appear as a complex mass with anechoic cystic area and/or septa [26]. It is often localized underneath the chorionic plate, usually close to the umbilical insertion; its aspect can change during the pregnancy. The Colour Doppler is usually helpful in identifying vascular channels contiguous to the fetal circulation and distinguishing the chorioangioma from other placental lesions as hematoma, teratomas or hydatiform partial mole [28 - 30].

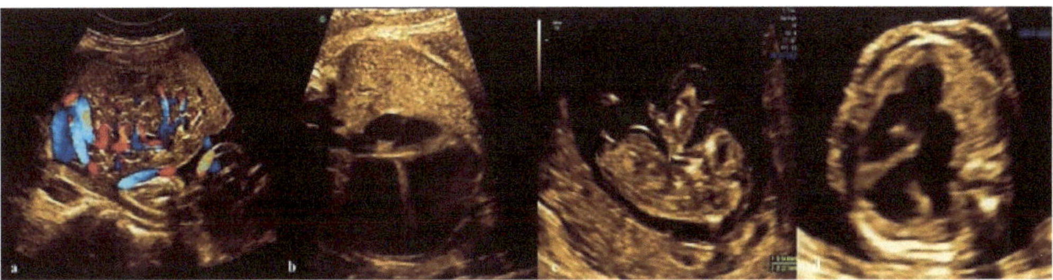

Fig. (1). Extra-cardiac anomalies leading to fetal heart failure. a and b: placental chorioangioma associated with cardiomegaly. c and d, twin reversed arterial perfusion (TRAP) sequence associated with cardiomegaly of the pump twin.

Cardiovascular Changes

The chorioangioma acts as a large arterio-venous malformation or shunt within the placenta: the increased blood flow through the shunts alters the fetal circulation leading to high output cardiac failure, similarly to teratomas or VCGAM.

The pathophysiology behind the association between chorioangioma and impaired fetal growth seems to be the consequence of placental insufficiency related to the decrease in the placental tissue area necessary for adequate nutrient exchange. Furthermore, there is a portion of non-oxygenated blood that bypasses the maternal circulation through the chorioangioma causing fetal anemia and high cardiac output. Therefore, when chorioangioma is detected longitudinal assessment of the PSV in the MCA is warranted in order to detect anemia [27, 31, 32].

Size of the mass remains the main determinant of perinatal outcome in pregnancies affected by chorioangioma. Cardiovascular changes associated to the presence of the mass includes cardiomegaly, tricuspid regurgitation and hydrops. Increased PSV in pregnancies complicated by chorioangioma should prompt intensive fetal monitoring in order to detect signs of cardiac compromise

Prenatal Management

The large majority of placental chorioangioma do not lead to *in utero* compromise requiring immediate intervention or delivery; conversely, large masses are associated with an increased risk of cardiac compromise, hydrops and eventually death. Serial ultrasound assessment through pregnancies in order to look for early signs of cardiac compromise (mainly cardiomegaly and increased PSV in the MCA) is the optimal approach when managing pregnancies complicated by chorioangioma. If fetal compromise is detected on the scan, the optimal approach largely depends upon the severity of fetal symptoms and gestational age at occurrence. In case of advanced gestational age, iatrogenic birth may be a reasonable option. Conversely, in cases far form viability intrauterine treatments should be considered, including laser coagulation or alcohol injection [32 - 35].

Post-natal outcome of placental chorioangioma is mainly determined by the gestational age at birth and signs of fetal compromise, with pregnancies complicated by fetal hydrops or requiring early delivery showing the higher risk of short- and long-term cardiovascular morbidity.

Teratoma

Teratomas are the most common fetal tumours diagnosed prenatally, with an estimated incidence of 1 in 40,000 births [36]. They most commonly involve the coccyx and the sacrum (sacrococcygeal teratomas), neck (cervical teratomas), mediastinum, brain, heart and abdomen. Teratomas derive from all three germ cell layers (endodermal, ectodermal and mesodermal) and are usually characterized by rapid growth *in utero* [37]. Size and location are the main determinants of perinatal outcome of fetal teratomas; cervical teratomas can cause airway compression while those located in the abdomen are usually characterized by a better prognosis [38 - 40].

Cardiovascular Changes

Teratomas are large, fast growing and highly vascularized fetal masses frequently associated with arterio-venous malformations. The pathophysiology of cardiac dysfunction related to teratomas is due to a persistence status of hyperdynamic circulation eventually leading to hydrops and death although direct compression of the heart exerted by the mass can contribute to heart dysfunction in those lesions located in the mediastinum. Furthermore, the increased venous return in large masses can contribute to diastolic dysfunction. Finally, intra-tumour bleeding may lead to fetal anemia worsening the cardiovascular function.

Treatment of Fetal Teratomas

Non-invasive fetal monitoring including serial ultrasound assessment through pregnancy is commonly the management of choice for the large majority of teratomas, especially if signs of cardiovascular compromise are detected at the scan. For tumours presenting with signs of haemodynamic compromise after viability, treatments options include iatrogenic preterm delivery or invasive fetal therapy. In the latter case, the treatment options include: amniodrainage for polyhydramnios in order to reduce the risk of preterm birth and attenuates maternal discomfort, drainage of the mass in order to reduce the volume of the tumour but only in cases where a cystic component is present and laser ablation of the feeding vessel in cases where it can be identified [13, 41]. When there is the suspicion of persistent airways obstructions (mainly polyhydramnios) a reasonable approach may be to perform ex-utero intrapartum treatment (EXIT) procedure. In such procedure, the fetus is partially delivered through the opening of the uterus but remains attached by its umbilical cord to the placenta, while a paediatric surgeon establishes an airway so the fetus can breathe. Once the EXIT is complete, the umbilical cord is clamped then cut and the infant is fully delivered [42].

Twin-to-twin Transfusion Syndrome

Twin-to-twin transfusion syndrome (TTTS) is the most common haemodynamic complications affecting monochorionic twin pregnancies. TTTS occurs in 10-15% of all monochorionic twin pregnancies and is associated with a high burden of perinatal mortality and morbidity, especially if untreated [43 - 46]. The anatomical rationale for the occurrence of TTTS is the presence of vascular communications, called anastomoses, between the two umbilical cords, which are virtually present in each monochorionic placenta [47].

Pathophysiology and Cardiovascular Changes

The pathophysiology of TTTS has not been completely elucidated yet; however, the current knowledge suggests that the abnormal vascular connections are responsible for a net transfer of volume between the donor that becomes hypovolemic and the recipient that becomes hypervolemic. The hypovolemia causes hypoperfusion of the donor's kidneys with consequent oliguria and oligohydramnios, triggering the activation of the renin-angiotensin-aldosterone system (RAAS) [47, 48]. The angiotensin II acts as a potent vasoconstrictor, sustaining the peripheral blood pressure through its direct action on vascular smooth cells [48], while the aldosterone is responsible for restoration of the blood volume through an increased tubular reabsorption of sodium and fluid [49]. The hypervolemia in the recipient should down-regulate the RAAS system, but the inter-twin connections are responsible for the transfer of the circulating angiotensin produced by the donor leading to hypertension and cardiomyopathy in the recipient [50].

In the initial stages of TTTS, the recipient shows an increased cardiac output compared to the donor; however, with the progression of the disease, the diastolic first and the systolic function later deteriorate so there is a decrease in the cardiac output. Usually the right heart shows changes in function at an earlier stage compared to the left heart. Severe right heart dysfunction may result in functional pulmonary stenosis/atresia which commonly resolves following laser therapy in most cases [51, 52] .

Signs of volume overload and congestive heart failure should be evaluated in the recipient; in particular, the diastolic dysfunction should be assessed evaluating the E:A ratio in the inflow patterns of the atrio-ventricular valves as well as signs of pulmonary insufficiency, pulmonary artery hypoplasia and right-ventricular outflow tract obstruction. Moreover, the umbilical artery flow should always be assessed as absence or reversed diastolic flow, resulting from elevated placental resistances, is risk factors for fetal demise [13].

The donor usually shows normal echocardiographic parameters in the initial stages of TTTS. With the progression of the disease, the persistent hypovolemia may lead to dilatation of DV inlet, allowing more shunting of blood through the DV. This promotes an increased transmission of the pulse wave into the umbilical vein [53 - 60].

Diagnosis, Staging and Treatment of Twin-to-twin Transfusion Syndrome

According to International Society of Ultrasound in Obstetrics & Gynecology (ISUOG) guidelines, TTTS should be diagnosed in the presence of significant imbalance in the amniotic fluid with oligohydramnios in the donor (diagnosed by a deepest vertical pool (DVP) < 2 cm) and polyhydramnios in the recipient (diagnosed by a DVP ≥ 8 cm or ≥ 10 cm respectively at ≤ 20 or > 20 weeks of gestation) [46].

Currently, TTTS is classified into V stages according to Quintero's staging system [22, 23]. Despite this several criticisms have been raised on the use of such staging system, especially because it does not seem to reflect the chronological evolution of the disease, does not incorporate the cardiac changes which are characteristics of such diseases and does not predict the survival after treatment [46].

Selective fetoscopic laser coagulation of placental anastomoses represents the treatment of choice for TTTS stage ≥ II [45, 46]. This technique disrupts the imbalance in the circulations of the twins and results in a rapid improvement of the cardiovascular function in the recipient with a normalization of function within a month [46].

Twin-Reversed Arterial Perfusion (TRAP) Sequence

Twin-reverse arterial perfusion (TRAP) sequence complicates 1% of all monochorionic-diamniotic twin pregnancies with an incidence of 1 in 35,000 pregnancies [46]. It is characterized by the presence of an acardiac twin (TRAP mass) perfused by a structurally normal twin ("pump twin"); this perfusion occurs through a reversed arterio-arterial anastomosis within the placenta which deliver deoxygenated blood by retrograde flow. The acardiac twin returns deoxygenated blood to the pump twin through a veno-venous anastomosis. This process is usually facilitated by a common cord insertion [56, 57]. This condition, if untreated, is characterized by a mortality rate of the pump twin of around 33-55% [56, 58].

Cardiovascular Changes in Twin-Reversed Arterial Perfusion Sequence

In TRAP sequence, the normal twin pumps blood to the placenta through the umbilical arteries; the presence of arterio-arterial anastomosis within the placenta allows the delivery of deoxygenated blood flow to the TRAP mass which returns it back to the pump twin through veno-venous connections within the placenta. As a consequence, deoxygenated blood from the acardiac twin reaches the pump twin, leading to a volume overload and higher workload. The pump twin initially develops biventricular hypertrophy trying to compensate the overload, while with advancing disease it develops cardiomegaly, heart failure and hydrops resulting in fetal demise [13].

Treatment of Twin-Reversed Arterial Perfusion Sequence

Careful monitoring with serial ultrasounds should be warranted in TRAP sequence in order to guarantee an intrauterine treatment in case of cardiac strain of the pump twin and/or increased perfusion and growth of TRAP mass [46]. The goal of intrauterine treatment is to interrupt the blood flow from the pump twin towards the acardiac mass. Treatment options includes interstitial fetal laser or endoscopic laser coagulation of umbilical cord vessels of TRAP mass. *In utero* treatment is associated with a significant improvement in the perinatal survival of the pump twin at approximately 80–92% [59 - 61].

Congenital Pulmonary Airway Malformations

Congenital Pulmonary Airway Malformations (CPAM) encompasses a wide spectrum of conditions characterized by a rare developmental anomaly of the lower respiratory tract and including congenital cystic adenomatoid malformation (CCAM), pulmonary intra and extralobar sequestrations (BPS), bronchial atresia, foregut cysts, and congenital lobar emphysema.

CPAMs result from abnormalities of branching morphogenesis of the lung and the different types variants are thought to originate at different levels of the tracheobronchial tree and at different stages of lung development. According to their sonographic appearance they are usually divided into macrocystic, microcystic (echogenic), and mixed lesions since histopathological different lesions can share the same ultrasonographic aspects. Their cumulative incidence is

30-42 cases per 100,000, accounting for 5–18% of all congenital anomalies, although their prevalence is likely to be underestimated due to undetected or asymptomatic lesions [62, 63]. These conditions can be characterized by very different outcomes mainly according to the dimensions of the lesions and their vascularization. Rarely, they can be of significant dimensions and act as occupying-space lesions.

Cardiovascular changes in Congenital Pulmonary Airway Malformations

The CPAM can determine heart failure when they act as occupying-space lesions. In particular, they can compress and impair the growth of the adjacent normal lungs, but also cause mediastinal shift of the heart towards the contralateral side and impair the venous return to the right heart. The decrease of the preload and the cardiac compression can cause a decrease in cardiac output [63]. The impaired venous return is due to both direct obstruction to the flow, increase in atrial pressure as well as systemic venous pressure causing right heart failure and fetal hydrops. Furthermore, the mediastinal shift and compression of the heart may lead to kinking and or obstruction of the inferior vena cava, causing a further decrease in the preload and resulting in ascites. The increased thoracic pressure may cause a compression of the oesophagus and reduce the swallowing activity, causing polyhydramnios [13].

On fetal echocardiography, the main findings are impaired filling of the heart and small cardiothoracic ratio. In case hydrops occurs, it can be associated with reverse flow in inferior vena cava with atrial contraction and umbilical vein pulsations. The ventricular function can be normal or affected by impairment of the diastolic function.

Treatment for Congenital Pulmonary Airway Malformations

The CPAM lesions are stable during fetal life or undergo regression. However, in about 10% of cases, the lesion can cause heart failure and hydrops, which may require prenatal intervention [51]. The possible interventions include: drainage cyst in cases associated with hydrops, placement of a thoraco-amniotic shunt, laser ablation of the feeding vessel in broncho-pulmonary sequestration and/or open fetal surgery with resection of the mass [64 - 66].

Most commonly and if asymptomatic at birth, these neonates undergo a postnatal assessment of the lesion and an elective excision of the mass at 6-8 weeks of life to decrease the risk of infections, pneumothorax or malignancy [67, 68].

CONSENT FOR PUBLICATION

Not applicable.

CONFLICT OF INTEREST

The authors confirm that the contents of this chapter have no conflict of interest.

ACKNOWLEDGEMENTS

Declare none.

REFERENCES

[1]   Guyton AC, Hall JE. Textbook of Medical Physiology. 11th ed., Philadelphia, PA: Elsevier Saunder 2006.

[2]   Jessup M, Abraham WT, Casey DE, *et al.* 2009 focused update: ACCF/AHA Guidelines for the Diagnosis and Management of Heart Failure in Adults: a report of the American College of Cardiology Foundation/American Heart Association Task Force on Practice Guidelines: developed in collaboration with the International Society for Heart and Lung Transplantation. Circulation 2009; 119(14): 1977-2016.
[http://dx.doi.org/10.1161/CIRCULATIONAHA.109.192064] [PMID: 19324967]

[3]   Huhta JC. Guidelines for the evaluation of heart failure in the fetus with or without hydrops. Pediatr Cardiol 2004; 25(3): 274-86.
[http://dx.doi.org/10.1007/s00246-003-0591-3] [PMID: 15360118]

[4]   Rychik J, Tian Z, Bebbington M, *et al.* The twin-twin transfusion syndrome: spectrum of cardiovascular abnormality and development of a cardiovascular score to assess severity of disease. Am J Obstet Gynecol 2007; 197(4): 392.e1-8.
[http://dx.doi.org/10.1016/j.ajog.2007.06.055] [PMID: 17904973]

[5]   Crispi F, Hernandez-Andrade E, Pelsers MM, *et al.* Cardiac dysfunction and cell damage across clinical stages of severity in growth-restricted fetuses. Am J Obstet Gynecol 2008; 199(3): 254.e1-8.
[http://dx.doi.org/10.1016/j.ajog.2008.06.056] [PMID: 18771973]

[6]   Opie LH, Commerford PJ, Gersh BJ, Pfeffer MA. Controversies in ventricular remodelling. Lancet 2006; 367(9507): 356-67.
[http://dx.doi.org/10.1016/S0140-6736(06)68074-4] [PMID: 16443044]

[7]   Crispi F, Gratacós E. Fetal cardiac function: technical considerations and potential research and clinical applications. Fetal Diagn Ther 2012; 32(1-2): 47-64.
[http://dx.doi.org/10.1159/000338003] [PMID: 22614129]

[8]   Jefferies J, Chang A, Rossano J, Shaddy R, Towbin J. Heart Failure in the Child and Young Adult, from Bench to Bed side. 1st ed., Cambridge, MA: Academic Press 2017.

[9]   Eckersley L, Hornberger LK. Cardiac function and dysfunction in the fetus. Echocardiography 2017; 34(12): 1776-87.
[http://dx.doi.org/10.1111/echo.13654] [PMID: 29287133]

[10]   Tei C, Ling LH, Hodge DO, *et al.* New index of combined systolic and diastolic myocardial performance: a simple and reproducible measure of cardiac function--a study in normals and dilated cardiomyopathy. J Cardiol 1995; 26(6): 357-66.
[PMID: 8558414]

[11]   Van Mieghem T, Klaritsch P, Doné E, *et al.* Assessment of fetal cardiac function before and after therapy for twin-to-twin transfusion syndrome. Am J Obstet Gynecol 2009; 200(4): 400.e1-7.

[http://dx.doi.org/10.1016/j.ajog.2009.01.051] [PMID: 19318149]

[12]   Hernandez-Andrade E, López-Tenorio J, Figueroa-Diesel H, *et al.* A modified myocardial performance (Tei) index based on the use of valve clicks improves reproducibility of fetal left cardiac function assessment. Ultrasound Obstet Gynecol 2005; 26(3): 227-32.
[http://dx.doi.org/10.1002/uog.1959] [PMID: 16116562]

[13]   Davey B, Szwast A, Rychik J. Diagnosis and management of heart failure in the fetus. Minerva Pediatr 2012; 64(5): 471-92.
[PMID: 22992530]

[14]   Mari G, Norton ME, Stone J, *et al.* Society for Maternal-Fetal Medicine (SMFM) Clinical Guideline #8: the fetus at risk for anemia--diagnosis and management. Am J Obstet Gynecol 2015; 212(6): 697-710.
[http://dx.doi.org/10.1016/j.ajog.2015.01.059] [PMID: 25824811]

[15]   Mari G, Deter RL, Carpenter RL, *et al.* Noninvasive diagnosis by Doppler ultrasonography of fetal anemia due to maternal red-cell alloimmunization. N Engl J Med 2000; 342(1): 9-14.
[http://dx.doi.org/10.1056/NEJM200001063420102] [PMID: 10620643]

[16]   Baschat AA, Muench MV, Gembruch U. Coronary artery blood flow velocities in various fetal conditions. Ultrasound Obstet Gynecol 2003; 21(5): 426-9.
[http://dx.doi.org/10.1002/uog.82] [PMID: 12768550]

[17]   Gailloud P, O'Riordan DP, Burger I, *et al.* Diagnosis and management of vein of galen aneurysmal malformations. J Perinatol 2005; 25(8): 542-51.
[http://dx.doi.org/10.1038/sj.jp.7211349] [PMID: 16015373]

[18]   Alvarez H, Garcia Monaco R, Rodesch G, Sachet M, Krings T, Lasjaunias P. Vein of galen aneurysmal malformations. Neuroimaging Clin N Am 2007; 17(2): 189-206.
[http://dx.doi.org/10.1016/j.nic.2007.02.005] [PMID: 17645970]

[19]   King WA, Wackym PA, Viñuela F, Peacock WJ. Management of vein of Galen aneurysms. Combined surgical and endovascular approach. Childs Nerv Syst 1989; 5(4): 208-11.
[http://dx.doi.org/10.1007/BF00271021] [PMID: 2790832]

[20]   Vijayaraghavan SB, Vijay S, Kala MR, Neha D. Prenatal diagnosis of thrombosed aneurysm of vein of Galen. Ultrasound Obstet Gynecol 2006; 27(1): 81-3.
[http://dx.doi.org/10.1002/uog.2660] [PMID: 16317769]

[21]   Hoang S, Choudhri O, Edwards M, Guzman R. Vein of Galen malformation. Neurosurg Focus 2009; 27(5): E8.
[http://dx.doi.org/10.3171/2009.8.FOCUS09168] [PMID: 19877798]

[22]   Paladini D, Deloison B, Rossi A, *et al.* Vein of Galen aneurysmal malformation (VGAM) in the fetus: retrospective analysis of perinatal prognostic indicators in a two-center series of 49 cases. Ultrasound Obstet Gynecol 2017; 50(2): 192-9.
[http://dx.doi.org/10.1002/uog.17224] [PMID: 27514305]

[23]   McSweeney N, Brew S, Bhate S, Cox T, Roebuck DJ, Ganesan V. Management and outcome of vein of Galen malformation. Arch Dis Child 2010; 95(11): 903-9.
[http://dx.doi.org/10.1136/adc.2009.177584] [PMID: 20605862]

[24]   Geibprasert S, Krings T, Armstrong D, Terbrugge KG, Raybaud CA. Predicting factors for the follow-up outcome and management decisions in vein of Galen aneurysmal malformations. Childs Nerv Syst 2010; 26(1): 35-46.
[http://dx.doi.org/10.1007/s00381-009-0959-7] [PMID: 19662427]

[25]   Guschmann M, Henrich W, Dudenhausen JW. Chorioangiomas--new insights into a well-known problem. II. An immuno-histochemical investigation of 136 cases. J Perinat Med 2003; 31(2): 170-5.
[http://dx.doi.org/10.1515/JPM.2003.023] [PMID: 12747234]

[26]   Benirschke K, Kaufmann P, Baergen RN. Benign tumors and chorangiosis.Pathology of Human

Placenta. 5th ed. New York, NY: Springer 2006; pp. 863-76.

[27]   Fan M, Skupski DW. Placental chorioangioma: literature review. J Perinat Med 2014; 42(3): 273-9.
       [http://dx.doi.org/10.1515/jpm-2013-0170] [PMID: 24334427]

[28]   Bromley B, Benacerraf BR. Solid masses on the fetal surface of the placenta: differential diagnosis
       and clinical outcome. J Ultrasound Med 1994; 13(11): 883-6.
       [http://dx.doi.org/10.7863/jum.1994.13.11.883] [PMID: 7837336]

[29]   Zalel Y, Weisz B, Gamzu R, Schiff E, Shalmon B, Achiron R. Chorioangiomas of the placenta:
       sonographic and Doppler flow characteristics. J Ultrasound Med 2002; 21(8): 909-13.
       [http://dx.doi.org/10.7863/jum.2002.21.8.909] [PMID: 12164576]

[30]   Zanardini C, Papageorghiou A, Bhide A, Thilaganathan B. Giant placental chorioangioma: natural
       history and pregnancy outcome. Ultrasound Obstet Gynecol 2010; 35(3): 332-6.
       [http://dx.doi.org/10.1002/uog.7451] [PMID: 19859897]

[31]   Wehrens XH, Offermans JP, Snijders M, Peeters LL. Fetal cardiovascular response to large placental
       chorioangiomas. J Perinat Med 2004; 32(2): 107-12.
       [http://dx.doi.org/10.1515/JPM.2004.020] [PMID: 15085884]

[32]   Haak MC, Oosterhof H, Mouw RJ, Oepkes D, Vandenbussche FP. Pathophysiology and treatment of
       fetal anemia due to placental chorioangioma. Ultrasound Obstet Gynecol 1999; 14(1): 68-70.
       [http://dx.doi.org/10.1046/j.1469-0705.1999.14010068.x] [PMID: 10461342]

[33]   Mendez-Figueroa H, Papanna R, Popek EJ, *et al.* Endoscopic laser coagulation following
       amnioreduction for the management of a large placental chorioangioma. Prenat Diagn 2009; 29(13):
       1277-8.
       [http://dx.doi.org/10.1002/pd.2400] [PMID: 19918962]

[34]   Nicolini U, Zuliani G, Caravelli E, Fogliani R, Poblete A, Roberts A. Alcohol injection: a new method
       of treating placental chorioangiomas. Lancet 1999; 353(9165): 1674-5.
       [http://dx.doi.org/10.1016/S0140-6736(99)00781-3] [PMID: 10335791]

[35]   Lau TK, Leung TY, Yu SC, To KF, Leung TN. Prenatal treatment of chorioangioma by microcoil
       embolisation. BJOG 2003; 110(1): 70-3.
       [http://dx.doi.org/10.1046/j.1471-0528.2003.02003.x] [PMID: 12504940]

[36]   Coppit GL III, Perkins JA, Manning SC. Nasopharyngeal teratomas and dermoids: a review of the
       literature and case series. Int J Pediatr Otorhinolaryngol 2000; 52(3): 219-27.
       [http://dx.doi.org/10.1016/S0165-5876(00)00288-3] [PMID: 10841951]

[37]   Peiró JL, Sbragia L, Scorletti F, Lim FY, Shaaban A. Management of fetal teratomas. Pediatr Surg Int
       2016; 32(7): 635-47.
       [http://dx.doi.org/10.1007/s00383-016-3892-3] [PMID: 27112491]

[38]   Moore SW, Satgé D, Sasco AJ, Zimmermann A, Plaschkes J. The epidemiology of neonatal tumours.
       Report of an international working group. Pediatr Surg Int 2003; 19(7): 509-19.
       [http://dx.doi.org/10.1007/s00383-003-1048-8] [PMID: 14523568]

[39]   Sbragia L, Paek BW, Feldstein VA, *et al.* Outcome of prenatally diagnosed solid fetal tumors. J
       Pediatr Surg 2001; 36(8): 1244-7.
       [http://dx.doi.org/10.1053/jpsu.2001.25785] [PMID: 11479867]

[40]   Peiro JL, Sbragia L, Scorletti F, Lim FY. Perinatal management of fetal tumors. Curr Pediatr Rev
       2015; 11(3): 151-63.
       [http://dx.doi.org/10.2174/1573396311666150714105727] [PMID: 26168946]

[41]   Kay S, Khalife S, Laberge JM, Shaw K, Morin L, Flageole H. Prenatal percutaneous needle drainage
       of cystic sacrococcygeal teratomas. J Pediatr Surg 1999; 34(7): 1148-51.
       [http://dx.doi.org/10.1016/S0022-3468(99)90587-0] [PMID: 10442611]

[42]   Liechty KW, Crombleholme TM, Flake AW, *et al.* Intrapartum airway management for giant fetal

neck masses: the EXIT (ex utero intrapartum treatment) procedure. Am J Obstet Gynecol 1997; 177(4): 870-4.
[http://dx.doi.org/10.1016/S0002-9378(97)70285-0] [PMID: 9369836]

[43]	Habli M, Lim FY, Crombleholme T. Twin-to-twin transfusion syndrome: a comprehensive update. Clin Perinatol 2009; 36(2): 391-416, x.
[http://dx.doi.org/10.1016/j.clp.2009.03.003] [PMID: 19559327]

[44]	Roberts D, Gates S, Kilby M, Neilson JP. Interventions for twin-twin transfusion syndrome: a Cochrane review. Ultrasound Obstet Gynecol 2008; 31(6): 701-11.
[http://dx.doi.org/10.1002/uog.5328] [PMID: 18504775]

[45]	Roberts D, Neilson JP, Kilby MD, Gates S. Interventions for the treatment of twin-twin transfusion syndrome. Cochrane Database Syst Rev 2014; (1): CD002073
[http://dx.doi.org/10.1002/14651858.CD002073.pub3] [PMID: 24482008]

[46]	Khalil A, Rodgers M, Baschat A, *et al.* ISUOG Practice Guidelines: role of ultrasound in twin pregnancy. Ultrasound Obstet Gynecol 2016; 47(2): 247-63.
[http://dx.doi.org/10.1002/uog.15821] [PMID: 26577371]

[47]	Wohlmuth C, Gardiner HM, Diehl W, Hecher K. Fetal cardiovascular hemodynamics in twin-twin transfusion syndrome. Acta Obstet Gynecol Scand 2016; 95(6): 664-71.
[http://dx.doi.org/10.1111/aogs.12871] [PMID: 26872246]

[48]	Gomez RA, El-Dahr S, Chevalier RL. Vasoactive hormones.Pediatric Nephrology. 4th ed., Baltimore, MD: Lippincott-Williams & Wilkins 1999.

[49]	Paul M, Poyan Mehr A, Kreutz R. Physiology of local renin-angiotensin systems. Physiol Rev 2006; 86(3): 747-803.
[http://dx.doi.org/10.1152/physrev.00036.2005] [PMID: 16816138]

[50]	Mahieu-Caputo D, Muller F, Joly D, *et al.* Pathogenesis of twin-twin transfusion syndrome: the renin-angiotensin system hypothesis. Fetal Diagn Ther 2001; 16(4): 241-4.
[http://dx.doi.org/10.1159/000053919] [PMID: 11399888]

[51]	Quintero RA, Morales WJ, Allen MH, Bornick PW, Johnson PK, Kruger M. Staging of twin-twin transfusion syndrome. J Perinatol 1999; 19(8 Pt 1): 550-5.
[http://dx.doi.org/10.1038/sj.jp.7200292] [PMID: 10645517]

[52]	Quintero RA, Dickinson JE, Morales WJ, *et al.* Stage-based treatment of twin-twin transfusion syndrome. Am J Obstet Gynecol 2003; 188(5): 1333-40.
[http://dx.doi.org/10.1067/mob.2003.292] [PMID: 12748508]

[53]	Barrea C, Alkazaleh F, Ryan G, *et al.* Prenatal cardiovascular manifestations in the twin-to-twin transfusion syndrome recipients and the impact of therapeutic amnioreduction. Am J Obstet Gynecol 2005; 192(3): 892-902.
[http://dx.doi.org/10.1016/j.ajog.2004.09.015] [PMID: 15746688]

[54]	Mahieu-Caputo D, Salomon LJ, Le Bidois J, *et al.* Fetal hypertension: an insight into the pathogenesis of the twin-twin transfusion syndrome. Prenat Diagn 2003; 23(8): 640-5.
[http://dx.doi.org/10.1002/pd.652] [PMID: 12913870]

[55]	Fesslova V, Villa L, Nava S, Mosca F, Nicolini U. Fetal and neonatal echocardiographic findings in twin-twin transfusion syndrome. Am J Obstet Gynecol 1998; 179(4): 1056-62.
[http://dx.doi.org/10.1016/S0002-9378(98)70215-7] [PMID: 9790398]

[56]	Moore TR, Gale S, Benirschke K. Perinatal outcome of forty-nine pregnancies complicated by acardiac twinning. Am J Obstet Gynecol 1990; 163(3): 907-12.
[http://dx.doi.org/10.1016/0002-9378(90)91094-S] [PMID: 2206078]

[57]	Wong AE, Sepulveda W. Acardiac anomaly: current issues in prenatal assessment and treatment. Prenat Diagn 2005; 25(9): 796-806.
[http://dx.doi.org/10.1002/pd.1269] [PMID: 16170844]

[58]   Lewi L, Valencia C, Gonzalez E, Deprest J, Nicolaides KH. The outcome of twin reversed arterial perfusion sequence diagnosed in the first trimester. Am J Obstet Gynecol 2010; 203(3): 213.e1-4.
[http://dx.doi.org/10.1016/j.ajog.2010.04.018] [PMID: 20522408]

[59]   Lee H, Wagner AJ, Sy E, *et al.* Efficacy of radiofrequency ablation for twin-reversed arterial perfusion sequence. Am J Obstet Gynecol 2007; 196(5): 459.e1-4.
[http://dx.doi.org/10.1016/j.ajog.2006.11.039] [PMID: 17466701]

[60]   Quintero RA, Chmait RH, Murakoshi T, *et al.* Surgical management of twin reversed arterial perfusion sequence. Am J Obstet Gynecol 2006; 194(4): 982-91.
[http://dx.doi.org/10.1016/j.ajog.2005.10.195] [PMID: 16580287]

[61]   Chaveeva P, Poon LC, Sotiriadis A, Kosinski P, Nicolaides KH. Optimal method and timing of intrauterine intervention in twin reversed arterial perfusion sequence: case study and meta-analysis. Fetal Diagn Ther 2014; 35(4): 267-79.
[http://dx.doi.org/10.1159/000358593] [PMID: 24751835]

[62]   Chowdhury MM, Chakraborty S. Imaging of congenital lung malformations. Semin Pediatr Surg 2015; 24(4): 168-75.
[http://dx.doi.org/10.1053/j.sempedsurg.2015.02.001] [PMID: 26051049]

[63]   Szwast A, Tian Z, McCann M, *et al.* Impact of altered loading conditions on ventricular performance in fetuses with congenital cystic adenomatoid malformation and twin-twin transfusion syndrome. Ultrasound Obstet Gynecol 2007; 30(1): 40-6.
[http://dx.doi.org/10.1002/uog.4032] [PMID: 17533619]

[64]   Schrey S, Kelly EN, Langer JC, *et al.* Fetal thoracoamniotic shunting for large macrocystic congenital cystic adenomatoid malformations of the lung. Ultrasound Obstet Gynecol 2012; 39(5): 515-20.
[http://dx.doi.org/10.1002/uog.11084] [PMID: 22223532]

[65]   Cavoretto P, Molina F, Poggi S, Davenport M, Nicolaides KH. Prenatal diagnosis and outcome of echogenic fetal lung lesions. Ultrasound Obstet Gynecol 2008; 32(6): 769-83.
[http://dx.doi.org/10.1002/uog.6218] [PMID: 18956429]

[66]   Adzick NS. Open fetal surgery for life-threatening fetal anomalies. Semin Fetal Neonatal Med 2010; 15(1): 1-8.
[http://dx.doi.org/10.1016/j.siny.2009.05.003] [PMID: 19540178]

[67]   Wong A, Vieten D, Singh S, Harvey JG, Holland AJ. Long-term outcome of asymptomatic patients with congenital cystic adenomatoid malformation. Pediatr Surg Int 2009; 25(6): 479-85.
[http://dx.doi.org/10.1007/s00383-009-2371-5] [PMID: 19404649]

[68]   Tsai AY, Liechty KW, Hedrick HL, *et al.* Outcomes after postnatal resection of prenatally diagnosed asymptomatic cystic lung lesions. J Pediatr Surg 2008; 43(3): 513-7.
[http://dx.doi.org/10.1016/j.jpedsurg.2007.10.032] [PMID: 18358291]

CHAPTER 6

Heart Failure in Fetuses

James C. Huhta[1,*] and Nathalie J. M. Bravo-Valenzuela[2,3]

[1] *Perinatal Cardiology, Mednax, St. Joseph Hospital, Tampa, FL, United States of America*

[2] *Department of Obstetrics, Discipline of Fetal Medicine, Paulista School of Medicine, Federal University of São Paulo (EPM-UNIFESP), São Paulo, SP, Brazil*

[3] *Discipline of Pediatrics (Pediatric Cardiology), Department of Medicine, Federal University of Rio de Janeiro (UFRJ), Rio de Janeiro-RJ, Brazil*

Abstract: Fetal echocardiography began in the late 1970's with the development of ultrasound imaging and has progressed to be able to make the diagnosis of many forms of structural and functional congenital heart disease. Coupled with the pulsed and color Doppler technique, echocardiography has made advances in determining the prognosis of individual fetuses *in utero*. The assessment of fetal cardiac function in fetuses continues to evolve including many markers of poor prognosis in the fetus. A tool for this clinical diagnosis is the Cardiovascular Profile Score. This score has become the "heart failure score" and combines echo markers of fetal cardiovascular functional deficits that have been correlated with perinatal mortality. The goal of this score is to detect signs of heart failure before they progress to non-immune-hydrops fetalis. The fetus with hydrops from noncardiac causes may improve spontaneously, or progress to develop heart failure and the score can be used in the early assessment of this fetal clinical picture development. This chapter presents the CVP score for use in fetuses who appear to have heart failure.

Keywords: Circulatory system, Doppler, Echocardiography, Fetus, Heart failure, Hemodynamic.

THE FETAL CIRCULATION AND HEART FAILURE

The fetal ventricles pump in parallel prior to birth rather than in series as is the case after birth. Left ventricle pumps to the aorta and upper body, and the right ventricle pumps to the ductus arteriosus and the lower body and placenta. The lungs have a high resistance *in utero* and the placenta fulfills the role of oxygenating the blood, providing nutrition, and ridding the body of the wastes.

---

[*] **Address Correspondence James C. Huhta:** Perinatal Cardiology, Mednax, St. Joseph Hospital, 3915 Americana Dr, Tampa, Florida 36334; USA; Tel: 727-322-4830; Fax: 727-821-2461; E-mail: aa4md@aol.com

Oxygenated blood returns from the placenta to the right atrium (RA) through the umbilical vein and through the ductus venosus (DV) and through the foramen ovale to the left atrium (LA). Then, his blood mixes with blood from the pulmonary veins, passing from the LA to the left ventricle (LV) and it is then ejected from it to the aorta.

Approximately third of the poorly oxygenated blood reaching the right ventricle (RV) from the inferior vena cava reaches the pulmonary artery. The remaining two thirds are passed to the descending aorta, placenta and lower half of the body, through the patent arterial duct.

Three shunts (ductus venosus, foramen ovale and ductus arteriosus) allow the fetal heart to work as a parallel rather than a series circulation. Atrial and ventricle pressures are almost equal because of the presence of the foramen ovale and the ductus arteriosus, respectively. The major determinant of cardiac output is the afterload of the fetal ventricles. Any influence which raises the impedance to ejection will inversely lower the ventricular stroke volume by the effect on both the systolic and diastolic function of the heart [1 - 3].

Causes of Fetal Heart Failure

1) Fetal arrhythmias;

2) Immune or infection related inflammation;

3) Congenital heart diseases (CHD) with valvular regurgitation;

4) Primary myocardial disease;

5) Non-cardiac malformations such as congenital diaphragmatic hernia, cystic adenomatoid pulmonary malformation CAPM, arteriovenous (AV) fistula with high cardiac output and extra-cardiac tumors;

6) Twin-to-twin transfusion syndrome;

7) Maternal diabetes;

8) Fetal growth restriction due to placental insufficiency;

Why Fetal Heart Failure?

The above listed diagnoses are related to a higher susceptibility of the fetus for the development of cardiac failure:

a) The compromised ability of the fetal cardiac muscle to contract and to generate force,

b) The altered diastolic relaxation kinetics of fetal cardiac ventricles early in gestation,

c) The lack of adrenoceptors.

Non-immune fetal hydrops or the excessive fluid accumulation in the tissue around heart, lungs, abdomen and under the skin, may be the result of fetal heart failure. Some of the factors that favor fluid movement into fetal tissue are:

i) the extracellular water content is higher and the tissue pressure is lower in younger fetuses.

ii) the membranes are more permeable for fluid and protein in fetuses.

iii) the albumin concentration, largely responsible for oncotic pressure, is lower *in utero*.

Non- immune hydrops fetalis can be due to cardiac, inflammatory, or metabolic causes as outlined above. There are several possibilities for the cause of heart failure in the fetus after ruling out fetal infection [2, 3].

Prognosis of Fetal Heart Failure-Markers of Fetal Mortality and the Cardiovascular Profile Score

Fetal echocardiographic approach to defining the prognosis of fetal congestive heart failure [2, 4 - 11]:

a) Cardio-thoracic (C/T) ratio: Cardiac divided by thoracic area ratio (normal 0.25-0.35) or C/T circumference ratio (normal <0.5).

b) Venous Doppler: inferior vena cava or hepatic venous (increased atrial reversal), ductus venosus (with a wave reversal), and umbilical cord vein (atrial pulsations).

c) Doppler evaluation of the inflow and outflow valves: any leak of the valve should be evaluated further.

The diagnosis of fetal congestive heart failure therefore must be addressed in a clinical fashion similar to that after birth. This clinical state in the fetus can be characterized by findings in at least five categories, which are obtained during the ultrasonographic examination. The following five categories are each worth 2 points in a ten-point scoring system to assess the cardiovascular system. Abnormalities in the cardiovascular profile score may occur prior to the clinical state of hydrops fetalis. The five categories are [2, 5, 6, 11, 12]:

1. Hydrops- Fluid collection in third spaces;

2. Venous Doppler- Transmission of atrial pressure changes into the venous circulation;

3. Heart size - General cardiac enlargement;

4. Abnormal myocardial function- Abnormal shortening of the ventricles or leak of any of the four valves;

5. Umbilical Arterial Doppler- Increases in pulsatility of this waveform are associated with placental disease or very low effective cardiac output.

Within specific disease entities, more emphasis is placed on certain areas by the attending physician to predict the prognosis. As always, this information can only comprise a portion of the total picture and must be integrated by the attending perinatologist into the diagnostic and treatment plan for the patient. The cardiovascular profile score gives a semiquantitative score of the condition of the fetus and uses known markers by ultrasound which have been correlated with poor fetal outcome (Fig. **1**). This profile is normal if the score is ten and signs of cardiac abnormalities result in a decrease of the score from normal. For example, if there is hydrops with ascites and no other abnormalities, there would be a deduction of one point for hydrops (ascites but no skin edema) and no deductions for the other categories for a score of 9 out of 10.

The cardiovascular profile (CVP) profile score is an amalgamation of five markers: two points for each of the five markers are used to provide a method of consistent physiological assessment [5]. This type of multifactorial score is an indirect indicator of fetal cardiac output [2, 3, 13].

CV profile score 10 points: normal. The heart failure score is 10 if there are no abnormal signs and reflects 2 points for each of 5 categories: Hydrops, Venous Doppler, Heart size, Cardiac function, and Arterial Doppler.

Clinical validation of the CVP score has been performed over the last 15 years in a variety of fetal conditions. In the case of hydrops fetalis, Falkensammer *et al.* [4] studied 23 normal fetuses and seven fetuses with hydrops (3 of them with CHD). Among fetuses with heart failure (hydropic), the myocardial performance indices (Tei-index) were significantly increased and correlated inversely with CVP score.

Hydrops	None (2 pts)	Ascites <u>or</u> Pleural effusion <u>or</u> Pericardial effusion	Skin edema
Venous Doppler **(Umbilical vein)** **(Ductus venosus)**	UV DV (2 pts)	UV DV	UV pulsations
Heart Size **(Heart Area /** **Chest Area)**	>0.20 and ≤ 0.35 (2 pts)	0.35 - 0.50	> 0.50 or <0.20
Cardiac Function	Normal TV & MV RV/LV S.F. > 0.28 Biphasic diastolic filling (2 pts)	Holosystolic TR <u>or</u> RV/LV S.F. < 0.28	Holosystolic MR <u>or</u> TR dP/dt < 400 <u>or</u> Monophasic filling
Arterial Doppler **(Umbilical artery)**	UA (2 pts)	UA (AEDV)	UA (REDV)

Fig. (1). Cardiovascular profile (CVP) score. AEDV: absent end diastolic velocity, dP/dt: change in pressure over time of TR jet, DV: ductus venosus, LV: left ventricle, MR: mitral valve regurgitation, MV: mitral valve, pts: points, SF: ventricular shortening fraction, TR: tricuspid valve regurgitation, TV: tricuspid valve, REDV: reversed end diastolic velocity, RV: right ventricle, UV: umbilical vein.

Hofstaetter *et al*. measured the CVP score in 102 fetuses with hydrops and concluded that the CVP score could be applied to the surveillance of hydrops for the prediction mortality [13]. In this study, the median CVP in fetuses who survived was 7.

Results from other studies showed that the average CVP score in the survivors was 6 to 7 and in those who died *in utero* or postnatally was 5 [13 - 17]. Studying fetuses with CHD, Miyoshi *et al*. demonstrated that there was an inverse correlation between 30 day mortality and the CVP score. This study showed that fetuses with CHD and a CVP score ≤7 were more likely to require urgent cesarean delivery due to acute intrapartum non-reassuring fetal status than those with CVP score ≥8 [15].

In the study of Makikallio *et al.* with 75 growth restricted fetuses there were 7 deaths/injuries with a median CVP score of 5 while those who survived had a score of 8 [18].

Other authors have validated its use in fetal cardiomyopathy, fetal sacrococcygeal teratoma, complete heart block and twin-to-twin transfusion syndrome [19 - 24]. In a meta-analysis of the CVP score, values of CVP score ≤6 were statistically significantly associated with fetal adverse outcome [24].

HOW TO ACCESS THE FETAL CARDIAC FUNCTION BY FETAL ECHOCARDIOGRAPHY/ CARDIAC ULTRASOUND?

a). Cardiac Biometry

The cardio-thoracic index (CTI) can be calculated by the ratio between the cardiac and chest circumferences (normal ≤ 0.5) or between their areas (normal ≤ 0.35) (Fig. **2**) [8, 25]. CTI is increased in situations with global cardiac enlargement such as fetal dilated cardiomyopathy/myocarditis, twin-to-twin transfusion syndrome, and infection. The thickness of the myocardium can be measured by M-mode, two-dimensional (2D) and four-dimensional (4D) ultrasonography/ echocardiography. Maternal diabetes mellitus is the most common cause of hypertrophic cardiomyopathy. Other possible causes of hypertrophic cardiomyopathy are genetic factors (familial, Noonan syndrome and chromosomal abnormalities), metabolic (mitochondrial) diseases, renal malformations and twin-to-twin transfusion syndrome [26].

b). Cardiac Output

The stroke volume (SV) or ejected volume can be calculated for each ventricle by the 2D echocardiography/cardiac ultrasound by multiplying the area of the ventricular outflow tract by the velocity time integral (VTI) of the ventricular outflow (Fig. **3**). It can also be calculated by the three-dimensional (3D) ultrasonography using the following formula: SV= end-diastolic ventricular volume (EDV) – end-systolic ventricular volume (ESV). The combined cardiac output (CCO) can be calculated by multiplying the sum of the SV of each ventricle by the heart rate (bpm) (CCO = RV + LVCO × heart rate). The CO increases in situations such as arteriovenous fistulas, teratomas, and twin-to-twin transfusion syndrome. On the other hand, CO decreases in cases in of systolic myocardial dysfunction [27, 28]. Z-Score reference ranges for Doppler indices of the fetal cardiac outflow tracts, which focus on velocity–time integral (VTI) and cardiac output (CO) have been developed [29, 30].

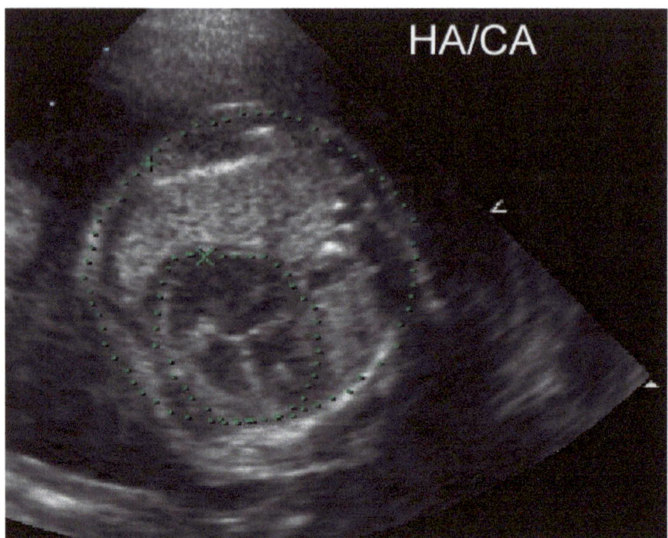

Fig. (2). Technique of cardiomegaly assessment by measuring the cardiac and chest areas. HA/CA = heart area over chest area ratio. The normal range is 0.25-0.35.

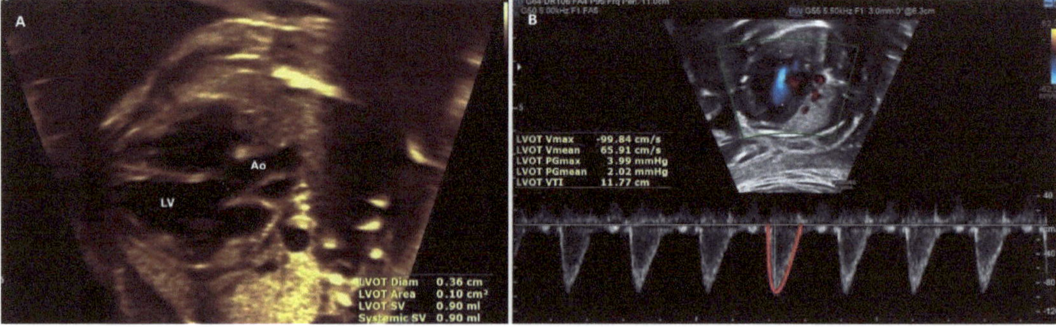

Fig. (3). Calculation of left ventricular (LV) cardiac output by 2D cardiac ultrasound/echocardiography: LV CO = area of the LVOT x VTI of LVOT. A) Diameter of left ventricular outflow tract (LVOT). B) VTI of left ventricular outflow tract. CO: cardiac output; LV: left ventricle; VTI: mean velocity time integral; Ao: aorta.

c). Ejection Fraction and Shortening Fraction

The shortening fraction (SF) corresponds to an index that evaluates the reduction of the ventricular diameter of the end-diastole (EDD) to end-systole (ESD). SF can be calculated separately for each ventricle by M-mode using the following formula: EDD - ESD/EDD (Fig. **4**). Values of SF below 0.28 are considered abnormal [3]. The ejection fraction (EF) reflects the percentage of blood ejected by the ventricles in each cardiac cycle. EF can be calculated using the 3D method and the following formula: end-diastolic ventricular (EDV) volume - end-systolic ventricular (ESV) volume / EDV volume [31]. EF and SF are applied to assess the systolic function (global radial contractility), and these parameters are usually abnormal in the late stages of fetal cardiac dysfunction.

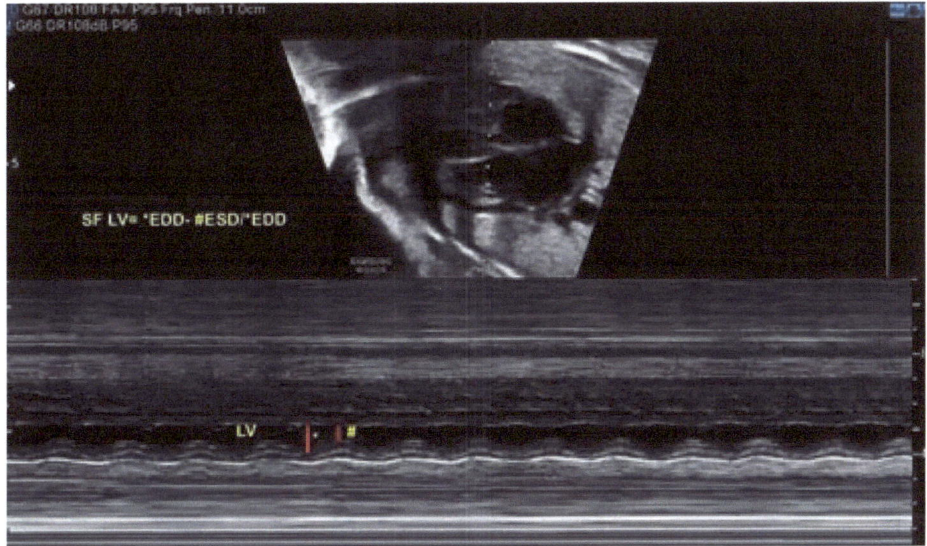

Fig. (4). Calculation of left ventricular (LV) shortening fraction (SF) using the M-mode at the four-chamber view. SF = *EDD – #ESD/*EDD. LV: left ventricle; SF: shortening fraction; *EDD: maximum ventricular or end-diastolic diameter; #ESD: minimum ventricular or end-systolic diameter.

d). Mitral, Tricuspid and Interventricular Septum Annular Plane Systolic Excursions

These allow the evaluation of the longitudinal systolic function by measuring the atrioventricular annular and interventricular septum movement using M-mode. For this purpose, it is necessary to obtain the four-chamber view. The M mode should be positioned at the junction between the mitral annulus (MAPSE), the tricuspid annulus (TAPSE) and the ventricular free wall to measure the maximum systolic excursion of the respective valves (Fig. **5**). To measure the maximum systolic excursion of the interventricular septum (SAPSE), M-mode should be positioned on the crux of the heart. These parameters are easy to obtain and can be altered in the early stages of cardiac dysfunction. The reference values for MAPSE (MAPSE: 2.5 ± 1.8 mm) and TAPSE increase with advancing gestational age, with TAPSE values are higher than MAPSE values (TAPSE: 3.6 ± 1.1 mm at

21 weeks and 8.3 ± 1.4 mm at 39 weeks) [32, 33].

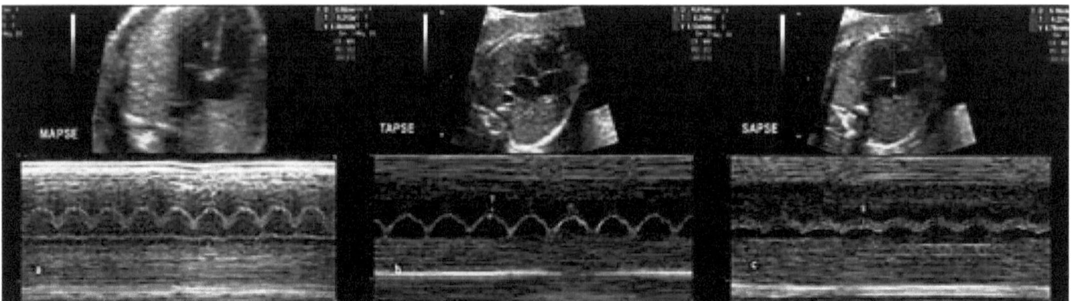

Fig. (5). Four-chamber view of the fetal heart, the M-mode image is positioned at the junction between the free ventricular wall and the atrioventricular valve, or between the ventricular wall and interventricular septum, to measure the maximum systolic excursion of the mitral valve (MAPSE), tricuspid valve (TAPSE), or interventricular septum (SAPSE), respectively. a) M: MAPSE; b) T: TAPSE; c) S: SAPSE.

e). Myocardial Performance Index or Tei Index

The myocardial performance index (MPI) or Tei index can be used to assess of systolic and diastolic cardiac function. The MPI is obtained for each ventricle in the five-chamber view by simultaneously recording of the ventricular inflow (either mitral or tricuspid) and ventricular outflow (aortic or pulmonary), either by either conventional Doppler or by tissue Doppler (TD), and it also allows for the measurement of each interval of the cardiac cycle. The MPI of the LV can be obtained at any gestational age and the MPI of the RV in up to 16 weeks, because of the increased distance between the tricuspid and pulmonary after this period valves (RV geometry). The MPI or Tei index can be calculated by the following formula: isovolumetric contraction time (IVF) + isovolumetric relaxation time (IVR) / ejection time (ET) (Fig. **6**). Myocardial dysfunction may lead to prolonged isovolumetric intervals and decreased ET, which increases MPI. Despite the variability of the results among the reference values for the modified MPI (Mod-MPI), different ultrasound equipment, in general, MPI values < 0.48 are considered normal [34 - 36]. MPI has been used for predicting perinatal morbidity and mortality in fetuses of pregnant women with diabetes mellitus, intrauterine growth restriction (IUGR) and twin-to-twin transfusion syndrome [37, 38].

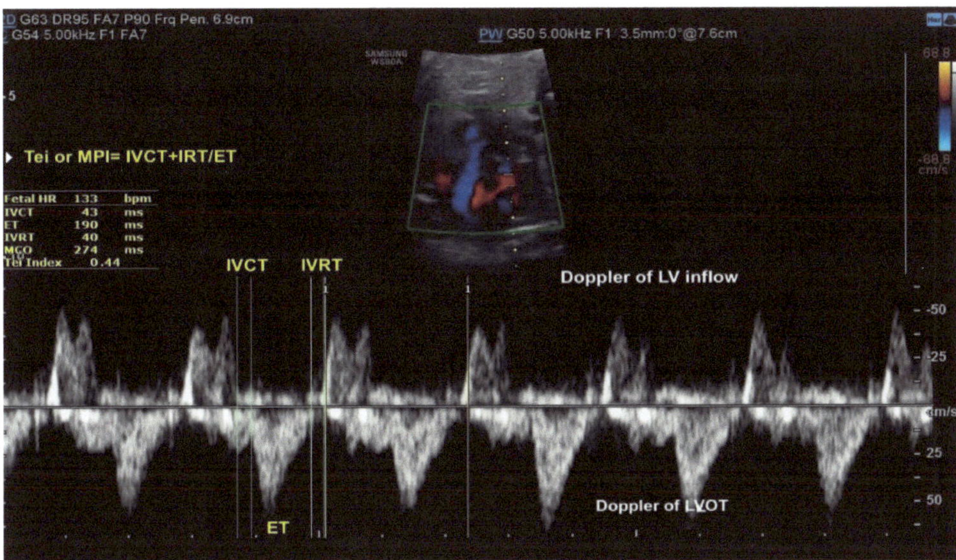

Fig. (6). The MPI or Tei index is obtained for left ventricle (LV) in the five-chamber view by simultaneous recording of LV inflow (mitral valve) and LV ventricular outflow (aortic flow) by conventional Doppler. The MPI can be calculated using the formula: isovolumetric contraction time (IVCT) + isovolumetric relaxation time (IVRT) / ejection time (ET). MPI= 0.44. HR= 133 bpm. IVCT= 43 ms. IVRT= 40ms. ET= 274 ms. LV= left ventricle; LVOT: LV ventricular outflow tract; IVCT: isovolumetric contraction time; IVRT: isovolumetric relaxation time; ET: ejection time; MPI: myocardial performance index.

f). E-A and E'/A' Relationship

The classical evaluation of fetal diastolic function uses the relationship between E (passive ventricular filling) and A (atrial contraction) waves of ventricular inflows, either mitral and tricuspid valves (Fig. **7**). During gestation, the normal values of the E/A ratio are lower than 1.0 [38]. The E/A ratio can be obtained by TD as well as classical spectral Doppler. The TD (E' and A' ratio and peak velocities) is a sensitive early parameter for detecting diastolic dysfunction and has been used to assess the cardiac function in fetuses from diabetic mothers and IUGR [39 - 43].

g). Venous Doppler: Umbilical Vein, Ductus venosus, and Pulmonary Vein

The increase in right atrial (RA) pressure can be transmitted retrogradely, generating biphasic, or triphasic pulsations in the umbilical vein, as a sign of hypoxemia and heart failure in hydropic fetuses [3, 5]. The ductus venosus (DV) reflects the RA dynamics and preload of the RV, being a parameter of evaluation of the diastolic function (RV relaxation). In several pathological conditions with fetal deterioration such as IUGR, there is an increase in its pulsatility index (PI) with a decrease (Fig. **8**) or reversal of its A wave (Fig. **9**) [44, 45].

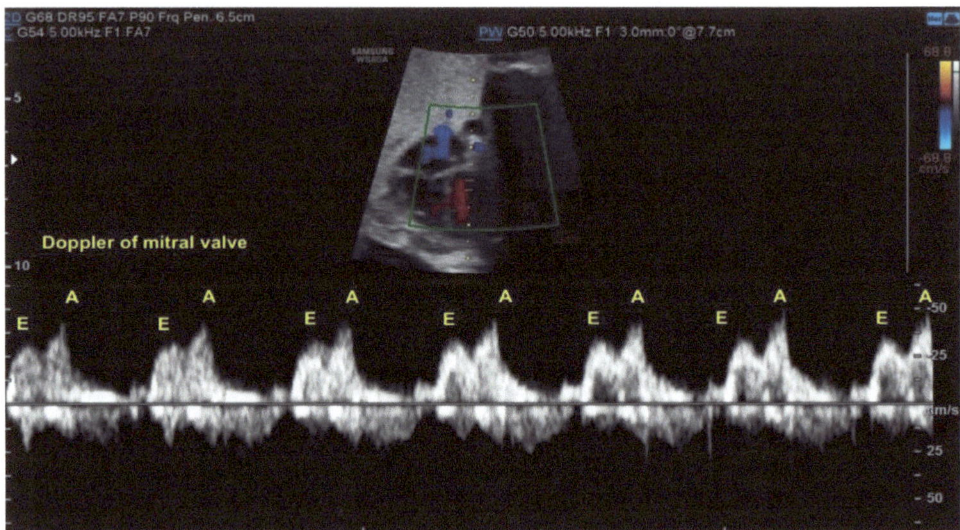

Fig. (7). E-A ratio assessed by pulsed Doppler of mitral valve. E-A: relationship between E and A (atrial contraction) waves of left ventricle (LV) ventricular inflow; E: E wave (passive LV ventricular filling) of mitral valve flow; A: A wave (atrial contraction) of mitral valve flow.

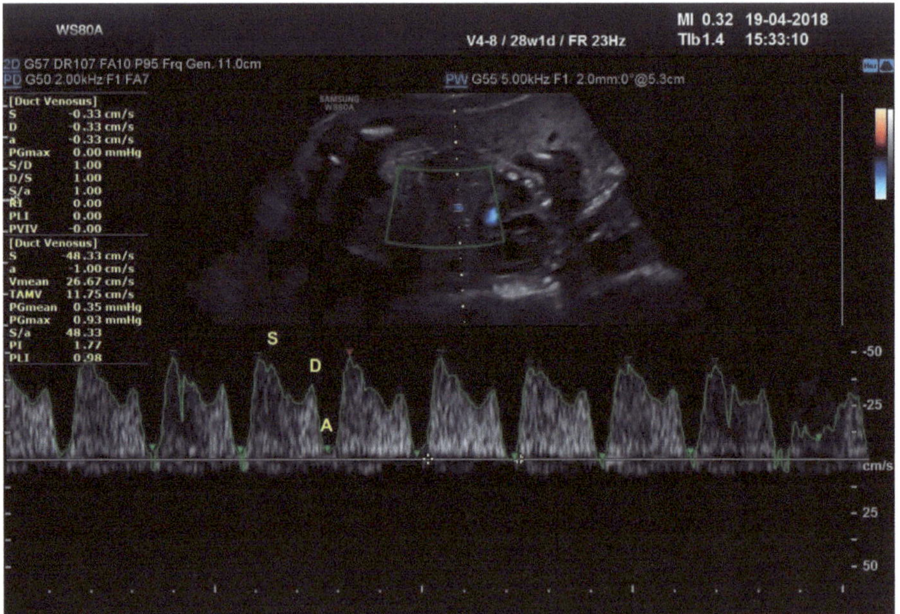

Fig. (8). Doppler of the ductus venosus obtained with the sample volume of the pulsed Doppler in the sagittal plane. Note the decreased A wave with an increased pulsatility index (PI= 1.77). DV: ductus venosus; PI: pulsatility index; S: systolic wave; D: diastolic wave; A: a pre-systolic wave.

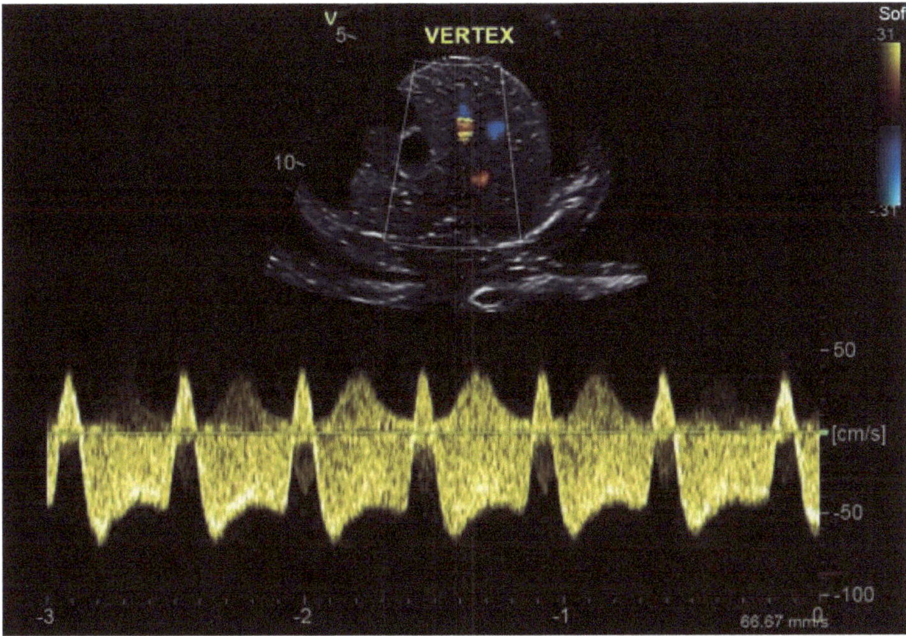

Fig. (9). Ductus venosus Doppler tracing by pulsed Doppler showing a reverse wave.

Similar to DV, the pattern of pulmonary vein (PV) Doppler is a triphasic flow. The flow of PV reflects the left atrial (LA) dynamics, being a parameter for evaluation of the LV diastolic function. In situations of lower LV compliance and an increased LA pressure (maternal diabetes mellitus, IUGR and hypoplastic left heart syndrome with restrictive atrial septum), an A-wave of PV is reduced or reversed with an increased PV PI (Fig. **10**) [46 - 48].

h). Advanced Techniques for Evaluation of Myocardial Function

Spatio-temporal Image Correlation (STIC)

Three (3D) and four (4D)-dimensional ultrasound using the Spatio-temporal Image Correlation (STIC) software enables a complete analysis of the cardiac cycle. This technology, initially described by De Vore *et al.*, allows the acquisition of cardiac volumes by means of a volumetric transducer during a single scan in a period of 7.5 to 15 seconds [49]. The measurements of diastolic and systolic ventricular volumes associated with the virtual organ computer-aided analyses software (VOCAL) enable calculations of CO and EF of each ventricle (Fig. **11**) [50, 51].

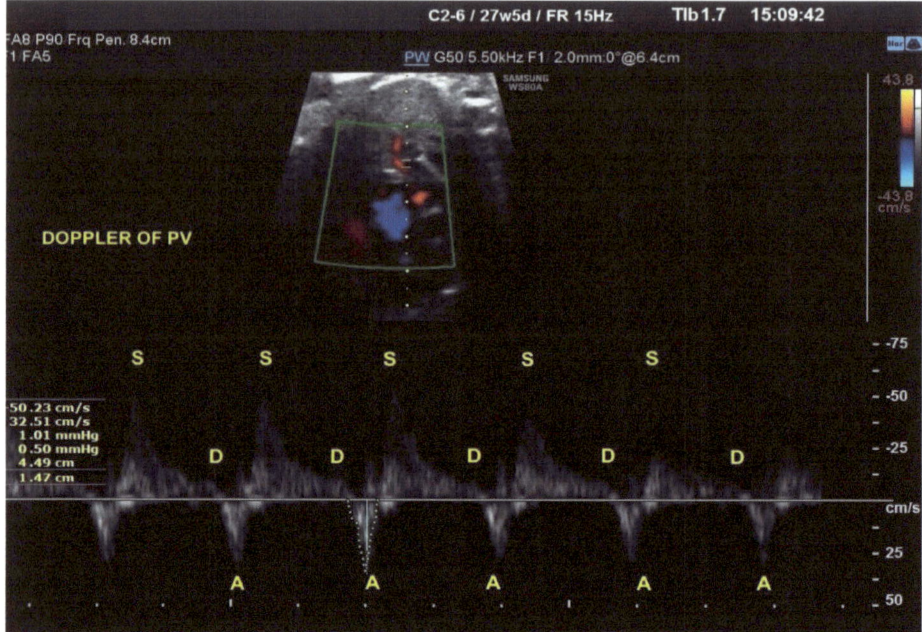

Fig. (10). Doppler of pulmonary vein (PV) obtained in a four-chamber view at the venoatrial junction, right superior pulmonary vein, and the left atrium, showing a reversed A wave in a fetus with hypoplastic left heart syndrome. PV: pulmonary vein; S: systolic wave; D: diastolic wave; A: A wave.

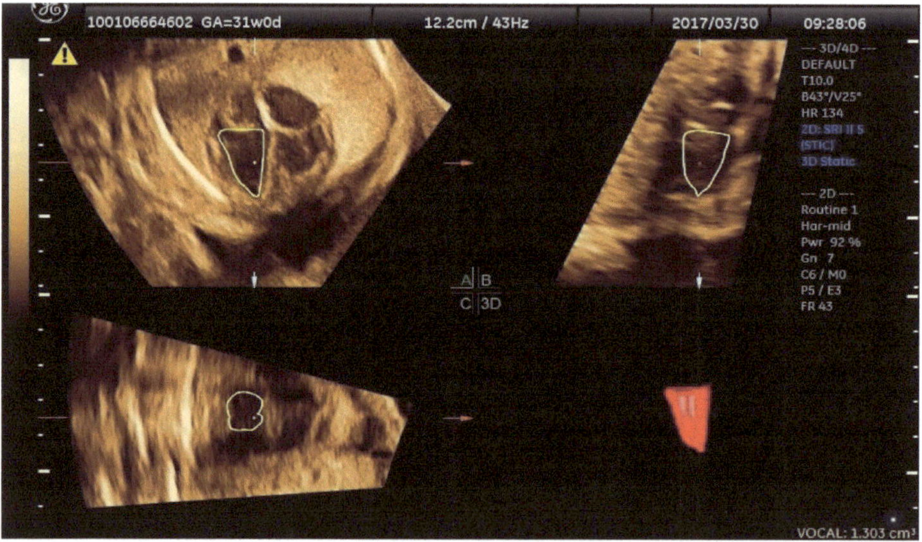

Fig. (11). Reconstruction of the left ventricular systolic volume from the acquisition by the STIC method using the VOCAL software for this calculation offline in a 31 weeks fetus. VOCAL= 1.303 cm³. HR= 134 bpm. STIC: spatio-temporal image correlation; VOCAL: virtual-organ computer-aided analysis; HR: heart rate.

2D SPECKLE TRACKING AND IMAGE OF STRAIN/STRAIN RATE

The strain is the degree of the regional myocardial deformation which achieves its maximum intensity at the end of the systole. Strain is usually described as a percentage. The strain rate is the velocity of the cardiac fiber deformation. Strain rate measurements derived from myocardial wall velocities are obtained by TD and more accurately by a non-Doppler technology: 2D-speckle tracking. The spectral tracking is based on the quantification of the myocardial deformation by using a frame-by-frame tracking of the acoustic markers (speckle) within the myocardium with 2D-echocardiography (Fig. **12**). These parameters have been proposed in the evaluation of cardiac deformity (remodeling) in IUGR. The limitations of the strain/strain rate and speckle tracking in fetuses are as follows: the impossibility of synchronization with electrocardiographic recording, being the correlation with the events of the cardiac cycle performed by alternative methods (valve movement), the interference of fetal movements and the lack of uniform software [52, 53].

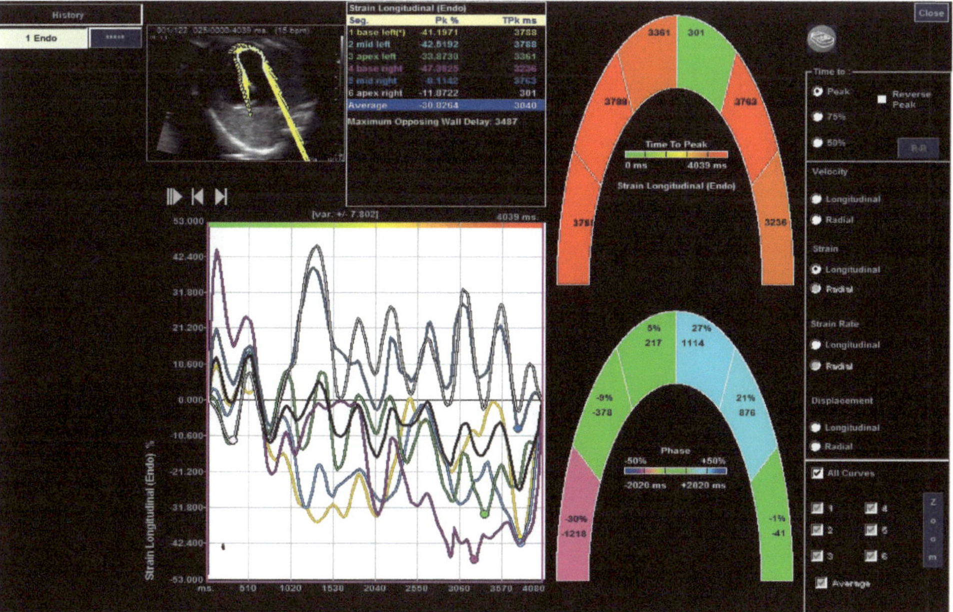

Fig. (12). Acquisition of a digital dynamics four-chamber view (5 seconds video clip) from a fetus for analysis of the left ventricle deformation by the technique of 2D-speckle tracking offline.

i). *A Score for the Evaluation of Fetal Heart Failure: Cardiovascular Score*

With the aim to optimize perinatal outcome and predict risk, a CVP score was developed and validated for evaluation of fetal heart failure [4]. This score, known as a 10-point score, includes some of the basic parameters of functional echocardiography described above, such as cardiac size/thoracic size ratio (CTR), atrioventricular valve Doppler, venous Doppler, ventricle SF added to the Doppler of the umbilical artery and signs of hydrops signs [5]. A score of 10 is considered normal and values < 7 are related to higher perinatal morbidity and mortality [25]. The CVP score is very useful during routine evaluation of fetal heart function and should be performed in fetuses with or at risk of heart failure [4, 5, 24, 25].

MEDICAL TREATMENT OF FETAL HEART FAILURE

a) Treatment of fetal cardiac failure can be classified into groups based on the etiology of congestive heart failure:

i) Abnormal peripheral impedances causing redistribution of flow and growth failure;

ii) High output due to anemia, arteriovenous fistula, absence of the ductus venosus with connection of the umbilical vein to a systemic vein, or acardiac twin pregnancy;

iii) Primary or secondary valvular regurgitation;

iv) Myocardial dysfunction;

v) Tachycardia/bradycardia.

b) Interventions aimed at improving the effective cardiac output are also aimed at prolonging the pregnancy and preventing prematurity and prenatal asphyxia.

c) Echocardiography has long depended on the shortening of the ventricles to assess the systolic function. However, it is known that the shortening is inversely proportional to the afterload of the heart and intense vasoconstriction and redistribution of flow are the rule in fetal congestive heart failure.

d) The usual treatment of placental dysfunction is designed to improve the vascular impedance of the placenta and to increase the flow of oxygenated blood to the fetus:

i) Bed rest, nutrition or maternal oxygen may improve placental function; Tocolytic medications may improve placental function and relax it.

ii) Myocardial support for advanced growth restriction has not been proposed, partly, because the validation of diagnostic methods is lacking. Studies of ventricular ejection force in growth restriction have shown that both ventricles have decreased ejection force. Advanced heart failure in this setting with severely decreased arterial paO2 and poor nutrition, is manifested by nonspecific signs of increased RV and RA size, atrial reversal in the venous Doppler pattern, and altered forward flow velocities;

iv) Treatment with digoxin for evidence of decreased ventricular shortening is controversial but recent data suggests that fetal cardiac heart failure may be improved by its use transplacentally [54, 55]. Digoxin is known to decrease the catecholamine response to congestive heart failure and if there is diastolic dysfunction in the fetus, then this may improve filling and lower filling pressures. If the afterload is high, then an increase in oxygen consumption could result from increased inotropy without improved myocardial perfusion. Digoxin has been used in such circumstances due to its antiadrenergic benefits and the significant experience that has been gained about its safety in pregnancy. We use maternal Lanoxin 0.25 mg orally two to three times per day based on maternal serum levels. We use a trough level of 1.0-2.0 to avoid any maternal side effects. In fetuses with high cardiac output such as arteriovenous fistula and heart failure, we also use digoxin at the same doses to support the fetal heart and circulation.

Currently, we use digoxin for fetal cardiac failure due to arrhythmias and high output states (fistula and anemia). Moreover, digoxin appeared to improve cardiac function of the normal twin in cases of acardiac twinning [5]. Fetoscopic laser coagulation is the optimal treatment for twin-to-twin transfusion syndrome [55].

The diagnosis of fetal anemia can be made using the middle cerebral artery peak velocity. With anemia, the cardiac output is increased with a reduced oxygen carrying capacity. When there is cardiomegaly, (see above for criteria), it is rational to use transplacental treatment of the fetus to support the myocardium if the pregnancy will be continuing for enough time to get medication levels to therapeutic levels. It is possible to transfuse the fetus with anemia by umbilical vein [55, 56].

When CHD is present with fetal valvular regurgitation, it could be useful to decrease the afterload of the fetal ventricles as is done in infants with a similar problem. However, medications that reduce the afterload such as angiotensin-converting enzyme (ACE) inhibitors are known to be dangerous to the fetus in pregnancy. Reduction of catecholamine levels could have a similar effect and digoxin could be useful in this situation.

In cases of right CHD with tricuspid valve regurgitation such as Ebstein's malformation or tricuspid valve dysplasia, the prognosis can be evaluated with an adaptation of the original CVP score. Two key markers of prognosis in these fetuses are estimated RV pressure and the peak velocity of flow from the aortic valve. Integrating these variables into the CVP score is shown in Fig. (**13**) [57].

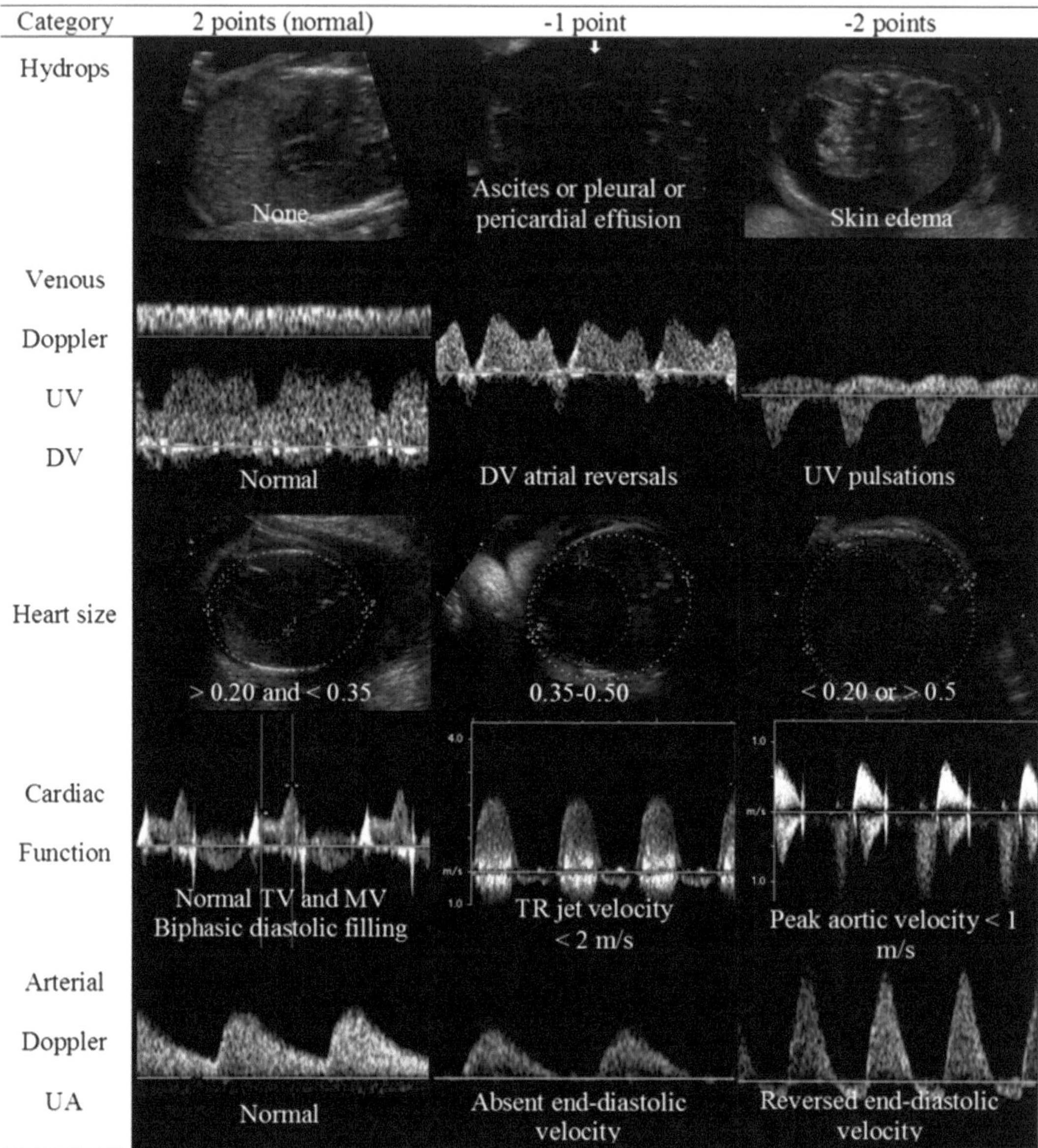

Fig. (13). Modified cardiovascular profile score for use in fetuses with right congenital heart diseases such as Ebstein, tricuspid valve dysplasia or critical pulmonary stenosis. Note the use in the cardiac function category of the tricuspid valve regurgitation (TR) jet to assess peak right ventricle pressure and the aortic peak velocity to assess the combined cardiac output. UV: umbilical vein; DV: ductus venosus; UA: umbilical artery; TV: tricuspid valve; MV: mitral valve; TR: tricuspid regurgitation.

In pregnancies where the mother has significant levels of anti-Rho and anti-La antibodies, we recommend dexamethasone 4 mg daily if there are signs of valvular regurgitation, heart block, valvulitis, myocardial dysfunction, myocardial echogenicity, or effusion. Early use of this medication may prevent progression of heart block and myocardial injury [55]. Additionally, use of IVIG may be considered.

When myocardial dysfunction (fetal cardiomyopathy) is seen without obvious reasons and fetal infection has been excluded, we consider that an inherited form of cardiomyopathy of either the left or right ventricle can present *in utero* [19]. We use digoxin for these patients as long as there is no sign of ventricular ectopy or tachycardia. This decision should be guided by the CVP score [24, 55 - 57].

CONCLUSIONS

The challenge of the diagnosis of fetal heart failure can be summarized as the difficulty in knowing how well the fetal myocardium is performing under changing loading conditions. By combining information from the obstetrical and cardiological evaluations, the perinatal cardiologist can assess whether it is likely that the function abnormality is transient or permanent. The etiology cannot always be known but the differential is between infectious, inherited, and congenital or toxin can be tested. The CVP score can be used to identify a cardiac cause of hydrops and to grade the severity of fetal heart failure. Serial studies using the CVP score are necessary to obtain the value from this test.

CONSENT FOR PUBLICATION

Not applicable.

CONFLICT OF INTEREST

The authors confirm that the contents of this chapter have no conflict of interest.

ACKNOWLEDGEMENTS

Declare none.

REFERENCES

[1]   Kiserud T, Acharya G. The fetal circulation. Prenat Diagn 2004; 24(13): 1049-59.
        [http://dx.doi.org/10.1002/pd.1062] [PMID: 15614842]

[2]   Thakur V, Fouron JC, Mertens L, Jaeggi ET. Diagnosis and management of fetal heart failure. Can J Cardiol 2013; 29(7): 759-67.
        [http://dx.doi.org/10.1016/j.cjca.2013.02.001] [PMID: 23664320]

[3]   Huhta JC. Fetal congestive heart failure. Semin Fetal Neonatal Med. 2005; 10: 542-52. 24.

[http://dx.doi.org/10.1016/j.siny.2005.08.005]

[4]   Falkensammer CB, Paul J, Huhta JC. Fetal congestive heart failure: correlation of Tei-index and Cardiovascular-score. J Perinat Med 2001; 29(5): 390-8.
        [http://dx.doi.org/10.1515/JPM.2001.055] [PMID: 11723840]

[5]   Huhta JC. Right ventricular function in the human fetus. J Perinat Med 2001; 29(5): 381-9.
        [http://dx.doi.org/10.1515/JPM.2001.054] [PMID: 11723839]

[6]   Respondek M, Respondek A, Huhta JC, Wilczynski J. 2D echocardiographic assessment of the fetal heart size in the 2nd and 3rd trimester of uncomplicated pregnancy. Eur J Obstet Gynecol Reprod Biol 1992; 44(3): 185-8.
        [http://dx.doi.org/10.1016/0028-2243(92)90096-H] [PMID: 1535053]

[7]   Gudmundsson S, Huhta JC, Wood DC, Tulzer G, Cohen AW, Weiner S. Venous Doppler ultrasonography in the fetus with nonimmune hydrops. Am J Obstet Gynecol 1991; 164(1 Pt 1): 33-7.
        [http://dx.doi.org/10.1016/0002-9378(91)90618-2] [PMID: 1986621]

[8]   Johnson P, Sharland G, Allan LD, Tynan MJ, Maxwell DJ. Umbilical venous pressure in nonimmune hydrops fetalis: correlation with cardiac size. Am J Obstet Gynecol 1992; 167(5): 1309-13.
        [http://dx.doi.org/10.1016/S0002-9378(11)91707-4] [PMID: 1442983]

[9]   Respondek ML, Kammermeier M, Ludomirsky A, Weil SR, Huhta JC. The prevalence and clinical significance of fetal tricuspid valve regurgitation with normal heart anatomy. Am J Obstet Gynecol 1994; 171(5): 1265-70.
        [http://dx.doi.org/10.1016/0002-9378(94)90144-9] [PMID: 7977531]

[10]   Tulzer G, Gudmundsson S, Rotondo KM, *et al.* Doppler in the evaluation and prognosis of fetuses with tricuspid regurgitation. J Matern Fetal Investig 1991; 1: 15-8.

[11]   Tulzer G, Gudmundsson S, Wood DC, Cohen AW, Weiner S, Huhta JC. Doppler in non-immune hydrops fetalis. Ultrasound Obstet Gynecol 1994; 4(4): 279-83.
        [http://dx.doi.org/10.1046/j.1469-0705.1994.04040279.x] [PMID: 12797161]

[12]   Mäkikallio K, Vuolteenaho O, Jouppila P, Räsänen J. Association of severe placental insufficiency and systemic venous pressure rise in the fetus with increased neonatal cardiac troponin T levels. Am J Obstet Gynecol 2000; 183(3): 726-31.
        [http://dx.doi.org/10.1067/mob.2000.106753] [PMID: 10992200]

[13]   Hofstaetter C, Hansmann M, Eik-Nes SH, Huhta JC, Luther SL. A cardiovascular profile score in the surveillance of fetal hydrops. J Matern Fetal Neonatal Med 2006; 19(7): 407-13.
        [http://dx.doi.org/10.1080/14767050600682446] [PMID: 16923695]

[14]   Huhta JC. Diagnosis and treatment of foetal heart failure: foetal echocardiography and foetal hydrops. Cardiol Young 2015; 25 (Suppl. 2): 100-6.
        [http://dx.doi.org/10.1017/S104795111500089X] [PMID: 26377716]

[15]   Miyoshi T, Katsuragi S, Neki R, *et al.* Cardiovascular profile score as a predictor of acute intrapartum non-reassuring fetal status in infants with congenital heart defects. J Matern Fetal Neonatal Med 2017; 30: 2831-7.

[16]   Miyoshi T, Umekawa T, Hosoda H, *et al.* Plasma natriuretic peptide levels in fetuses with congenital heart defect and/or arrhythmia. Ultrasound Obstet Gynecol 2018; 52(5): 609-16.
        [http://dx.doi.org/10.1002/uog.18925] [PMID: 29024133]

[17]   Miyoshi T, Hosoda H, Umekawa T, *et al.* Amniotic fluid natriuretic peptide levels in fetuses with congenital heart defects or arrhythmias. Circ J 2018; 82(10): 2619-26.
        [http://dx.doi.org/10.1253/circj.CJ-18-0235] [PMID: 29998930]

[18]   Mäkikallio K, Räsänen J, Mäkikallio T, Vuolteenaho O, Huhta JC. Human fetal cardiovascular profile score and neonatal outcome in intrauterine growth restriction. Ultrasound Obstet Gynecol 2008; 31(1): 48-54.
        [http://dx.doi.org/10.1002/uog.5210] [PMID: 18069700]

[19]   Weber R, Kantor P, Chitayat D, *et al.* Spectrum and outcome of primary cardiomyopathies diagnosed during fetal life. JACC Heart Fail 2014; 2(4): 403-11.
[http://dx.doi.org/10.1016/j.jchf.2014.02.010] [PMID: 25023818]

[20]   Byrne FA, Lee H, Kipps AK, Brook MM, Moon-Grady AJ. Echocardiographic risk stratification of fetuses with sacrococcygeal teratoma and twin-reversed arterial perfusion. Fetal Diagn Ther 2011; 30(4): 280-8.
[http://dx.doi.org/10.1159/000330762] [PMID: 22086180]

[21]   Zielinski R, Respondek-Liberska M. Cardiovascular profile score in 44 fetuses with cervicofacial tumors. J Perinat Med 2015; 43(5): 591-5.
[http://dx.doi.org/10.1515/jpm-2014-0304] [PMID: 25503861]

[22]   Statile CJ, Cnota JF, Gomien S, Divanovic A, Crombleholme T, Michelfelder E. Estimated cardiac output and cardiovascular profile score in fetuses with high cardiac output lesions. Ultrasound Obstet Gynecol 2013; 41(1): 54-8.
[http://dx.doi.org/10.1002/uog.12309] [PMID: 23001941]

[23]   Shah AD, Border WL, Crombleholme TM, Michelfelder EC. Initial fetal cardiovascular profile score predicts recipient twin outcome in twin-twin transfusion syndrome. J Am Soc Echocardiogr 2008; 21(10): 1105-8.
[http://dx.doi.org/10.1016/j.echo.2008.05.004] [PMID: 18558475]

[24]   Li Y, Fang J, Zhou K, *et al.* Prediction of fetal outcome without intrauterine intervention using a cardiovascular profile score: a systematic review and meta-analysis. J Matern Fetal Neonatal Med 2015; 28(16): 1965-72.
[http://dx.doi.org/10.3109/14767058.2014.974536] [PMID: 25308207]

[25]   Huhta JC. Guidelines for the evaluation of heart failure in the fetus with or without hydrops. Pediatr Cardiol 2004; 25(3): 274-86.
[http://dx.doi.org/10.1007/s00246-003-0591-3] [PMID: 15360118]

[26]   Nardozza LM, Rolo LC, Araujo Júnior E, *et al.* Reference range for fetal interventricular septum area by means of four-dimensional ultrasonography using spatiotemporal image correlation. Fetal Diagn Ther 2013; 33(2): 110-5.
[http://dx.doi.org/10.1159/000345650] [PMID: 23295684]

[27]   Van Mieghem T, Hodges R, Jaeggi E, Ryan G. Functional echocardiography in the fetus with non-cardiac disease. Prenat Diagn 2014; 34(1): 23-32.
[http://dx.doi.org/10.1002/pd.4254] [PMID: 24122932]

[28]   Mielke G, Benda N. Cardiac output and central distribution of blood flow in the human fetus. Circulation 2001; 103: 1662-8.26.
[http://dx.doi.org/10.1161/01.CIR.103.12.1662]

[29]   Gagnon C, Bigras JL, Fouron JC, Dallaire F. Reference values and Z scores for pulsed-wave Doppler and M-Mode measurements in fetal echocardiography. J Am Soc Echocardiogr 2016; 29(5): 448-460.e9.
[http://dx.doi.org/10.1016/j.echo.2016.01.002] [PMID: 26971082]

[30]   Rocha LA, Rolo LC, Nardozza LMM, Tonni G, Araujo Júnior E. Z-score reference ranges for fetal heart functional measurements in a large brazilian pregnant women sample. Pediatr Cardiol 2019; 40(3): 554-62.
[http://dx.doi.org/10.1007/s00246-018-2026-1] [PMID: 30415382]

[31]   Hamill N, Yeo L, Romero R, *et al.* Fetal cardiac ventricular volume, cardiac output, and ejection fraction determined with 4-dimensional ultrasound using spatiotemporal image correlation and virtual organ computer-aided analysis. Am J Obstet Gynecol 2011; 205(1): 76.e1-76.e10.
[http://dx.doi.org/10.1016/j.ajog.2011.02.028] [PMID: 21531373]

[32]   Mao YK, Zhao BW, Wang B. Z-score reference ranges for angular m-mode displacement at 22-40

weeks' gestation. Fetal Diagn Ther 2017; 41(2): 115-26.
[http://dx.doi.org/10.1159/000446071] [PMID: 27255287]

[33] Messing B, Gilboa Y, Lipschuetz M, Valsky DV, Cohen SM, Yagel S. Fetal tricuspid annular plane systolic excursion (f-TAPSE): evaluation of fetal right heart systolic function with conventional M-mode ultrasound and spatiotemporal image correlation (STIC) M-mode. Ultrasound Obstet Gynecol 2013; 42(2): 182-8.
[http://dx.doi.org/10.1002/uog.12375] [PMID: 23288668]

[34] Hernandez-Andrade E, Figueroa-Diesel H, Kottman C, *et al.* Gestational-age-adjusted reference values for the modified myocardial performance index for evaluation of fetal left cardiac function. Ultrasound Obstet Gynecol 2007; 29(3): 321-5.
[http://dx.doi.org/10.1002/uog.3947] [PMID: 17290412]

[35] Van Mieghem T, Gucciardo L, Lewi P, *et al.* Validation of the fetal myocardial performance index in the second and third trimesters of gestation. Ultrasound Obstet Gynecol 2009; 33(1): 58-63.
[http://dx.doi.org/10.1002/uog.6238] [PMID: 18973212]

[36] Peixoto AB, Bravo-Valenzuela NJM, Martins WP, Mattar R, Moron AF, Araujo Júnior E. Reference ranges for the left ventricle modified myocardial performance index, respective time periods, and atrioventricular peak velocities between 20 and 36 + 6 weeks of gestation. J Matern Fetal Neonatal Med 2019; 2: 1-10. Epub ahead of print
[http://dx.doi.org/10.1080/14767058.2019.1609933] [PMID: 30999802]

[37] Hernandez-Andrade E, Figueroa-Diesel H, Kottman C, *et al.* Gestational-age-adjusted reference values for the modified myocardial performance index for evaluation of fetal left cardiac function. Ultrasound Obstet Gynecol 2007; 29(3): 321-5.
[http://dx.doi.org/10.1002/uog.3947] [PMID: 17290412]

[38] Naujorks AA, Zielinsky P, Klein C, *et al.* Myocardial velocities, dynamics of the septum primum, and placental dysfunction in fetuses with growth restriction. Congenit Heart Dis 2014; 9: 138-43.
[http://dx.doi.org/10.1111/chd.12099]

[39] Hernandez-Andrade E, Benavides-Serralde JA, Cruz-Martinez R, Welsh A, Mancilla-Ramirez J. Evaluation of conventional Doppler fetal cardiac function parameters: E/A ratios, outflow tracts, and myocardial performance index. Fetal Diagn Ther 2012; 32(1-2): 22-9.
[http://dx.doi.org/10.1159/000330792] [PMID: 22677618]

[40] Vyas HV, Eidem BW, Cetta F, *et al.* Myocardial tissue Doppler velocities in fetuses with hypoplastic left heart syndrome. Ann Pediatr Cardiol 2011; 4(2): 129-34.
[http://dx.doi.org/10.4103/0974-2069.84650] [PMID: 21976871]

[41] Comas M, Crispi F. Assessment of fetal cardiac function using tissue Doppler techniques. Fetal Diagn Ther 2012; 32(1-2): 30-8.
[http://dx.doi.org/10.1159/000335028] [PMID: 22626950]

[42] Hatém MA, Zielinsky P, Hatém DM, *et al.* Assessment of diastolic ventricular function in fetuses of diabetic mothers using tissue Doppler. Cardiol Young 2008; 18(3): 297-302.
[http://dx.doi.org/10.1017/S1047951108002138] [PMID: 18405423]

[43] Naujorks AA, Zielinsky P, Beltrame PA, *et al.* Myocardial tissue Doppler assessment of diastolic function in the growth-restricted fetus. Ultrasound Obstet Gynecol 2009; 34(1): 68-73.
[http://dx.doi.org/10.1002/uog.6427] [PMID: 19565528]

[44] Baschat AA, Turan OM, Turan S. Ductus venosus blood-flow patterns: more than meets the eye? Ultrasound Obstet Gynecol 2012; 39(5): 598-9.
[http://dx.doi.org/10.1002/uog.10151] [PMID: 22223470]

[45] Turan OM, Turan S, Berg C, *et al.* Duration of persistent abnormal ductus venosus flow and its impact on perinatal outcome in fetal growth restriction. Ultrasound Obstet Gynecol 2011; 38(3): 295-302.
[http://dx.doi.org/10.1002/uog.9011] [PMID: 21465604]

[46]   Bravo-Valenzuela NJ, Zielinsky P, Huhta JC, *et al.* Dynamics of pulmonary venous flow in fetuses with intrauterine growth restriction. Prenat Diagn 2015; 35(3): 249-53.
[http://dx.doi.org/10.1002/pd.4529] [PMID: 25388941]

[47]   Zielinsky P, Piccoli AL Jr. Myocardial hypertrophy and dysfunction in maternal diabetes. Early Hum Dev 2012; 88(5): 273-8.
[http://dx.doi.org/10.1016/j.earlhumdev.2012.02.006] [PMID: 22445568]

[48]   Michelfelder E, Gomez C, Border W, Gottliebson W, Franklin C. Predictive value of fetal pulmonary venous flow patterns in identifying the need for atrial septoplasty in the newborn with hypoplastic left ventricle. Circulation 2005; 112(19): 2974-9.
[http://dx.doi.org/10.1161/CIRCULATIONAHA.105.534180] [PMID: 16260632]

[49]   DeVore GR, Falkensammer P, Sklansky MS, Platt LD. Spatio-temporal image correlation (STIC): new technology for evaluation of the fetal heart. Ultrasound Obstet Gynecol 2003; 22(4): 380-7.
[http://dx.doi.org/10.1002/uog.217] [PMID: 14528474]

[50]   Molina FS, Faro C, Sotiriadis A, *et al.* Heart stroke volume and cardiac output by four-dimensional ultrasound in normal fetuses. Ultrasound Obstet Gynecol 2008; 32: 181-7. 28.
[http://dx.doi.org/10.1002/uog.5374]

[51]   Messing B, Cohen SM, Valsky DV, *et al.* Fetal heart ventricular mass obtained by STIC acquisition combined with inversion mode and VOCAL. Ultrasound Obstet Gynecol 2011; 38(2): 191-7.
[http://dx.doi.org/10.1002/uog.8980] [PMID: 21370304]

[52]   Germanakis I, Gardiner H. Assessment of fetal myocardial deformation using speckle tracking techniques. Fetal Diagn Ther 2012; 32(1-2): 39-46.
[http://dx.doi.org/10.1159/000330378] [PMID: 22626849]

[53]   DeVore GR, Polanco B, Satou G, Sklansky M. Two-dimensional speckle tracking of the fetal heart: a practical step-by-step approach for the fetal sonologist. J Ultrasound Med 2016; 35(8): 1765-81.
[http://dx.doi.org/10.7863/ultra.15.08060] [PMID: 27353066]

[54]   Patel D, Cuneo B, Viesca R, Rassanan J, Leshko J, Huhta J. Digoxin for the treatment of fetal congestive heart failure with sinus rhythm assessed by cardiovascular profile score. J Matern Fetal Neonatal Med 2008; 21(7): 477-82.
[http://dx.doi.org/10.1080/14767050802073790] [PMID: 18570128]

[55]   Donofrio MT, Moon-Grady AJ, Hornberger LK, *et al.* American Heart Association Adults With Congenital Heart Disease Joint Committee of the Council on Cardiovascular Disease in the Young and Council on Clinical Cardiology, Council on Cardiovascular Surgery and Anesthesia, and Council on Cardiovascular and Stroke Nursing. Diagnosis and treatment of fetal cardiac disease: a scientific statement from the American Heart Association. Circulation 2014; 129(21): 2183-242.
[http://dx.doi.org/10.1161/01.cir.0000437597.44550.5d] [PMID: 24763516]

[56]   Wieczorek A, Hernandez-Robles J, Ewing L, Leshko J, Luther S, Huhta J. Prediction of outcome of fetal congenital heart disease using a cardiovascular profile score. Ultrasound Obstet Gynecol 2008; 31(3): 284-8.
[http://dx.doi.org/10.1002/uog.5177] [PMID: 18253925]

[57]   Neves AL, Mathias L, Wilhm M, *et al.* Evaluation of prenatal risk factors for prediction of outcome in right heart lesions: CVP score in fetal right heart defects. J Matern Fetal Neonatal Med 2014; 27(14): 1431-7.
[http://dx.doi.org/10.3109/14767058.2013.878695] [PMID: 24392847]

CHAPTER 7

Extra Cardiac Defects in Fetuses with Congenital Heart Diseases

Alberto Borges Peixoto[1,2,*] and **Edward Araujo Júnior**[3,4]

[1] *Discipline of Gynecology and Obstetrics, University of Uberaba (UNIUBE), Uberaba-MG, Brazil*

[2] *Department of Gynecology and Obstetrics, Federal University of Triângulo Mineiro (UFTM), Uberaba-MG, Brazil*

[3] *Discipline of Fetal Medicine, Department of Obstetrics, Paulista School of Medicine –Federal University of São Paulo (EPM-UNIFESP), São Paulo-SP, Brazil*

[4] *Medical Course, Municipal University of São Caetano do Sul (USCS), Bela Vista Campus, São Paulo-SP, Brazil*

Abstract: Extracardiac malformations (ECMs) and chromosomal abnormalities are common in fetuses with some congenital heart defects (CHD). The frequency and type of ECMs and chromosomal abnormalities vary according to the type of CHD and the studied population. The detection rate of CHD and ECMs depends on the first-trimester screening through nuchal translucence (NT) measurement, second trimester anomaly scan, and fetal echocardiography. The CHDs most frequently associated with ECMs are atrioventricular septal defect (AVSD), ventricular septal defect (VSD), tetralogy of Fallot (TOF), hypoplastic left heart syndrome (HLHS), tricuspid atresia (TA), aortic arch, coarctation of the aorta (CoA) and interruption of the aortic arch (IAA). Conversely, the association of ECMs and chromosomal abnormalities with the transposition of the great arteries (TGA) is low. CHD such as: Ebstein's anomaly, left ventricular outflow tract obstruction (aortic stenosis) and obstruction of the right ventricular outflow tract (atresia and pulmonary stenosis) are associated with extremely low ECMs and chromosomal abnormalities, and are limited to a few sporadic cases.

Keywords: Chromosomal abnormalities, Congenital heart defects, Genetic syndromes, Non-cardiac anomalies.

INTRODUCTION

Congenital heart defects (CHDs) are one of the most common congenital anomalies diagnosed during prenatal care; they account for approximately 45% of

---

* **Address Correspondence Alberto Borges Peixoto:** Discipline of Gynecology and Obstetrics, University of Uberaba (UNIUBE), Av. Da Saudade, 550, Apto. 602, Uberaba, Minas Gerais, Brazil, Zip code:38061-00; Tel/Fax: +55 34-99781-0107; E-mail: albertobpeixoto@gmail.com

diagnoses assessed within the uterus [1]. At birth, the prevalence of CHDs is 1:100 live births whereas it is 1:500 during ultrasonographic evaluation [2, 3].

The causes of CHDs include chromosomal anomalies, dominant or recessive genes (determined by a single gene), family inheritance in the absence of a determinant gene, exposure to teratogens (ethanol, sodium valproate, retinoic acid, lithium), congenital infections (cytomegalovirus, rubella), diabetes mellitus, and unknown causes [4]. CHDs are frequently associated with fetal extracardiac malformations (ECMs); however, their incidence and the type of associated ECMs vary greatly between studies [5].

Stoll *et al.* analyzed 346,831 pregnancies with known postnatal outcomes including live births, intrauterine fetal demise, and therapeutic abortions due to fetal malformations regardless of gestational age [6]. This study reported that 26.3% of the fetuses with CHDs had major ECMs, 8.8% were associated with chromosomal anomalies, and 2.5% were associated with some dysmorphic condition not related to chromosomal anomalies. Trisomy 21 was the most frequent chromosomal abnormality associated with CHDs (62%), followed by trisomy 18 (15%) and trisomy 13 (6%). Among the cases not related to numerical chromosome alterations, VACTREL syndrome (23%), Noonan syndrome (8%), fetal alcohol syndrome (7%), and skeletal dysplasias (6%) were the most frequent abnormalities. Renal malformations (20%) were the most frequently associated with CHDs, followed by skeletal anomalies (18%), digestive system abnormalities (16%), ocular and lip and palate abnormalities (14%), central nervous system (CNS) abnormalities, genital abnormalities (5%), and abdominal wall abnormalities (4%).

The molecular basis for CHDs remains unknown. Tonni *et al.* performed a systematic review to evaluate the presence of genetic abnormalities using array-comparative genomic hybridization (a-CGH) in fetuses with structural malformations and normal karyotype [7]. The authors determined that abnormalities in a-CGH occurred more frequently in fetuses with CHDs (30.3%), multiple malformations (28.6%), and CNS abnormalities (18.8%). Lanini *et al.* identified 55 copy variants (CNVs) > 50 kb in length that were present in subjects with CHDs and extracardiac abnormalities but were absent in controls. Several knockout studies performed on rats have identified more than 300 genes that may be present in offspring and mimic the presence of CHDs in humans, including NR2F2, TBX5, TBX1, TBX3, NKX2-5, GATA 4, and ADAP2 [8, 9].

The prenatal diagnostic capacity of CHDs is better when they are associated with ECMs [3, 10]. In this context, first-trimester screening plays an important role in the diagnosis of CHDs and ECMs. The increase in nuchal translucency (NT) measurement is an important extracardiac abnormality that improves the diagnosis of CHDs and ECMs since it carefully assesses the fetal anatomy during the first and second trimester; moreover, fetal echocardiography and invasive procedures are necessary to determine karyotype and fetal gene abnormalities [11]. Detecting the association of CHDs with ECMs and chromosomal abnormalities is important for counseling during pregnancy since it is related to a worse perinatal prognosis [3, 10].

Some CHDs have a clear association with ECMs and chromosomal abnormalities, whereas others lack this association. In this chapter, we will address which ECMs are most associated with the presence of specific CHDs.

FIRST-TRIMESTER SCREENING FOR FETAL ABNORMALITIES

The increase in NT measurements is related to the increased risk of chromosomal disorders, CHDs, structural abnormalities, and genetic syndromes (Fig. **1**) [12]. In individuals with increased NT and a normal karyotype, the increased risk for CHDs and ECMs is directly related to the NT measurement (Table **1**) [13].

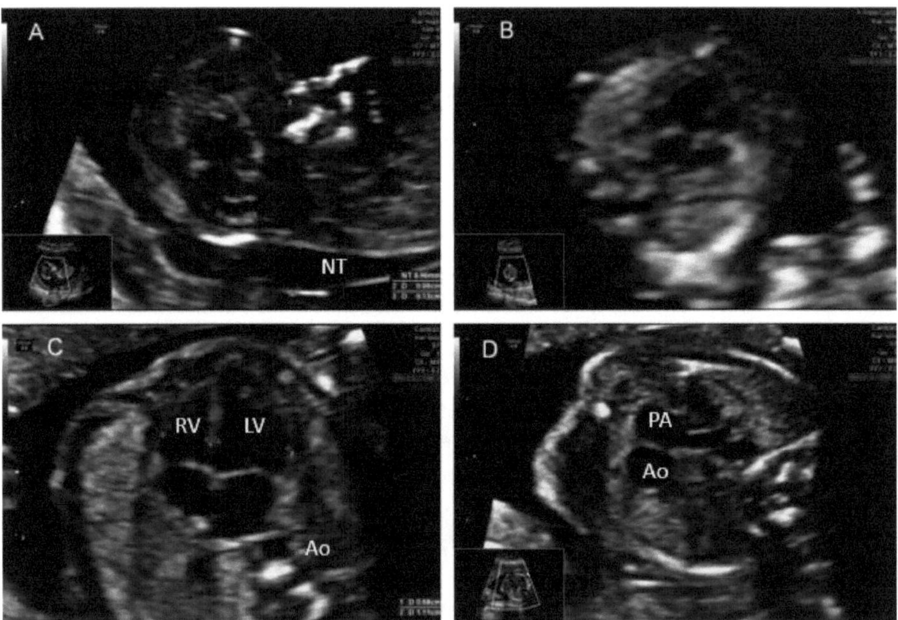

Fig. (1). Ultrasound images of a fetus with increased nuchal translucency (NT) showing disproportion between right ventricle (RV) and left ventricle (LV) on first and second trimester examination. (A) Increased nuchal translucency (NT: 5.96 mm); (B) transverse view of the thorax at the level of the four-chamber view during the first trimester, evidencing disproportion between RV and LV; (C) transverse view of the thorax at the level of the four-chamber view during the second trimester, evidencing a disproportion between RV and LV; (D) 3 vessels view, demonstrating disproportion between the aorta (Ao) and pulmonary artery (PA).

Table 1. Relationship of nuchal translucency measurement and risk of congenital heart defects (CHD) and extracardiac fetal abnormalities (ECMs) in individuals with normal karyotype.

Nuchal Translucence Measurement (mm)	ECMs	CHD
< 95%	1.5%	0.3%
95-99%	2.5%	1.5%
3.5-4.4 mm	10%	3.0%
4.5-5.4 mm	20%	6.5%
5.5-6.4 mm	25%	10%
> 6.5 mm	45%	20%

There is no ideal NT cut-off value from which the presence of cardiac abnormalities is more likely because it depends on the sensitivity and false positive rate desired [13]. Ghi *et al.* reported that for NT measurements between 2.5 and 2.9 mm, CHDs had an incidence of 2.4%, which is comparable to the risk of heart disease due to family history or diabetes mellitus [4, 14, 15]; an NT value in or above this range indicates the need for a fetal echocardiogram between 20 and 24 weeks. Therefore, it is justifiable to perform a fetal echocardiogram for all cases with NT measurements greater than 2.5 mm, even though this includes 5% of all pregnant women submitted to first-trimester screening [13]. Alanen *et al.* evaluated the capacity to detect major CHD in 31,144 pregnant women submitted to first-trimester screening [16]. This study observed that the detection rate and the false positive rate varied according to the NT cut-off value used. For NT cut-off values of 1.5, 2.0, and 3.5 mm, the highest CHD detection rates were 46.8%, 25.3%, and 17.7%, respectively. For the same NT cut-off values, the false positive rates were 18.5%, 3.3%, and 0.4%, respectively.

There is an association between the increase in NT measurement and the presence of abnormalities such as congenital diaphragmatic hernia (CDH), omphalocele, body stalk anomalies, fetal akinesia deformity sequence, skeletal dysplasias, and genetic syndromes [17, 18]. First-trimester screening can diagnose up to 43.8% of non-chromosomal origin anomalies; its association with the second trimester exam increases this detection rate to as high as 97.4% [18].

Therefore, the association of first-trimester screening through NT measurements, the second-trimester morphological examinations, and fetal echocardiography may improve the detection of CHDs and ECMs, which aids in perinatal counseling and management.

CONGENITAL HEART DISEASE AND ASSOCIATION WITH EXTRA-FETAL FETAL ABNORMALITIES

Atrioventricular Septal Defect (AVSD)

Atrioventricular septal defect (AVSD) is the most frequently identified CHD during the perinatal period; it accounts for 15-20% of all CHDs diagnosed. Its incidence in the postnatal series is lower, ranging from 5.5% to 8.0% [19 - 21]. AVSD is characterized by a change in the formation of the atrioventricular valves, interatrial septum, and the interventricular septum as a result of abnormal endocardial cushion development.

According to the degree of the defect, it may be classified as complete AVSD (single atrioventricular valve) or partial/incomplete AVSD (presence of a common valve ring with two valvular orifices). In most cases, there is an alignment between the interatrial septum and the interventricular septum that favors a symmetrical opening of the valve ring and thus homogeneous growth of the ventricles (balanced AVSD). When there is poor alignment of the septa, there is asymmetric opening of the common valve ring and unequal ventricular growth (unbalanced AVSD).

AVSD can be isolated or associated with heterotaxia, extracardiac abnormalities, genetic syndromes, or chromosomal abnormalities [22]. The prognosis is directly associated with the presence of associated cardiac and extracardiac abnormalities. Isolated AVSD cases that are not associated with cardiac and extracardiac defects are those most associated with chromosomal abnormalities, with trisomy 21 being the most frequent abnormality [23]. Huggon *et al.* found 35% association between AVSD and chromosomal abnormalities, with trisomy 21 in 80.4% of cases, trisomy 18 in 12.1%, trisomy 13 in 3.7%, and other trisomies in 3.8% [24]. Conversely, Hartman *et al.* confirmed the presence of trisomy 21 in 52.9% of AVSD cases [25]. The association with genetic syndromes is also common, particularly with Ellis Van Creveld syndrome (shortening of limbs, short ribs, polydactyly, nail abnormalities, dental abnormalities, cardiac defects), Holt-Oram syndrome (upper limb and hand anomalies, heart defects), Cornelia de Lange syndrome (growth abnormality, mental retardation, abnormalities of arms, hands and fingers, arched eyebrows, long eyelashes, cardiac defects), Goldenhar syndrome (facial asymmetry, preauricular or facial folds, ear abnormalities, microphthalmia, cardiac defects), VACTREL complex (vertebral anomalies, anal atresia, cardiac defects, tracheoesophageal fistula, renal abnormalities, limb abnormalities), and CHARGE syndrome (coloboma of the eyes, cardiac defects, choanal atresia, restriction of fetal growth, genital abnormalities and/or urinary disorders, ear abnormalities) [24, 26].

Isolated balanced AVSDs not associated with chromosomal abnormalities have a greater association with ECMs [24, 26]. A retrospective analysis of 72 cases without other associated heart defects reported that in 38% of cases, AVSD coexisted with ECMs that did not require postnatal surgery whereas AVSD coexisted with 52% of ECMs that did require postnatal surgical treatment (20). The isolated ECMs most commonly associated with AVSD include CNS (5.3-22.5%), gastrointestinal (6.3-31.4%), skeletal (8.6-17.7%), facial (3.6-9.6%), genitourinary (6.3-13.5%), and respiratory (2.3-3.9%) abnormalities [25, 27] (Fig. 2).

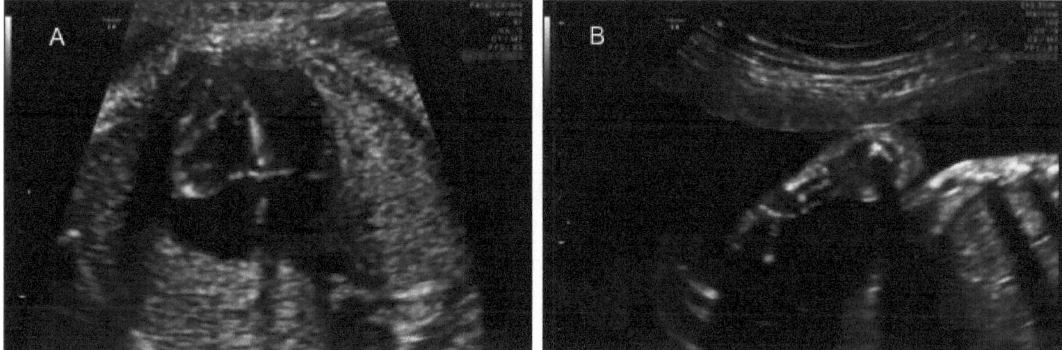

Fig. (2). Image representing the association between euploid fetus with 26 weeks with atrioventricular septal defect (AVSD) and extra-fetal malformation. (A) Partial balanced AVSD; (B) shortening of radius and ulna (mesomelia).

Ventricular Septal Defect (VSD)

Ventricular septal defect (VSD) is poorly diagnosed through prenatal ultrasound evaluation, but it is the most diagnosed CHD during the first year of life [5]. Tegnander *et al.* showed that 75-100% of the different types of VSD were identified only in the postnatal period [3]. The low intrauterine diagnostic capacity may be related to the low resolution of the devices used to study the fetal heart, evaluation of only the four-chamber apical view during the ultrasound screening, and the non-use of color Doppler during the second trimester examination.

The prognosis of small VSD is very favorable, generally with little hemodynamic repercussion on fetal circulation, and with spontaneous closure in 60% of cases during the first year of life [28]. Despite the good prognosis, a prenatal VSD diagnosis is important because of its high association with chromosomal abnormalities, genetic syndromes, and ECMs. There is a greater association between chromosomal disorders and ECMs during fetal life than during postnatal life since many cases progress to the end of gestation. During prenatal evaluation, Tegnander *et al.* showed evidence that 67% of VSDs were associated with chromosomal anomalies and 33% were associated with ECMs [3]. Chaoui *et al.* also evaluated prenatal diagnoses of CHDs and showed that 43% of VSDs were associated with chromosomal anomalies and 90% were associated with ECMs. Paladini *et al.* reported associations of VSD with chromosomal abnormalities and ECMs in 47% and 33% of cases, respectively [29, 30]. In a study of birth registrations, Stoll *et al.* reported that 10.2% of VSDs were associated with chromosomal anomalies and 19.5% were associated with multiple ECMs [6].

According to Soto *et al.*, there are four types of VSDs: perimembranous (70-80%), entry (5%), muscular (15-20%), and infundibular (5%) [31]. They can be isolated (62%), associated with conotruncal anomalies (CATs) (11%), small (24%), and large (3%) [3]. The association rate of VSDs with chromosomal disorders and ECMs also depends on the location and size of the interventricular septum defects (Table **2**).

The most frequent chromosomal abnormalities are trisomy 21, trisomy 18, trisomy 13, and microdeletion 22q11. The most common ECMs are CNS, neural tube, abdominal wall, and skeletal abnormalities [29] (Figs. **3** to **5**).

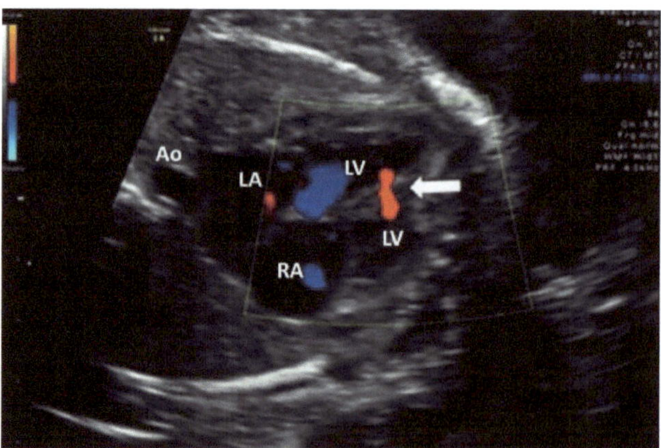

Fig. (3). Ultrasound image of fetal four-chamber view with color Doppler, demonstrating trabecular muscular ventricular septal defect (arrow). Ao: aorta; LA: left atrium; RA: right atrium; RV: right ventricle; LV: left ventricle.

Table 2. Association between ventricular septal defects (VSD), chromosomal abnormalities and extracardiac anomalies according to size and location.

Type of Defect	Chromosomal Abnormalities	Extracardiac Abnormalities
Muscular VSD	1%	5%
Isolated VSD	1.2%	4.4%
Small perimembranous VSD	23.5%	8.8%
Conotruncal abnormalities + VSD	30%	23%

(Table 2) cont.....

Type of Defect	Chromosomal Abnormalities	Extracardiac Abnormalities
Large VSD	44%	22%
Perimembranous VSD + muscular VSD	50%	17%

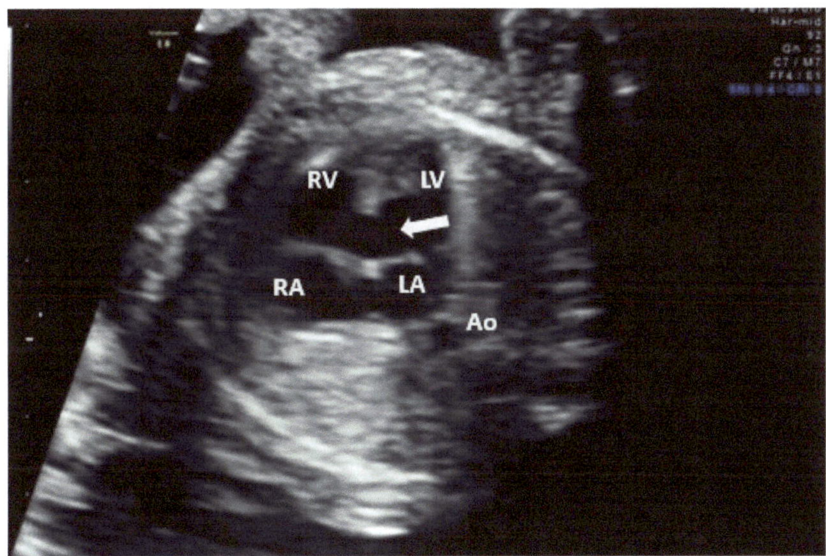

Fig. (4). Ultrasound image of the four-chamber view of the heart, demonstrating large inlet perimembranous ventricular septal defect (arrow). Ao: aorta; LA: left atrium; RA: right atrium; RV: right ventricle; LV: left ventricle.

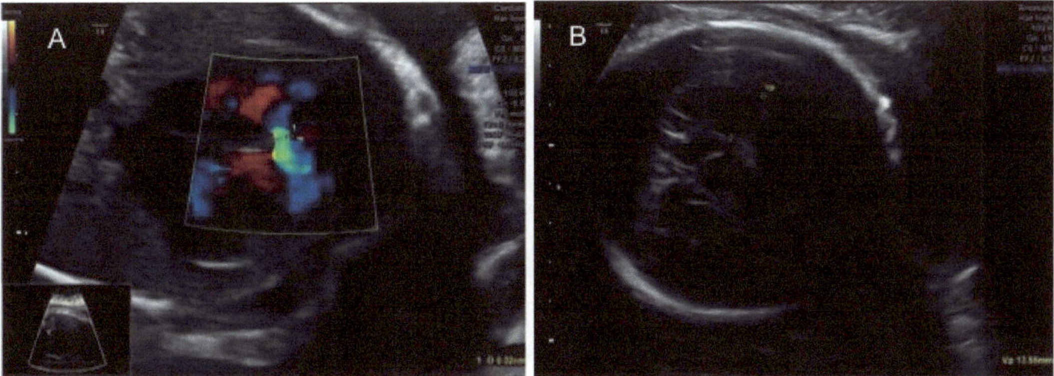

Fig. (5). Ultrasound images of fetus with ventricular septal defect (VSD) and ventriculomegaly. (A) trabecular muscular VSD (defect measurement: 3.2 mm); (B) moderate unilateral ventriculomegaly (measured as posterior lateral ventricle (13.56 mm).

Conotruncal Anomalies

Conotruncal anomalies (CTAs) are a category of cardiac abnormalities characterized by alterations in the conotruncal septum originating from the abnormal migration of cardiac neural crest cells. CTAs include truncus arteriosus, transposition of the great arteries, tetralogy of Fallot (TOF), and double outlet right ventricle [32]. The incidence of CTAs varies between prenatal series (10-12% of all CHDs) and studies performed during the postnatal period (19-30% of all CHDs) [33 - 36]. CTAs, except for the transposition of the great arteries, are associated with extracardiac abnormalities and chromosomal abnormalities, particularly trisomy 13 [37].

Tetralogy of Fallot

Tetralogy of Fallot (TOF) is a CTA whose anatomical basis is the antero-superior displacement of the infundibular septum. It consists of a combination of four cardiac abnormalities: right ventricle outflow tract obstruction, poorly aligned VSD, overriding aorta and right ventricular hypertrophy (mainly in the postnatal period) [38]. TOF presents a low rate of prenatal detection and represents 3-7% of CHD diagnosed intrauterine cases [3]. After birth, TOF has a frequency of 2 to 3 cases / 10,000 live births [38].

The three main modalities of TOF are pulmonary stenosis (2.78/10,000 live births) (Fig. **6**), pulmonary atresia (0.7/10,000 live births), and the absence of the pulmonary valve (0.2/10,000 live births) [39]. The prognosis depends on the severity of the disease, coexistence with intra- and extracardiac anomalies, and postnatal treatment [40] (Fig. **6**).

A careful ultrasonographic assessment is necessary in TOF cases because 25-40% of cases are associated extracardiac abnormalities [32, 41]. ECMs vary in type and severity, with the most frequent being omphalocele, renal anomalies, CNS, skeletal muscle, esophageal tracheal fistula, labial cleft, and single umbilical artery abnormalities [32, 41, 42].

Chromosomal abnormalities are present in 25-30% of TOF cases and vary according to the TOF subtype [40] (Table **3**). The association with the microdeletion of the long arm of chromosome 22 (22q11) becomes greater as pulmonary valve involvement likewise increases. Moreover, it is important to note that the 22q11 microdeletion is not detected by a conventional karyotype, and FISH or a-CGH is required for its detection [7, 43].

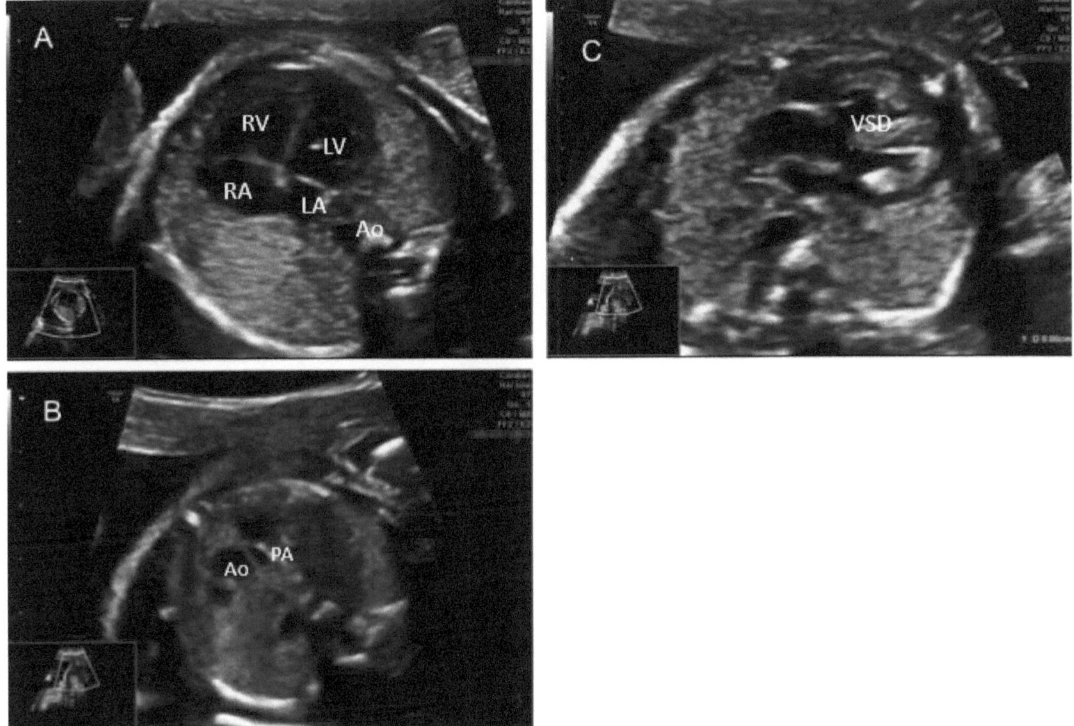

Fig. (6). Ultrasound image of tetralogy of Fallot (TOF) with pulmonary artery (PA) stenosis. **(A)** Four chamber view of the heart demonstrating left cardiac axis deviation; **(B)** 3 vessels view with disproportion between aorta (Ao) and PA; **(C)** septal view of the heart demonstrating the presence of a large ventricular septal defect (VSD) with overriding aorta (Ao). LV: left ventricle; RV: right ventricle; RA: right atrium; LA: left atrium.

Table 3. Comparison between the type of tetralogy of Fallot (TOF) and chromosomal abnormalities.

Chromosomal Abnormality	TOF	TOF with PS	TOF with PA	TOF with APV
T21	4.3%	5.9%	0.8%	2.2%
T18	3.4%	5.4%	0.0%	0.0%
T13	3.9%	3.8%	6.6%	1.1%
Microdeletion 22q11	17.4%	8.8%	24.2%	32.3%

PS: pulmonary valve stenosis; PA: pulmonary valve atresia; APV: absence of pulmonary valve.

Double Outlet Right Ventricle (DORV)

Double outlet right ventricle (DORV) is an anomaly of the arterial ventricle connections in which the great arteries originate from the morphologically right ventricle. The incidence of DORV in childhood ranges from 0.003 to 0.2/1,000 live births [44]. DORV presents a high degree of complexity and numerous variations, making the diagnosis difficult and challenging [33]. The incidence of a prenatal diagnosis of DORV comprises from 1.9-3.0% of CHDs [45, 46].

The physiology of DORV after birth depends on the location of the VSD, the relationship of the great arteries to one another, and the presence of outlet obstruction [45]. The classification of DORV according to the position of the VSD and the great vessels is described as follows [45] (Fig. 7):

1- DORV with subaortic VSD (55-70%) may be associated with poor anterior alignment of the infundibular septum with the normalized arteries. Pulmonary artery stenosis is common (50% of cases).
2- DORV with subpulmonary VSD (10-30%) may be associated with poor posterior alignment of the infundibular septum. The great arteries are usually in transposition. The presence of subaortic stenosis is frequent. This type of DORV is also known as *Taussig-Bing*.
3- DORV with double related VSD (5%), in which the VSD is related to both semilunar valves. The aortic and pulmonary valves are contiguous due to lack or hypoplasia of the infundibular septum.
4- DORV with unrelated or remote VSD (10%), in which the defect is located in the perimembranous portion of the inlet or the trabecular portion of the interventricular septum.

According to the spatial relationship of the great arteries, DORV can be classified into five subgroups:

1- Posterior aortic artery and located to the right (normal positioning);
2- Aortic artery and trunk of the pulmonary artery located side by side;
3- Aortic artery located anterior and to the right;
4- Right aortic artery;
5- Aortic artery located left and anterior.

The incidence of chromosomal abnormalities and ECMs varies considerably between studies (Table **4**).

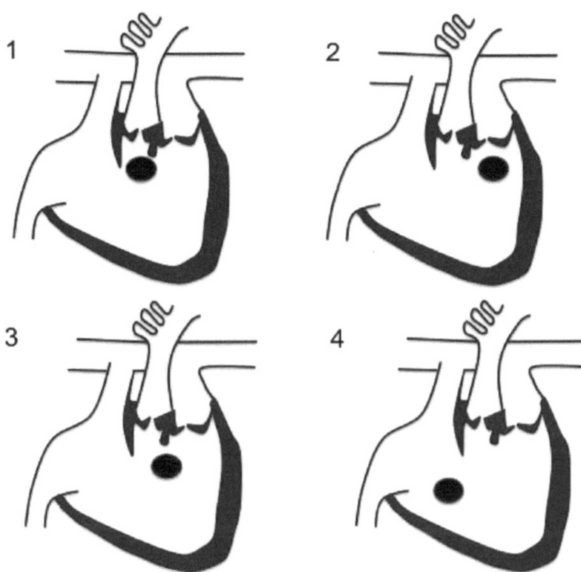

Fig. (7). Types of double outlet right ventricle (DORV) according to the positioning of the ventricular septal defect (VSD). (1) DORV with subaortic VSD; (2) DORV with subpulmonary VSD; (3) DORV with doubly related VSD; (4) DORV with unrelated or remote VSD.

Table 4. Incidence of chromosomal abnormalities and extracardiac abnormalities in fetuses with double outlet right ventricle.

Authors	Chromosomal Abnormality	Extracardiac Abnormality
Tometzki *et al.* 1999 [48]	14%	14%
Fesslova *et al.* 1999 [49]	45%	19%
Kim *et al.* 2006 [46]	21%	50%
Gedkibasi *et al.* 2008 [45]	21,4%	43,7%

Trisomy 18 (26%), trisomy 13 (13%), deletions, duplications, and reorganizations are more common in Fallot-type DORV but rarer in major artery transposition defects [32]. Associations with trisomy 21 are less common (10%) [32]. The 22q11 microdeletion is more frequently observed in cases with only the conotruncal defect [32].

The most common ECMs are CDH, cleft lip, cleft palate, CNS anomalies, skeletal abnormalities (Figs. **8** and **9**), and urogenital abnormalities [32, 45, 46].

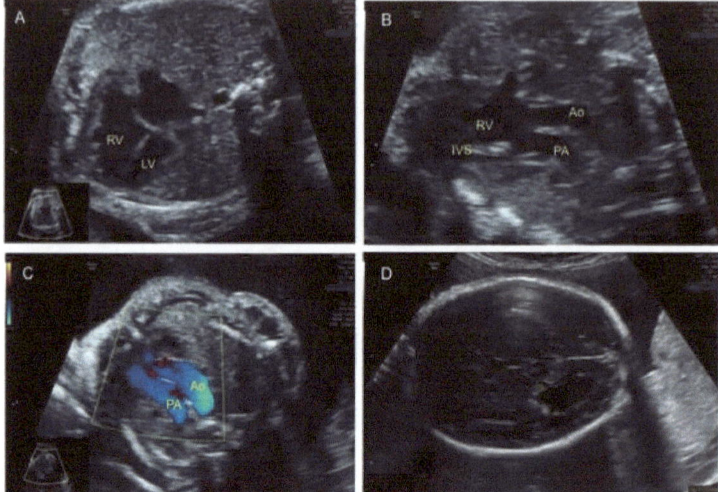

Fig. (8). Ultrasound image of fetus with double outlet right ventricle (DORV) associated with central nervous system abnormality. **(A)** Axial view of the thorax at level of four chamber view, demonstrating disproportion between right ventricle (RV) and left ventricle (LV); **(B)** Axial view of the thorax showing DORV with abnormal position of the great arteries - Taussig-Bing; **(C)** Color Doppler demonstrating blood flow in parallel through the aorta (Ao) and pulmonary artery (PA) from the RV; **(D)** Axial view of the cephalic pole at the level of the transventricular level, demonstrating mild ventriculomegaly (posterior horn of the lateral ventricle: 12.9 mm). IVS: interventricular septum.

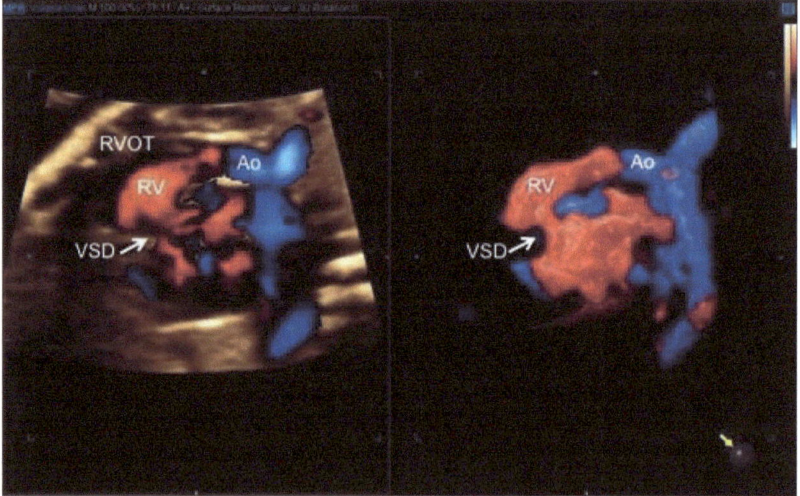

Fig. (9). Ultrasound image of the double outlet right ventricle - Taussig-Bing type, using color Doppler and 3D reconstruction, demonstrating ventricular septal defect (VSD) (arrows) associated with transposition of the great arteries. RV: right ventricle; Ao: aorta; RVOT: right ventricle outflow tract.

Common Arterial Trunk

Common arterial trunk (CAT) or truncus arteriosus is a rare CHD that comprises 0.7-1.4% of CHDs [50]. A single arterial trunk originating from the base of both ventricles characterizes CAT, riding a large VSD, through which a single valve is responsible for systemic, pulmonary, and coronary irrigation [50]. This fetal CHD has an unknown etiology and a very limited prognosis [51].

According to Collet and Edwards, CAT can be subdivided into four types (Fig. **10**) [52]:

I- Pulmonary trunk with two branches originating from the truncus arteriosus (Fig. **11**) (60%).
II- Branches of the pulmonary artery originating posteriorly and at the same level as the truncus arteriosus (35%).
III- Branches of the pulmonary artery originating in different levels of the same truncus arteriosus (laterally) (5%).
IV- Branches of the pulmonary artery originating from the aortic arch or descending aorta (5%).

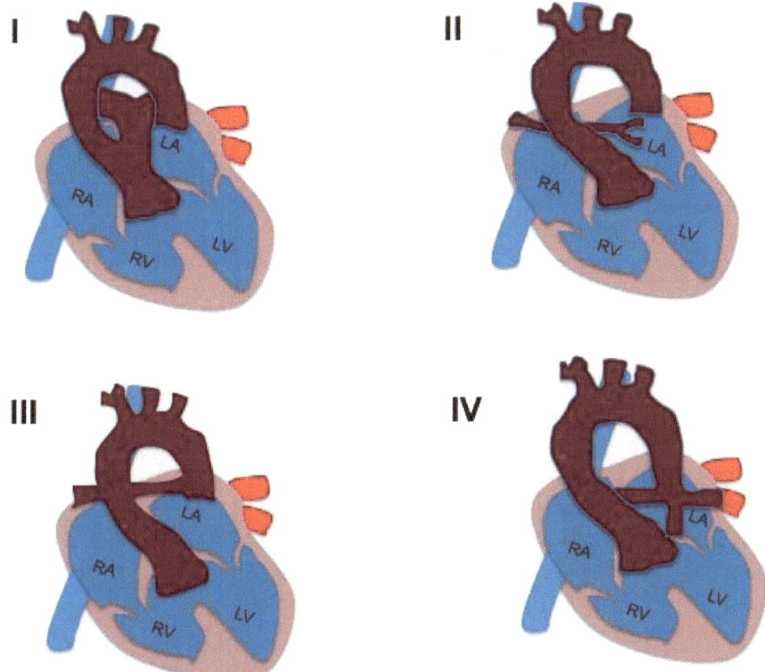

Fig. (10). Types of common arterial trunk, according to Collet e Edwards. RA: right atrium, LA: left atrium; RV: right ventricle; LV: left ventricle.

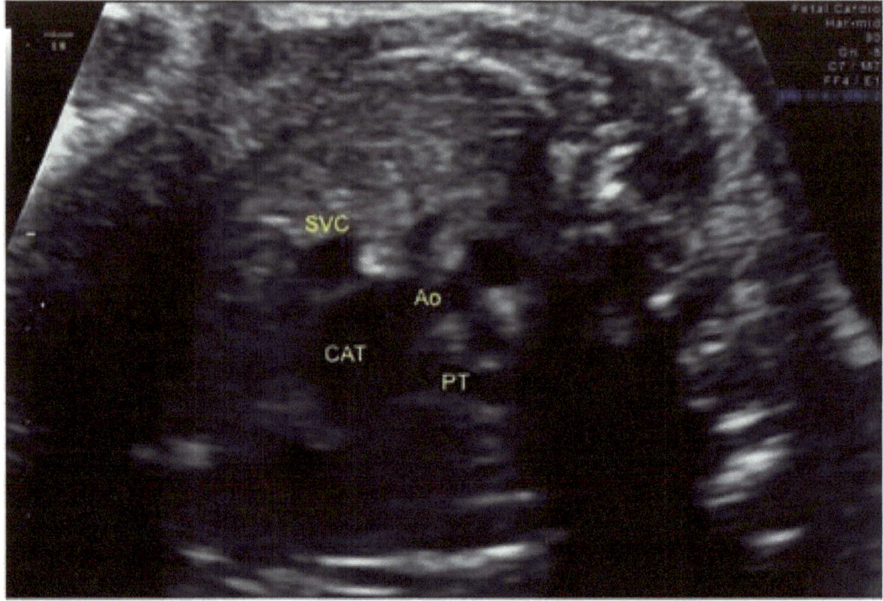

Fig. (11). Ultrasound image of fetus with common arterial trunk (CAT) type I. The vessel corresponding to the CTA where the pulmonary trunk (PT) is originated. SVC: superior vena cava; Ao: aorta.

CAT is often associated with chromosomal abnormalities and ECMs. In a series of 14 CAT cases, Fessolova *et al.* [49] reported that 29% had aneuploidies and 21% had ECMs. Similarly, Tometzki *et al.* [48] performed a cohort study and found that 33% of fetuses had aneuploidies and 33% had ECMs. The 22q11 microdeletion was present in 30% of CAT cases [53]. The main chromosomal disorders associated with CAT were trisomy 13 and trisomy 18 [48]. ECMs in euploid fetuses include omphalocele, cerebral ventriculomegaly, duodenal atresia, imperforate anus, and CHARGE associations [54].

Transposition of the Great Arteries

Transposition of the great arteries (TGA) is the most frequent congenital cyanosis heart disease at birth and the major cause of infant mortality [33, 55]. It is characterized by a ventriculo-arterial discordance secondary to a conotruncal rotation anomaly in which the aorta arises from the right ventricle and the pulmonary artery originates from the left ventricle. The etiology is multifactorial, although there are some risk factors such as diabetes mellitus, exposure to teratogenic drugs, herbicides, and rodenticides [56].

In the classic form of TGA (simple transposition), the aortic valve is located to the right of the pulmonary valve, and for this reason it is also known as d TGA. In this case, there is a correct atrioventricular position. In the congenitally corrected

TGA, there is a double discordance, atrioventricular and ventriculo-arterial, constituting a different entity and treated independently (Fig. **12**) [57]. Both variants are highly associated with additional cardiac malformations but are rarely associated with aneuploidies and ECMs [58].

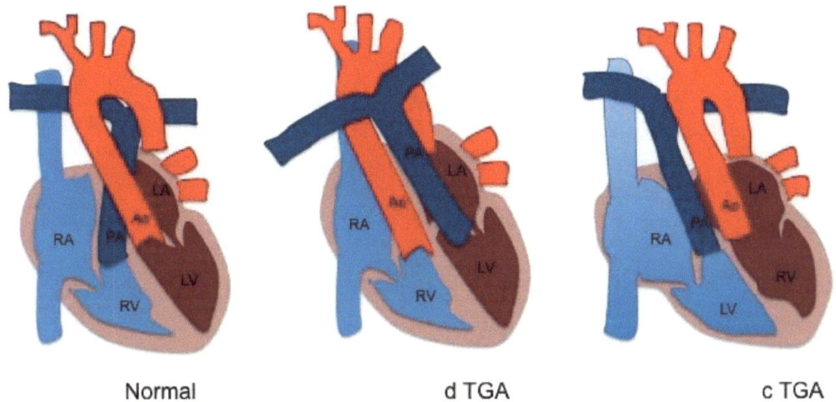

Fig. (12). Types of transposition of the great arteries (TGA). In the simple TGA (d TGA), there is atrioventricular concordance with the aorta (Ao) arising from the right ventricle (RV) and pulmonary artery (PA) originating from the left ventricle (LV). In the congenitally corrected TGA (c TGA), there is atrioventricular and ventriculo-arterial discordance. In this case, PA arises from the morphologically LV and Ao originates from the morphologically RV. LA: left atrium; RA: right atrium.

Despite the rare relationship between TGA and ECMs, the incidence of this association varies greatly between studies. In a retrospective study, Ravi *et al.* [59] observed an increase in the diagnostic capacity of TGA in Canada from 14% between 2003 and 2010 to 50% between 2011 and 2013 and 77% between 2014 and 2015. In this study, 127 TGA cases were found in the pre- and / or postnatal period. The association with ECMs was evident in 2.4% of the cases, including two cases with intestinal obstruction (duodenal atresia and jejunal atresia) and one case with cerebral ventriculomegaly. However, Khoshnood *et al.* [60] showed an association with ECMs in 9.3% of the d TGA cases. According to Domíngues-Manzano *et al.* [61], ECMs were present in 12.8% of fetuses with chromosomally normal d TGA. The ECMs were single umbilical artery (3.2%), intrahepatic persistence of the right umbilical vein (1.1%), hypospadia (4.2%), renal dysplasia (1.1%), choroid plexus cyst (1,1%), choledochal cyst (1.1%), and choanal atresia (1.1%). Most prenatal series report that the incidence of aneuploidies in TGA cases ranges from 0-7% (Fig. **13**) [49, 62]. Fesslova *et al.* [49] reported one case of trisomy 21 and one case of trisomy 18 in their series of 39 fetuses with d TGA. There is a negative correlation between TGA and abnormal karyotypes, particularly among fetuses with c TGA [63].

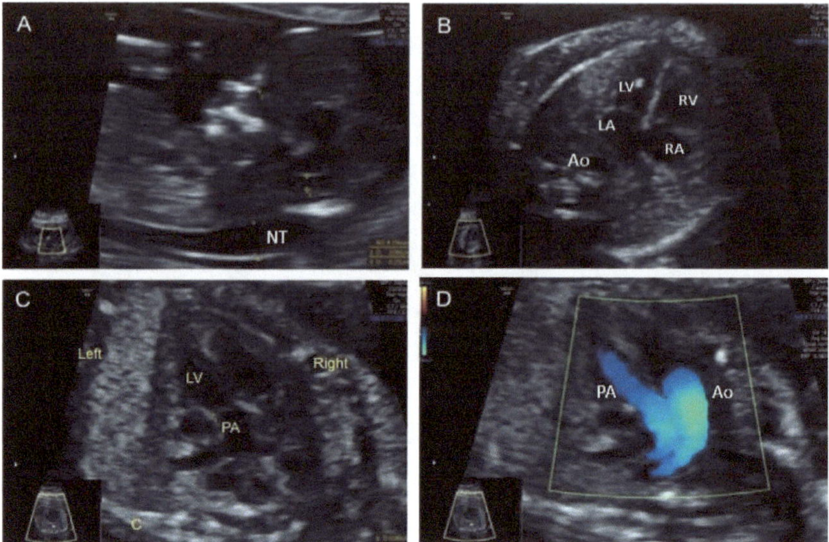

Fig. (13). Ultrasound image of chromosomally normal fetus with increased nuchal translucency (NT) and simple transposition of the great arteries (d TGA) diagnosed during second trimester scan. (A) First trimester examination demonstrating increased NT (NT: 4.79 mm); (B) Second trimester scan demonstrating normal 4-chamber view of the heart; (C) Ventricular outflow tract, demonstrating ventriculo-arterial discordance; (D) ventricular outflow tract with color Doppler, demonstrating aorta (Ao) and pulmonary artery (PA) in parallel. LA: left atrium; RA: right atrium; RV: right ventricle; LV: left ventricle.

Hypoplastic Left Heart Syndrome

Hypoplastic left heart syndrome (HLHS) is one of the CHDs most commonly diagnosed during the prenatal period because of the abnormal appearance of the heart in the four-chamber view during routine ultrasound examination [64]. HLHS includes a set of heart diseases characterized by severe hypoplasia of the left ventricle and all of its outflow tract, secondary to a severe obstruction at one or more levels of the inlet (mitral valve) or outlet tract (aortic valve) [65] (Fig. **14**).

The spectrum of HLHS includes a varied degree of aortic valve and mitral valve obstructions [64]:

- aortic atresia with mitral atresia,
- aortic atresia with mitral stenosis,
- aortic stenosis with mitral stenosis,
- aortic stenosis with mitral atresia.

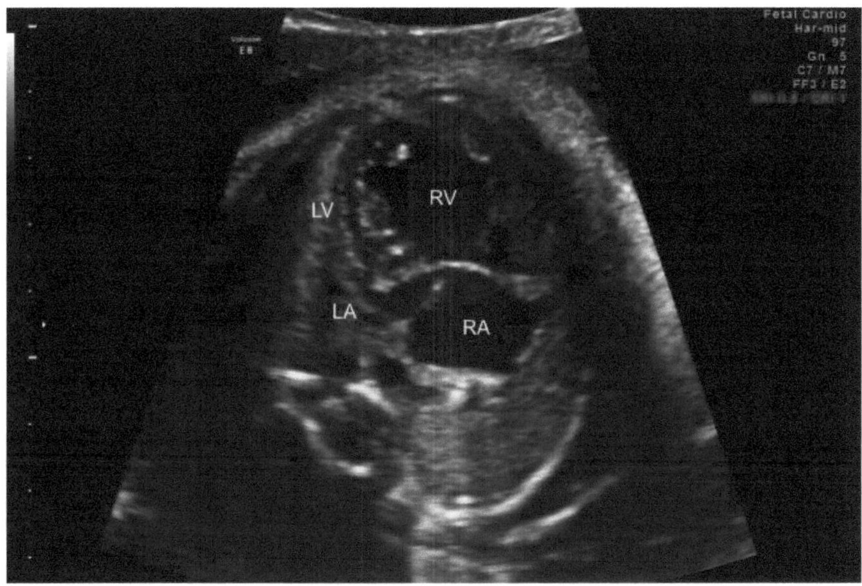

Fig. (14). Ultrasound image demonstrating the four chambers view with hypoplastic left heart syndrome due to mitral atresia and aortic atresia. The left ventricle (LV) cavity is not observed; the left atrium (LA), dilation of the right atrium (RA) and right ventricle (RV) are noted. The hyperechoic mitral valve is constantly closed.

The classic form of HLHS consists of aortic atresia, with atresia or severe hypoplasia of the mitral valve [66]. In these cases, the incidence of chromosomal abnormalities ranges from 4-10% [67 - 69]. The most frequently associated chromosomal anomalies are monosomy X, trisomy 18, trisomy 13, and some partial deletions [70]. ECMs are estimated to be present in 15-20% of cases, with the most frequent being gastrointestinal, omphalocele, urinary, CNS, and musculoskeletal abnormalities [70].

Tricuspid Atresia

Tricuspid atresia (TA) is a rare CHD whose prevalence at birth is 1 / 15,000 [3]. In prenatal series, the incidence of TA is low, ranging from 2-4% [49, 71]. TA is characterized by complete agenesis, or more rarely, by an imperforate atrioventricular connection, causing the absence of communication between the right atrium and right ventricle [72]. In this case, there is hypoplasia of the right ventricle, and often the presence of a VSD, whose quantity and size will condition the degree of development of the right ventricle and pulmonary artery. In color Doppler study, no blood flow from the right atrium to the right ventricle is observed. The vessel that originates from the small right ventricle is generally hypoplastic [73].

There are three types of TA that are distinguished according to the relationship with the output [74, 75]:

1- Type I: normorelated vessels (50-70%)
2- Type II: D-transposition of TGA (28-46%)
3- Type III: L-transposition of TGA (3%)

In turn, these types are further subdivided according to the existence of pulmonary valve atresia or stenosis [74, 75].

The association of TA with aneuploidies and ECMs has been reported between 2-9% [49, 67] and 19-34% [37, 75] of cases. The most frequent chromosomal abnormalities are trisomy 13 (16.5%), trisomy 18 (8.3%), and partial tetrasomy 22q11 (16.5%) [74]. The most common ECMs are renal abnormalities, hypospadias, congenital crooked foot, hydrothorax, venous duct agenesis, microcephaly, and substernal cyst [74, 76].

Abnormalities of the Aortic Arch

Aortic arch abnormalities are present in 1-2% of the population [77, 78]. Most of these changes (up to 50%) have been reported to be associated with CHDs, which indicates that the presence of an isolated vascular ring is uncommon (1-1.6 / 1,000 pregnancies) [79].

The most common types of aortic arch abnormalities are:

4- left aortic arch with aberrant right subclavian artery,
5- right aortic arch with aberrant left subclavian artery (Fig. **15**),
6- aortic arch on the right with supra-aortic mirror-image branching pattern,
7- double aortic arch [79, 80].

Although there is no clinical importance for the neonate, the prenatal diagnosis of aortic arch abnormalities is an important marker of CHDs and chromosomal abnormalities, including the 22q11 microdeletion [81, 82]. The presence of an aberrant right or left subclavian artery, independent of the laterality of the aortic arch, has been associated with increase in the incidence of chromosomal anomalies, particularly when there is association with ECMs [82, 83]. Thus, the detection of aortic arch abnormalities is important for the counseling and management of pregnancies.

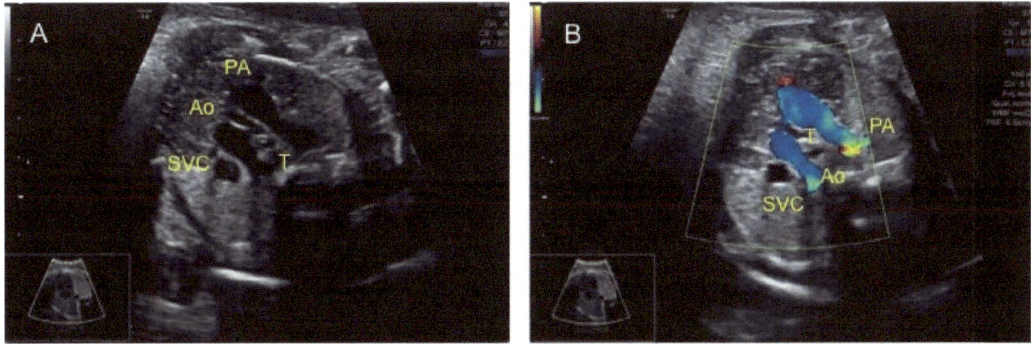

Fig. (15). Three vessels and trachea view in mode B (A) and color Doppler (B), of a fetus with right aortic arch. The aorta (Ao) is seen to the right of the trachea (T) and pulmonary artery (PA) to the left. SVC: superior vena cava.

The risk of CHDs concomitant to the right aortic arch (with a supra-aortic mirror pattern) is approximately 90%, whereas it is only 10% in the presence of a right aortic arch with an aberrant left subclavian artery [84]. A double aortic arch is usually an isolated finding [85, 86].

The most common association with right aortic arch (mirror-image branching type) is TOF (13-55%) [87]. Other common associations with right aortic arch are VSD (31-36%) and CAT (15-36%) [87]. In a series of cases with right aortic arch, 39% (28/71) had ECMs, such as polyhydramnios, atresia of the esophagus, cleft lip and palate, spina bifida, and congenital club foot [85].

Aorta Coarctation

Aorta coarctation (CoA) is a narrowing of the aortic lumen that obstructs the blood flow. It corresponds to approximately 8% of CHDs and is significantly associated with chromosomal abnormalities and ECMs [49, 62].

In most cases, aorta narrowing occurs in the portion between the left subclavian artery and the ductus arteriosus (pre-ductal). Aorta narrowing may also occur at the level of the ductus arteriosus (ductal) or distal to the ductus arteriosus (post-ductal) [88]. Pre-ductal CoA (2%) is the most diagnosed type during prenatal evaluation and is usually associated with other cardiac abnormalities. Ductal and post-ductal CoA correspond to 98% of cases, and the diagnosis generally occurs during childhood or adult life. They are usually isolated defects or associated with valvular diseases [88]. From the surgical point of view, CoA can be classified into three categories: isolated CoA, CoA associated with VSD, and CoA associated with complex cardiac abnormalities [89].

In total, 29% and 18% of CoA cases are associated chromosomal abnormalities and ECMs, respectively. The most common aneuploidies are monosomy X, trisomy 21, trisomy 18, trisomy 13, and microdeletion 22q11. The ECMs most frequently associated with CoA include skeletal anomalies (achondroplasia, chondrodysplasia punctata, congenital club foot, osteogenesis imperfecta), anomalies of the CNS (corpus callosum agenesis, encephalocele), esophageal atresia, anorectal atresia, renal anomalies (pyelectasis, polycystic kidneys, renal agenesis), hypospadias, ocular and ear abnormalities, and CDH [90] (Fig. **16**).

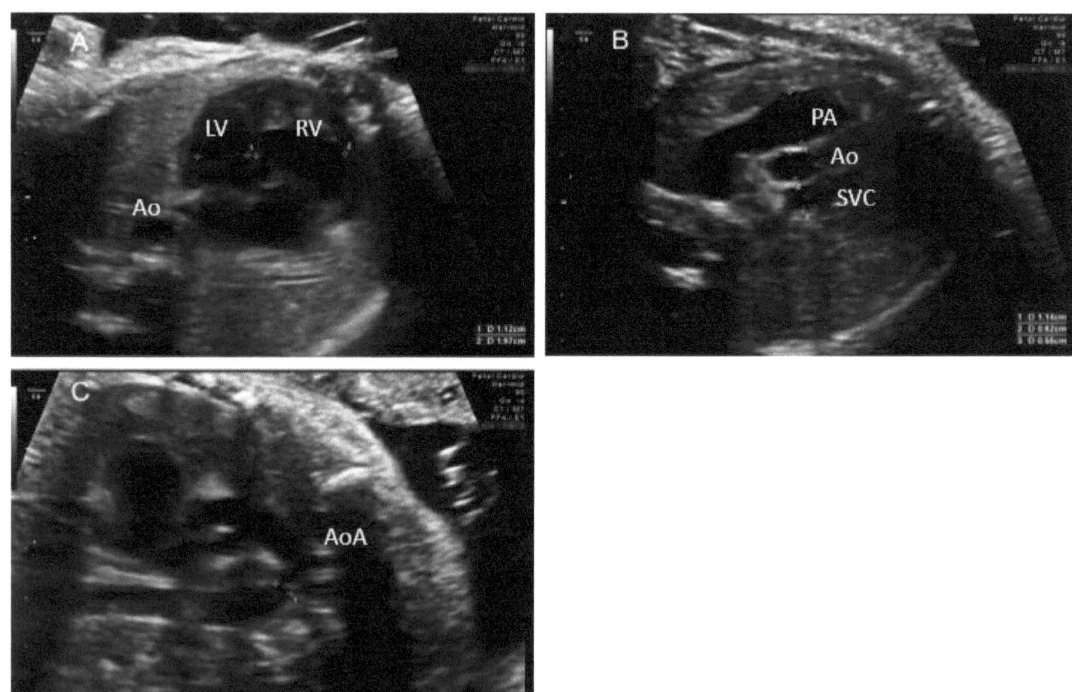

Fig. (16). Ultrasound image showing indirect (A and B) and direct (C) signs of aortic coarctation at 38 weeks gestation. (A) Asymmetry of the cardiac chambers (right ventricle - RV / left ventricle – LV ratio > 1.4 (RV/LV ratio = 1.75); (B) Asymmetry of the great vessels, with increased relation pulmonary artery (PA) trunk/aorta (Ao) (PA/Ao ratio = 1.8); (C) Sagittal section of the aortic arch (AoA) with measurement of the normal aortic isthmus (Isthmus: 3.5 mm, Z score: -1.6). SVC: superior vena cava.

Interrupted Aortic Arch

Interrupted aortic arch (IAA) is a rare heart disease that corresponds to 0.2-1% of all CHDs. Its incidence at birth is 2-3 cases per 1,000,000 births. It is characterized by an atresia located between the ascending and the descending aorta, with a lack complete anatomical continuity or an atresic cord between both extremes of the aorta [91]. Most IAA cases are associated with a subaortic VSD of variable size [92].

IAA can be subdivided into three groups: type A, distal interruption to the left subclavian artery (30%); type B, interruption between the carotid artery and left subclavian artery (50-60%); and type C, interruption between the brachiocephalic trunk and the left carotid artery (10%). The IAA is always pre-ductal, ensuring systemic perfusion to the lower body through the connection between the ductus arteriosus and descending aorta [91].

IAA type A is rarely associated with chromosomal abnormalities. However, IAA type B is associated with the 22q11 microdeletion and ECMs in 50-80% of cases [93]. The ECMs most associated with IAA type B include CNS, urinary, gastrointestinal, and skeletal anomalies [94].

CONCLUSION

The presence of ECMs and chromosomal abnormalities are common in fetuses with CHDs. We describe the main associations between ECMs and chromosomal abnormalities in fetuses with CHDs. We believe that this information may improve the prenatal management and counseling of patients affected by these conditions.

CONSENT FOR PUBLICATION

Not applicable.

CONFLICT OF INTEREST

The authors confirm that the contents of this chapter have no conflict of interest.

ACKNOWLEDGEMENTS

Declare none.

REFERENCES

[1]   Stoll C, Garne E, Clementi M. EUROSCAN Study Group. Evaluation of prenatal diagnosis of associated congenital heart diseases by fetal ultrasonographic examination in Europe. Prenat Diagn 2001; 21(4): 243-52.
       [http://dx.doi.org/10.1002/pd.34] [PMID: 11288111]

[2]   Meberg A, Hals J, Thaulow E. Congenital heart defects--chromosomal anomalies, syndromes and extracardiac malformations. Acta Paediatr 2007; 96(8): 1142-5.
       [http://dx.doi.org/10.1111/j.1651-2227.2007.00381.x] [PMID: 17590185]

[3]   Tegnander E, Williams W, Johansen OJ, Blaas HG, Eik-Nes SH. Prenatal detection of heart defects in a non-selected population of 30,149 fetuses--detection rates and outcome. Ultrasound Obstet Gynecol 2006; 27(3): 252-65.
       [http://dx.doi.org/10.1002/uog.2710] [PMID: 16456842]

[4]   Brennan P, Young ID. Congenital heart malformations: aetiology and associations. Semin Neonatol 2001; 6(1): 17-25.
       [http://dx.doi.org/10.1053/siny.2000.0032] [PMID: 11162282]

[5] Ferencz C, Rubin JD, McCarter RJ, *et al*. Congenital heart disease: prevalence at livebirth. The Baltimore-Washington Infant Study. Am J Epidemiol 1985; 121(1): 31-6.
[http://dx.doi.org/10.1093/oxfordjournals.aje.a113979] [PMID: 3964990]

[6] Stoll C, Dott B, Alembik Y, Roth MP. Associated noncardiac congenital anomalies among cases with congenital heart defects. Eur J Med Genet 2015; 58(2): 75-85.
[http://dx.doi.org/10.1016/j.ejmg.2014.12.002] [PMID: 25497206]

[7] Tonni G, Palmisano M, Perez Zamarian AC, *et al*. Phenotype to genotype characterization by array-comparative genomic hybridization (a-CGH) in case of fetal malformations: A systematic review. Taiwan J Obstet Gynecol 2019; 58(1): 15-28.
[http://dx.doi.org/10.1016/j.tjog.2018.11.003] [PMID: 30638470]

[8] Blue GM, Kirk EP, Sholler GF, Harvey RP, Winlaw DS. Congenital heart disease: current knowledge about causes and inheritance. Med J Aust 2012; 197(3): 155-9.
[http://dx.doi.org/10.5694/mja12.10811] [PMID: 22860792]

[9] Al Turki S, Manickaraj AK, Mercer CL, *et al*. UK10K Consortium. Rare variants in NR2F2 cause congenital heart defects in humans. Am J Hum Genet 2014; 94(4): 574-85.
[http://dx.doi.org/10.1016/j.ajhg.2014.03.007] [PMID: 24702954]

[10] Tegnander E, Eik-Nes SH, Johansen OJ, Linker DT. Prenatal detection of heart defects at the routine fetal examination at 18 weeks in a non-selected population. Ultrasound Obstet Gynecol 1995; 5(6): 372-80.
[http://dx.doi.org/10.1046/j.1469-0705.1995.05060372.x] [PMID: 7552797]

[11] Carvalho JS, Mavrides E, Shinebourne EA, Campbell S, Thilaganathan B. Improving the effectiveness of routine prenatal screening for major congenital heart defects. Heart 2002; 88(4): 387-91.
[http://dx.doi.org/10.1136/heart.88.4.387] [PMID: 12231598]

[12] Nicolaides KH. Turning the pyramid of prenatal care. Fetal Diagn Ther 2011; 29(3): 183-96.
[http://dx.doi.org/10.1159/000324320] [PMID: 21389681]

[13] Ghi T, Huggon IC, Zosmer N, Nicolaides KH. Incidence of major structural cardiac defects associated with increased nuchal translucency but normal karyotype. Ultrasound Obstet Gynecol 2001; 18(6): 610-4.
[http://dx.doi.org/10.1046/j.0960-7692.2001.00584.x] [PMID: 11844199]

[14] Burn J, Brennan P, Little J, *et al*. Recurrence risks in offspring of adults with major heart defects: results from first cohort of British collaborative study. Lancet 1998; 351(9099): 311-6.
[http://dx.doi.org/10.1016/S0140-6736(97)06486-6] [PMID: 9652610]

[15] Meyer-Wittkopf M, Simpson JM, Sharland GK. Incidence of congenital heart defects in fetuses of diabetic mothers: a retrospective study of 326 cases. Ultrasound Obstet Gynecol 1996; 8(1): 8-10.
[http://dx.doi.org/10.1046/j.1469-0705.1996.08010008.x] [PMID: 8843611]

[16] Alanen J, Leskinen M, Sairanen M, *et al*. Fetal nuchal translucency in severe congenital heart defects: experiences in Northern Finland. J Matern Fetal Neonatal Med 2019; 32(9): 1454-60.
[http://dx.doi.org/10.1080/14767058.2017.1408067] [PMID: 29157037]

[17] Blaas HG, Eik-Nes SH, Kiserud T, Hellevik LR. Early development of the abdominal wall, stomach and heart from 7 to 12 weeks of gestation: a longitudinal ultrasound study. Ultrasound Obstet Gynecol 1995; 6(4): 240-9.
[http://dx.doi.org/10.1046/j.1469-0705.1995.06040240.x] [PMID: 8590186]

[18] Syngelaki A, Chelemen T, Dagklis T, Allan L, Nicolaides KH. Challenges in the diagnosis of fetal non-chromosomal abnormalities at 11-13 weeks. Prenat Diagn 2011; 31(1): 90-102.
[http://dx.doi.org/10.1002/pd.2642] [PMID: 21210483]

[19] van der Linde D, Konings EE, Slager MA, *et al*. Birth prevalence of congenital heart disease worldwide: a systematic review and meta-analysis. J Am Coll Cardiol 2011; 58(21): 2241-7.
[http://dx.doi.org/10.1016/j.jacc.2011.08.025] [PMID: 22078432]

[20]   Słodki M, Soroka M, Rizzo G, Respondek-Liberska M. Prenatal Atrioventricular Septal Defect (AVSD) as a planned congenital heart disease with different outcome depending on the presence of the coexisting extracardiac abnormalities (ECA) and / or malformations (ECM). J Matern Neonatal Med 4:1-191. [Epub ahead of print]
[http://dx.doi.org/10.1080/14767058.2018.1556254]

[21]   Dolk H, Loane M, Garne E. European Surveillance of Congenital Anomalies (EUROCAT) Working Group. Congenital heart defects in Europe: prevalence and perinatal mortality, 2000 to 2005. Circulation 2011; 123(8): 841-9.
[http://dx.doi.org/10.1161/CIRCULATIONAHA.110.958405] [PMID: 21321151]

[22]   Allan LD. Atrioventricular septal defect in the fetus. Am J Obstet Gynecol 1999; 181(5 Pt 1): 1250-3.
[http://dx.doi.org/10.1016/S0002-9378(99)70117-1] [PMID: 10561654]

[23]   Latson LA, Jones TK, Jacobson J, Zahn E, Rhodes JF. Analysis of factors related to successful transcatheter closure of secundum atrial septal defects using the HELEX septal occluder. Am Heart J 2006; 151(5): 1129.e7-1129.e11.
[http://dx.doi.org/10.1016/j.ahj.2006.01.005] [PMID: 16644351]

[24]   Huggon IC, Cook AC, Smeeton NC, Magee AG, Sharland GK. Atrioventricular septal defects diagnosed in fetal life: associated cardiac and extra-cardiac abnormalities and outcome. J Am Coll Cardiol 2000; 36(2): 593-601.
[http://dx.doi.org/10.1016/S0735-1097(00)00757-9] [PMID: 10933376]

[25]   Hartman RJ, Riehle-Colarusso T, Lin A, *et al.* National Birth Defects Prevention Study. Descriptive study of nonsyndromic atrioventricular septal defects in the National Birth Defects Prevention Study, 1997-2005. Am J Med Genet A 2011; 155A(3): 555-64.
[http://dx.doi.org/10.1002/ajmg.a.33874] [PMID: 21337694]

[26]   Pajkrt E, Weisz B, Firth HV, Chitty LS. Fetal cardiac anomalies and genetic syndromes. Prenat Diagn 2004; 24(13): 1104-15.
[http://dx.doi.org/10.1002/pd.1067] [PMID: 15614851]

[27]   Sanapo L, Pruetz JD, Słodki M, Goens MB, Moon-Grady AJ, Donofrio MT. Fetal echocardiography for planning perinatal and delivery room care of neonates with congenital heart disease. Echocardiography 2017; 34(12): 1804-21.
[http://dx.doi.org/10.1111/echo.13672] [PMID: 29287132]

[28]   Minette MS, Sahn DJ. Ventricular septal defects. Circulation 2006; 114(20): 2190-7.
[http://dx.doi.org/10.1161/CIRCULATIONAHA.106.618124] [PMID: 17101870]

[29]   Chaoui R, Körner H, Bommer C, Göldner B, Bierlich A, Bollmann R. [Prenatal diagnosis of heart defects and associated chromosomal aberrations]. Ultraschall Med 1999; 20(5): 177-84.
[PMID: 10595385]

[30]   Paladini D, Palmieri S, Lamberti A, Teodoro A, Martinelli P, Nappi C. Characterization and natural history of ventricular septal defects in the fetus. Ultrasound Obstet Gynecol 2000; 16(2): 118-22.
[http://dx.doi.org/10.1046/j.1469-0705.2000.00202.x] [PMID: 11117079]

[31]   Soto B, Becker AE, Moulaert AJ, Lie JT, Anderson RH. Classification of ventricular septal defects. Br Heart J 1980; 43(3): 332-43.
[http://dx.doi.org/10.1136/hrt.43.3.332] [PMID: 7437181]

[32]   Paladini D, Rustico M, Todros T, *et al.* Conotruncal anomalies in prenatal life. Ultrasound Obstet Gynecol 1996; 8(4): 241-6.
[http://dx.doi.org/10.1046/j.1469-0705.1996.08040241.x] [PMID: 8916376]

[33]   Hoffman JI, Kaplan S. The incidence of congenital heart disease. J Am Coll Cardiol 2002; 39(12): 1890-900.
[http://dx.doi.org/10.1016/S0735-1097(02)01886-7] [PMID: 12084585]

[34]   Samánek M, Vorísková M. Congenital heart disease among 815,569 children born between 1980 and

1990 and their 15-year survival: a prospective Bohemia survival study. Pediatr Cardiol 1999; 20(6): 411-7.
[http://dx.doi.org/10.1007/s002469900502] [PMID: 10556387]

[35]   Rustico MA, Benettoni A, D'Ottavio G, *et al.* Fetal heart screening in low-risk pregnancies. Ultrasound Obstet Gynecol 1995; 6(5): 313-9.
[http://dx.doi.org/10.1046/j.1469-0705.1995.06050313.x] [PMID: 8590200]

[36]   Grandjean H, Larroque D, Levi S. The performance of routine ultrasonographic screening of pregnancies in the Eurofetus Study. Am J Obstet Gynecol 1999; 181(2): 446-54.
[http://dx.doi.org/10.1016/S0002-9378(99)70577-6] [PMID: 10454699]

[37]   Harris JA, Francannet C, Pradat P, Robert E. The epidemiology of cardiovascular defects, part 2: a study based on data from three large registries of congenital malformations. Pediatr Cardiol 2003; 24(3): 222-35.
[http://dx.doi.org/10.1007/s00246-002-9402-5] [PMID: 12632214]

[38]   Apitz C, Webb GD, Redington AN. Tetralogy of Fallot. Lancet 2009; 374(9699): 1462-71.
[http://dx.doi.org/10.1016/S0140-6736(09)60657-7] [PMID: 19683809]

[39]   Abuhamad AZ, Chaoui R. A Practical Guide to Fetal Echocardiography: Normal and Abnormal Hearts. Philadelphia, PA: Lippincott Williams & Wilkins 2010.

[40]   Zhao Y, Abuhamad A, Fleenor J, *et al.* Prenatal and postnatal survival of fetal tetralogy of fallot: A meta-analysis of perinatal outcomes and associated genetic disorders. J Ultrasound Med 2016; 35(5): 905-15.
[http://dx.doi.org/10.7863/ultra.15.04055] [PMID: 27022172]

[41]   Galindo A, Mendoza A, Arbues J, Grañeras A, Escribano D, Nieto O. Conotruncal anomalies in fetal life: accuracy of diagnosis, associated defects and outcome. Eur J Obstet Gynecol Reprod Biol 2009; 146(1): 55-60.
[http://dx.doi.org/10.1016/j.ejogrb.2009.04.032] [PMID: 19481856]

[42]   Poon LC, Huggon IC, Zidere V, Allan LD. Tetralogy of Fallot in the fetus in the current era. Ultrasound Obstet Gynecol 2007; 29(6): 625-7.
[http://dx.doi.org/10.1002/uog.3971] [PMID: 17405110]

[43]   Trainer AH, Morrison N, Dunlop A, Wilson N, Tolmie J. Chromosome 22q11 microdeletions in tetralogy of Fallot. Arch Dis Child 1996; 74(1): 62-3.
[http://dx.doi.org/10.1136/adc.74.1.62] [PMID: 8660052]

[44]   Keane JF, Fyler D. Double-outlet right ventricle.Nadas' Pediatric Cardiology. 2nd ed., Philadelphia, PA: Elsevier 2006.

[45]   Gedikbasi A, Oztarhan K, Gul A, Sargin A, Ceylan Y. Diagnosis and prognosis in double-outlet right ventricle. Am J Perinatol 2008; 25(7): 427-34.
[http://dx.doi.org/10.1055/s-0028-1083840] [PMID: 18720325]

[46]   Kim N, Friedberg MK, Silverman NH. Diagnosis and prognosis of fetuses with double outlet right ventricle. Prenat Diagn 2006; 26(8): 740-5.
[http://dx.doi.org/10.1002/pd.1500] [PMID: 16807954]

[47]   Galindo AI, Gratacós ES, Martínez JM. Ventrículo derecho de doble salida.Cardiología Fetal. 1st ed. Madrid: Marbán 2015; p. 629.

[48]   Tometzki AJ, Suda K, Kohl T, Kovalchin JP, Silverman NH. Accuracy of prenatal echocardiographic diagnosis and prognosis of fetuses with conotruncal anomalies. J Am Coll Cardiol 1999; 33(6): 1696-701.
[http://dx.doi.org/10.1016/S0735-1097(99)00049-2] [PMID: 10334445]

[49]   Fesslova' V, Nava S, Villa L. Fetal Cardiology Study Group of the Italian Society of Pediatric Cardiology. Evolution and long term outcome in cases with fetal diagnosis of congenital heart disease: Italian multicentre study. Heart 1999; 82(5): 594-9.

[http://dx.doi.org/10.1136/hrt.82.5.594] [PMID: 10525516]

[50]   Allan L, Hornberger L, Sharland GK. Textbook of fetal cardiology. London: Greenwich Medical Media 2000; pp. 288-304.

[51]   Mărginean C, Gozar L, Mărginean CO, *et al*. Prenatal diagnosis of the fetal common arterial trunk. A case series. Med Ultrason 2018; 1(1): 100-4.
[http://dx.doi.org/10.11152/mu-1084] [PMID: 29400376]

[52]   Collett RW, Edwards JE. Persistent truncus arteriosus; a classification according to anatomic types. Surg Clin North Am 1949; 29(4): 1245-70.
[http://dx.doi.org/10.1016/S0039-6109(16)32803-1] [PMID: 18141293]

[53]   Boudjemline Y, Fermont L, Le Bidois J, Lyonnet S, Sidi D, Bonnet D. Prevalence of 22q11 deletion in fetuses with conotruncal cardiac defects: a 6-year prospective study. J Pediatr 2001; 138(4): 520-4.
[http://dx.doi.org/10.1067/mpd.2001.112174] [PMID: 11295715]

[54]   Volpe P, Paladini D, Marasini M, *et al*. Common arterial trunk in the fetus: characteristics, associations, and outcome in a multicentre series of 23 cases. Heart 2003; 89(12): 1437-41.
[http://dx.doi.org/10.1136/heart.89.12.1437] [PMID: 14617557]

[55]   Lee K, Khoshnood B, Chen L, Wall SN, Cromie WJ, Mittendorf RL. Infant mortality from congenital malformations in the United States, 1970-1997. Obstet Gynecol 2001; 98(4): 620-7.
[http://dx.doi.org/10.1097/00006250-200110000-00017] [PMID: 11576578]

[56]   Martins P, Castela E. Transposition of the great arteries. Orphanet J Rare Dis 2008; 3: 27.
[http://dx.doi.org/10.1186/1750-1172-3-27] [PMID: 18851735]

[57]   Allan L. Transposition of great arteries.Textbook of fetal cardiology. London: Greenwich Medical Media 2000; pp. 261-74.

[58]   Pradat P, Francannet C, Harris JA, Robert E. The epidemiology of cardiovascular defects, part I: a study based on data from three large registries of congenital malformations. Pediatr Cardiol 2003; 24(3): 195-221.
[http://dx.doi.org/10.1007/s00246-002-9401-6] [PMID: 12632215]

[59]   Ravi P, Mills L, Fruitman D, *et al*. Population trends in prenatal detection of transposition of great arteries: impact of obstetric screening ultrasound guidelines. Ultrasound Obstet Gynecol 2018; 51(5): 659-64.
[http://dx.doi.org/10.1002/uog.17496] [PMID: 28436133]

[60]   Khoshnood B, Lelong N, Houyel L, *et al*. EPICARD Study group. Impact of prenatal diagnosis on survival of newborns with four congenital heart defects: a prospective, population-based cohort study in France (the EPICARD Study). BMJ Open 2017; 7(11)e018285
[http://dx.doi.org/10.1136/bmjopen-2017-018285] [PMID: 29122798]

[61]   Domínguez-Manzano P, Mendoza A, Herraiz I, *et al*. Transposition of the Great Arteries in Fetal Life: Accuracy of Diagnosis and Short-Term Outcome. Fetal Diagn Ther 2016; 40(4): 268-76.
[http://dx.doi.org/10.1159/000444296] [PMID: 26943122]

[62]   Paladini D, Russo M, Teodoro A, *et al*. Prenatal diagnosis of congenital heart disease in the Naples area during the years 1994-1999 -- the experience of a joint fetal-pediatric cardiology unit. Prenat Diagn 2002; 22(7): 545-52.
[http://dx.doi.org/10.1002/pd.356] [PMID: 12124685]

[63]   Paladini D, Volpe P, Marasini M, *et al*. Diagnosis, characterization and outcome of congenitally corrected transposition of the great arteries in the fetus: a multicenter series of 30 cases. Ultrasound Obstet Gynecol 2006; 27(3): 281-5.
[http://dx.doi.org/10.1002/uog.2715] [PMID: 16485324]

[64]   Nguyen T, Miller M, Gonzalez J, *et al*. Echocardiography of hypoplastic left heart syndrome. Cardiol Young 2011; 21 (Suppl. 2): 28-37.
[http://dx.doi.org/10.1017/S1047951111001557] [PMID: 22152526]

[65]   Arbués J, Herraiz I, Galindo A. Síndrome del ventrículo izquierdo hipoplásico.Cardiología Fetal. Madrid: Márban 2015; pp. 298-316.

[66]   Simpson JM. Hypoplastic left heart syndrome. Ultrasound Obstet Gynecol 2000; 15(4): 271-8. [http://dx.doi.org/10.1046/j.1469-0705.2000.00086.x] [PMID: 10895443]

[67]   Allan LD, Sharland GK, Milburn A, *et al.* Prospective diagnosis of 1,006 consecutive cases of congenital heart disease in the fetus. J Am Coll Cardiol 1994; 23(6): 1452-8. [http://dx.doi.org/10.1016/0735-1097(94)90391-3] [PMID: 8176106]

[68]   Raymond FL, Simpson JM, Sharland GK, Ogilvie Mackie CM. Fetal echocardiography as a predictor of chromosomal abnormality. Lancet 1997; 350(9082): 930. [http://dx.doi.org/10.1016/S0140-6736(05)63265-5] [PMID: 9314874]

[69]   Allan LD, Apfel HD, Printz BF. Outcome after prenatal diagnosis of the hypoplastic left heart syndrome. Heart 1998; 79(4): 371-3. [http://dx.doi.org/10.1136/hrt.79.4.371] [PMID: 9616345]

[70]   Brackley KJ, Kilby MD, Wright JG, *et al.* Outcome after prenatal diagnosis of hypoplastic left-heart syndrome: a case series. Lancet 2000; 356(9236): 1143-7. [http://dx.doi.org/10.1016/S0140-6736(00)02756-2] [PMID: 11030293]

[71]   Tennstedt C, Chaoui R, Körner H, Dietel M. Spectrum of congenital heart defects and extracardiac malformations associated with chromosomal abnormalities: results of a seven year necropsy study. Heart 1999; 82(1): 34-9. [http://dx.doi.org/10.1136/hrt.82.1.34] [PMID: 10377306]

[72]   Freedom RM, Yoo SJ. Tricuspid atresia.The Natural and Modified History of Congenital Heart Disease. New York: Blackwell Publishing 2004.

[73]   Allan L, Sharland G. Tricuspid valve abnormalities.Textbook of Fetal Cardiology. London: Greenwich Medical Media 2000; pp. 133-47.

[74]   Berg C, Lachmann R, Kaiser C, *et al.* Prenatal diagnosis of tricuspid atresia: intrauterine course and outcome. Ultrasound Obstet Gynecol 2010; 35(2): 183-90. [http://dx.doi.org/10.1002/uog.7499] [PMID: 20101636]

[75]   Wald RM, Tham EB, McCrindle BW, *et al.* Outcome after prenatal diagnosis of tricuspid atresia: a multicenter experience. Am Heart J 2007; 153(5): 772-8. [http://dx.doi.org/10.1016/j.ahj.2007.02.030] [PMID: 17452152]

[76]   Wolter A, Nosbüsch S, Kawecki A, *et al.* Prenatal diagnosis of functionally univentricular heart, associations and perinatal outcomes. Prenat Diagn 2016; 36(6): 545-54. [http://dx.doi.org/10.1002/pd.4821] [PMID: 27061183]

[77]   De León-Luis J, Gámez F, Bravo C, *et al.* Second-trimester fetal aberrant right subclavian artery: original study, systematic review and meta-analysis of performance in detection of Down syndrome. Ultrasound Obstet Gynecol 2014; 44(2): 147-53. [http://dx.doi.org/10.1002/uog.13336] [PMID: 24585513]

[78]   Yoo SJ, Min JY, Lee YH, Roman K, Jaeggi E, Smallhorn J. Fetal sonographic diagnosis of aortic arch anomalies. Ultrasound Obstet Gynecol 2003; 22(5): 535-46. [http://dx.doi.org/10.1002/uog.897] [PMID: 14618670]

[79]   Tuo G, Volpe P, Bava GL, *et al.* Prenatal diagnosis and outcome of isolated vascular rings. Am J Cardiol 2009; 103(3): 416-9. [http://dx.doi.org/10.1016/j.amjcard.2008.09.100] [PMID: 19166700]

[80]   Galindo A, Nieto O, Nieto MT, *et al.* Prenatal diagnosis of right aortic arch: associated findings, pregnancy outcome, and clinical significance of vascular rings. Prenat Diagn 2009; 29(10): 975-81. [http://dx.doi.org/10.1002/pd.2327] [PMID: 19603384]

[81]   McElhinney DB, Clark BJ III, Weinberg PM, *et al.* Association of chromosome 22q11 deletion with

isolated anomalies of aortic arch laterality and branching. J Am Coll Cardiol 2001; 37(8): 2114-9.
[http://dx.doi.org/10.1016/S0735-1097(01)01286-4] [PMID: 11419896]

[82]   Bravo C, Gámez F, Pérez R, Álvarez T, De León-Luis J. Fetal aortic arch anomalies: key sonographic views for their differential diagnosis and clinical implications using the cardiovascular system sonographic evaluation protocol. J Ultrasound Med 2016; 35(2): 237-51.
[http://dx.doi.org/10.7863/ultra.15.02063] [PMID: 26715656]

[83]   Rauch R, Rauch A, Koch A, *et al.* Laterality of the aortic arch and anomalies of the subclavian artery-reliable indicators for 22q11.2 deletion syndromes? Eur J Pediatr 2004; 163(11): 642-5.
[http://dx.doi.org/10.1007/s00431-004-1518-6] [PMID: 15300432]

[84]   Berg C, Gembruch U, Geipel A. Associated anomalies in congenital heart disease.Fetal Cardiology. 2nd ed. New York, NY: Informa Healthcare USA, Inc 2009; pp. 635-58.

[85]   Berg C, Bender F, Soukup M, *et al.* Right aortic arch detected in fetal life. Ultrasound Obstet Gynecol 2006; 28(7): 882-9.
[http://dx.doi.org/10.1002/uog.3883] [PMID: 17086578]

[86]   Valletta EA, Pregarz M, Bergamo-Andreis IA, Boner AL. Tracheoesophageal compression due to congenital vascular anomalies (vascular rings). Pediatr Pulmonol 1997; 24(2): 93-105.
[http://dx.doi.org/10.1002/(SICI)1099-0496(199708)24:2<93::AID-PPUL4>3.0.CO;2-J]   [PMID: 9292900]

[87]   Glew D, Hartnell GG. The right aortic arch revisited. Clin Radiol 1991; 43(5): 305-7.
[http://dx.doi.org/10.1016/S0009-9260(05)80534-3] [PMID: 2036753]

[88]   Gómez-Monte E, Escribano AG. Coartación de aorta.Cardiología Fetal. 1ˢᵗ ed. Madrid: Marbán 2015; pp. 316-33.

[89]   Backer CL, Mavroudis C. Congenital Heart Surgery Nomenclature and Database Project: vascular rings, tracheal stenosis, pectus excavatum. Ann Thorac Surg 2000; 69(4) (Suppl.): S308-18.
[http://dx.doi.org/10.1016/S0003-4975(99)01279-5] [PMID: 10798437]

[90]   Gabbay-Benziv R, Cetinkaya Demir B, Crimmins S, Esin S, Turan OM, Turan S. Retrospective case series examining the clinical significance of subjective fetal cardiac ventricular disproportion. Int J Gynaecol Obstet 2016; 135(1): 28-32.
[http://dx.doi.org/10.1016/j.ijgo.2016.03.016] [PMID: 27350224]

[91]   Celoria GC, Patton RB. Congenital absence of the aortic arch. Am Heart J 1959; 58: 407-13.
[http://dx.doi.org/10.1016/0002-8703(59)90157-7] [PMID: 13808756]

[92]   Achiron R, Rotstein Z, Heggesh J, *et al.* Anomalies of the fetal aortic arch: a novel sonographic approach to in-utero diagnosis. Ultrasound Obstet Gynecol 2002; 20(6): 553-7.
[http://dx.doi.org/10.1046/j.1469-0705.2002.00850.x] [PMID: 12493043]

[93]   Rauch A, Hofbeck M, Leipold G, *et al.* Incidence and significance of 22q11.2 hemizygosity in patients with interrupted aortic arch. Am J Med Genet 1998; 78(4): 322-31.
[http://dx.doi.org/10.1002/(SICI)1096-8628(19980724)78:4<322::AID-AJMG4>3.0.CO;2-N] [PMID: 9714433]

[94]   Volpe P, Marasini M, Caruso G, *et al.* 22q11 deletions in fetuses with malformations of the outflow tracts or interruption of the aortic arch: impact of additional ultrasound signs. Prenat Diagn 2003; 23(9): 752-7.
[http://dx.doi.org/10.1002/pd.682] [PMID: 12975788]

CHAPTER 8

Genetics and Congenital Heart Disease

Patricia Santana Correia[1,2,*]

[1] *Department of Medical Genetics, Fernandes Figueira, Institute, Oswaldo Cruz Foundation (IFF-FIOCRUZ), Rio de Janeiro-RJ, Brazil*

[2] *Department of Pediatrics, Bonsucesso Federal Hospital (HFB-MS), Rio de Janeiro-RJ, Brazil*

Abstract: Congenital defects are frequent, occurring in 2-3% of live births, with high morbidity and mortality. Congenital heart defects are the most frequent, occurring in 1% of all live births. Most occur as isolated malformations, but approximately 1/3 are part of a syndrome, usually of genetic etiology. The correct etiological diagnosis is important for useful clinical follow-up and genetic counseling. Children born with congenital heart defects should be carefully examined for other malformations and dysmorphia.

Keywords: Congenital heart defects, Genetics, Investigation.

INTRODUCTION

The main objective of this chapter is to draw attention from non-geneticist doctors and other health professionals to the importance of investigating the etiology of congenital heart diseases to identify genetic causes and other associated congenital defects. The investigation of other associated congenital defects and complications improves patient care, even though the heart may be the main concern at the moment. In most cases, the treatment of heart disease will not be modified with the etiological diagnosis but knowing the cause of the baby's problems is always important for the family. Depending on the diagnosis, the prognosis may be poor in relation to survival, regardless of the severity of the heart defect, and this should be considered when establishing the patient's therapeutic plan. Often, a critically ill baby dies without being fully investigated, and the opportunity to make the etiological diagnosis is missed, making genetic counseling for the family more difficult.

[*] **Address for correspondence Patricia Santana Correia:** Department of Medical Genetics, Fernandes Figueira, Institute, Oswaldo Cruz Foundation (IFFFIOCRUZ), Av. Rui Barbosa, 716 . Flamengo, Rio de Janeiro – RJ zip code 22520-020; Tel/Fax: +55 21 2554-1709; E-mail: correia.pat@gmail.com

Congenital anomalies have a high prevalence and significant morbidity and mortality rate, and it is estimated that 2 to 3% of live births present some type of major congenital defect [1]. Although the prevalence and mortality of congenital defects have remained stable or even decreased in recent decades, their importance as a cause of mortality in children under 5 years of age became more significant due to a decrease in other causes, such as infections and perinatal causes. In Brazil, a developing country, congenital anomalies were the fifth cause of mortality in children under the age of 5 in 1990 and the second in 2015 [2].

CLASSIFICATION OF CONGENITAL ANOMALIES

Type of Problem in Morphogenesis

- Malformations (defective formation) - when a primary problem occurs in the morphogenesis of a tissue. Congenital heart defects and neural tube defects are examples of malformation.
- Deformities (mechanical alteration) - when a normal tissue response occurs as a result of abnormal mechanical forces. These are observed in the presence of olygohydramnios, in small or malformed uterus, in some cases of twinning, and in fetal akinesia or hypokinesia. Deformities may be associated with malformations, such as olygohydramnios secondary to renal malformation or fetal akinesia secondary to the malformation of the central nervous system.
- Disruptions (destructive alteration) - when there is a breakdown of a previously normal tissue of vascular, infectious or mechanical etiology, as in the sequence of amniotic bands.
- Dysplasia (disorganization) - when the primary defect is the lack of organization of cells in tissues, as occurs in bone dysplasias.
- Presence of other associated anomalies.
- Isolated anomaly - when there is only one congenital defect not associated with dysmorphia, short stature or developmental delay. It is important to note that there may be short stature and/or delay as a sequela of clinical complications such as hypoxemia, malnutrition or central nervous system bleeding.
- Sequence - multiple anomalies occur secondarily to a primary congenital defect, which explains the entire clinical picture. The primary defect may be a malformation, deformity, disruption, or dysplasia. Example: myelomeningocele sequence, where hydrocephalus, congenital clubfoot and neurogenic bladder are secondary to the neural tube defect.
- Syndrome - there are several structural defects that cannot be explained by a single primary defect and its consequences. There seem to be multiple defects in different tissues, usually with a single etiology, which may be genetic or environmental (although it cannot always be established).
- Association - when two or more anomalies occur together at a frequency greater

than expected by chance but without an established cause (usually the causes are heterogeneous). This is a diagnosis of exclusion after ruling out the possibility of a malformative sequence or syndrome. Often, the discovery of the genetic basis of what was considered an association changes its classification, as in the case of CHARGE (Coloboma, Heart defects, Atresia choanae, growth and mental Retardation, Genital abnormalities, and Ear abnormalities) syndrome, whose molecular basis was discovered in 2004 [3].

The most frequent association of congenital defects that includes cardiopathy is the VATER/VACTERL association, meaning V - vertebral anomalies, A - anal atresia, C- cardiovascular anomalies, T- tracheoesophageal fistula, E- esophageal atresia, and L- preaxial limb anomalies. Three of the defects are necessary for the diagnosis. This association is frequent in children of diabetic mothers and may be present in many syndromes, which should be excluded [4, 5].

It is not always possible to distinguish between sequences, syndromes and associations in the perinatal period, but it is important to try to do so for a better definition of the prognosis, therapeutic limits and genetic counseling/risk of recurrence. Unlike the syndromes, where developmental delay and intellectual deficiency are quite frequent, in isolated defects and associations, these do not occur unless there is an involvement of the central nervous system.

ETIOLOGY OF BIRTH DEFECTS

- Multifactorial - due to small variations in multiple genes, confers a genetic predisposition in association with environmental factors that trigger, accelerate or exacerbate the disease. It is the etiology of most isolated congenital defects and common diseases of adulthood, such as diabetes and hypertension. The diagnosis is always clinical, and in some cases, it is made after the exclusion of other causes.
- Monogenic - due to mutation in a single gene, may have an autosomal dominant, autosomal recessive or X-linked inheritance. The diagnosis is usually based on clinical findings and can be confirmed by molecular biology methods in cases where the gene involved has already been identified.
- Chromosomal anomaly - due to a change in the number — trisomy or monosomy — or in the structure of one or more chromosomes — deletions, duplications, translocations. Structural chromosome abnormalities may or may not be cytogenetically visible. In the latter case, they are called microaberrations (microdeletions / microduplications). Diagnosis is clinical in the most common conditions, such as Down syndrome. The complementary tests indicated are cytogenetic analysis (karyotype) and, in cases of microaberrations, or for better definition of major structural abnormalities, techniques such as FISH, MLPA

and CGH array.

- Environmental - due to the action of a teratogenic substance or an intrauterine condition, including maternal systemic diseases. Diagnosis is made through evaluating history, a physical examination and the exclusion of other causes [3].

CONGENITAL HEART DEFECTS

Congenital heart defects are the most frequent malformations in the human species, occurring in approximately 1% of live births (2% if bicuspid aortic valve is included). In most cases, they are isolated defects, but approximately 1/3 are part of a malformative syndrome. Isolated heart diseases are usually of multifactorial inheritance with low familial recurrence, and specific genetic investigation is not necessary. However, some families who inherited the defects as monogenic traits have been described. Some genes that may be involved in isolated heart diseases include *ELN, JAG1, ZIC3, TFAP2B, GATA4* and *CRELD1* [1].

Some Syndromes with Cardiopathy Identified in the Perinatal Period

Cytogenetically Visible Chromosomal Abnormalities

<u>*Down Syndrome*</u>

It is the most common malformative syndrome in live births, with an incidence of 1:600–700. The etiology is the trisomy of chromosome 21, the most frequent karyotype being free trisomy (47, XX or XY, +21), in approximately 95% of the cases. Free trisomy results from a nondisjunction in gametogenesis, which is usually maternal and is related to advanced maternal age. In approximately 3% of cases, there is a translocation involving chromosome 21 and in 2%, mosaicism [3]. Most often, the diagnosis can be made clinically, and the karyotype is important in atypical cases and for genetic counseling. Diagnosis is often suspected during pregnancy when an ultrasound study shows increased nuchal translucency measurement or some malformation, usually cardiac or gastrointestinal.

The main physical features of Down syndrome are a round and flattened face, brachycephaly, upslanting palpebral fissures, epicanthus, a small nose with a low nasal bridge, anteverted nostrils, a protuberant tongue, small round ears, a short neck with loose folds of skin, small hands with short fingers, clinodactyly of fifth finger, single palmar crease, and a wide gap between first and second toes. Developmental impairment is variable, but all individuals with Down syndrome have some degree of hypotonia (which improves with age), and motor and speech delay, and they can develop intellectual disabilities, which are usually mild or moderate [3].

Congenital heart disease is present in approximately 40-50% of cases and is responsible, either directly or indirectly, for most deaths in Down syndrome, making its investigation a priority when the diagnosis of the syndrome is made. The most frequent cardiac malformations are atrial septal defect (ASD), ventricular septal defect (VSD), ASD+VSD, atrioventricular septal defect (AVSD), persistence of ductus arteriosus (PDA) and tetralogy of Fallot. AVSD is the most typical heart disease in Down syndrome, but its frequency varies considerably in the literature (8-40%, depending on the population studied) and may or may not be the most common [3, 6 - 8]. A Brazilian study in 2015 with more than 1,000 patients showed ASD as the most frequent heart disease, at 42.1%. AVSD occurred in approximately only 15% of the sample [9].

The second most common group of malformations is gastrointestinal (12%), such as esophageal and duodenal atresia and congenital megacolon. Complications in the neonatal period include congenital hypothyroidism and biliary lithiasis [3] (Fig. **1**).

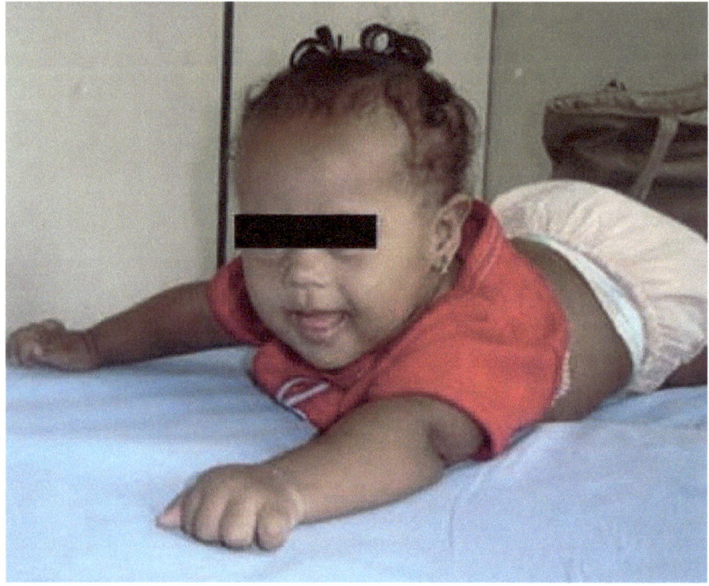

Fig. (1). Trisomy of chromosome 21 (Down syndrome).

Edwards Syndrome

Edward syndrome is the second most frequent malformative syndrome, with incidences of approximately 0.3:1,000 live births and a predominance of 3:1, females to males. The etiology is the trisomy of chromosome 18, usually free trisomy (47, XX or XY, +18), whose risk increases with advanced maternal age. There may be mosaicism and translocations involving chromosome 18. The diagnosis may be clinically suspected, but confirmation by karyotype is required.

Intrauterine growth restriction is quite characteristic; there may be polyhydramnios, and most babies have at least one malformation. Physical examination shows a prominent occipital area, short palpebral fissures, a small mouth, micrognathia, dysplastic ears, a short sternum, clenched hands with an overlapping index finger over the third and the fifth over the fourth finger, and a prominent calcaneus. There may be initial hypotonia, followed by hypertonia.

Congenital heart disease is the most frequent malformation, occurring in more than 50% of cases, and the most common are VSD, ASD and PDA. Gastrointestinal, renal, limb and central nervous system malformations may also occur.

The prognosis of Edwards syndrome is poor, with an average survival time of 14.5 days. Approximately 50% die in the first week of life, and only 5-10% survive the first year. The psychomotor development is quite late, and many patients require gastrostomy. Cognitive impairment is severe, but most are able to interact with their families. In cases where there is mosaicism and partial trisomy 18, longer survival is more frequent [3] (Fig. **2**).

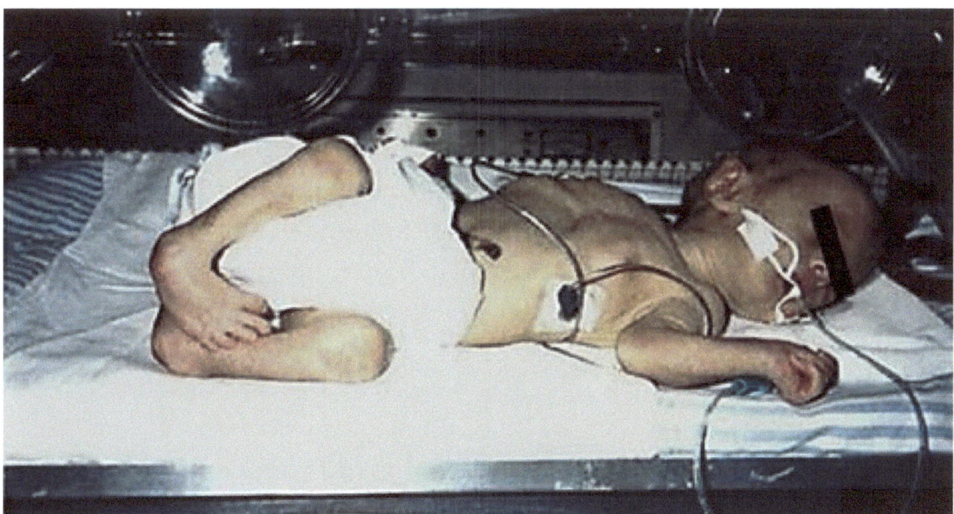

Fig. (2). Trisomy of chromosome 18 (Edwards syndrome).

Patau Syndrome

It occurs in 1:5,000 live births, and the etiology is the trisomy of chromosome 13. Free trisomy is also the most frequent, and there is also a relation with maternal age. There may be mosaicism and structural changes.

The diagnosis can be clinically suspected in cases with typical malformations and should always be confirmed by karyotype. The most characteristic malformation is holoprosencephaly (HPE), and there may be ocular and nasal defects and lip-palate clefts as part of the HPE sequence. Polydactyly (in hands and, less frequently, in feet) is common, and sometimes there is aplasia cutis vertex. Congenital heart disease occurs in 80% of cases, the most common being VSD, PDA and ASD.

As in Edwards' syndrome, the prognosis for survival and neuropsychomotor development is poor [3].

Turner Syndrome

Turner syndrome is a rare condition in live births — 1:2,500 females, but occurs quite frequently in first trimester abortions, where it is estimated that 98-99% of pregnancies of fetuses with Turner syndrome are aborted spontaneously. Approximately 50% of the patients have a karyotype 45,X; 12-20% have an Xq isochromosome (long arm duplication of one of the X with a short arm deletion), and approximately 40% are mosaics 45, X/46, XX, 45, X/46, XY or 45, X / other karyotypes with structural abnormalities of X. There is no relation to advanced maternal or paternal age, and the risk of recurrence in future pregnancies is the same as in the general population.

Intrauterine diagnosis may be suspected in the presence of increased nuchal translucency measurement, cystic hygroma or fetal hydrops. At birth, most patients go unnoticed, as phenotypic changes may only be short stature, ears with protruding lobes and mild lymphedema of the hands and feet. In some cases, especially in those with a history of cystic hygroma or hydrops, the clinical features can be quite marked, with lymphedema of varying severity, a short or webbed neck and low posterior hairline, epicanthus, ptosis, widely spaced nipples, cubitus valgus and hypoplastic or hyperconvex nails. When there is mosaicism 45, X/46, XY, there may be varying degrees of virilization. These cases are at risk for gonadoblastoma.

The two systems most affected by malformations in Turner's syndrome are the urinary and cardiovascular systems. More than 60% of Turner syndrome girls have some kidney defects, such as horseshoe kidney, double or cleft renal pelvis and other minor changes [3]. The most common cardiac defects are bicuspid aorta (30%) and coarctation of the aorta (10%). In adulthood, aortic dilatation occurs in up to 40% of cases, with a risk of dissection; therefore, even females without congenital heart disease should be observed by a cardiologist [3, 10].

As the phenotype of Turner syndrome may be quite mild in some cases, it is recommended that any females with a short stature without a definite cause be investigated with a karyotype. It is also important to mention that isolated coarctation of the aorta is much more frequent in males, and its presence in a female should lead to the suspicion of Turner syndrome even in the absence of other characteristics (Fig. **3**).

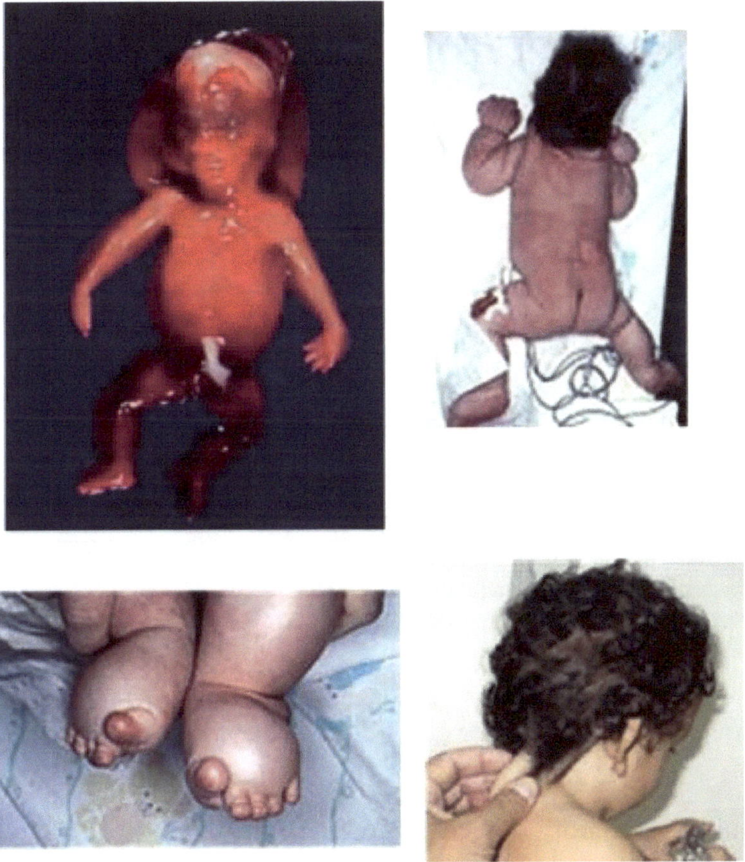

Fig. (3). Turner syndrome findings.

Microdeletion Syndromes

22q11.2 Deletion Syndrome - DiGeorge's Syndrome, Velo-cardio-facial Syndrome

DiGeorge's syndrome is the most common microdeletion in the human species, with great phenotypic variability, ranging from very little symptoms in some individuals to patients with dysmorphia, severe heart disease, cleft palate, immunodeficiency and hypocalcemia. Intellectual disability is variable, and there is an increased risk of psychiatric problems. The deleted region contains at least 30 genes, including *TBX1*, which plays an important role in embryogenesis. The diagnosis is made by *in situ* hybridization with fluorescence (FISH) with a probe specific for the region (Fig. **4**). Parents should be screened for subtle signs of the syndrome and investigated with FISH if suspected of having the microdeletion.

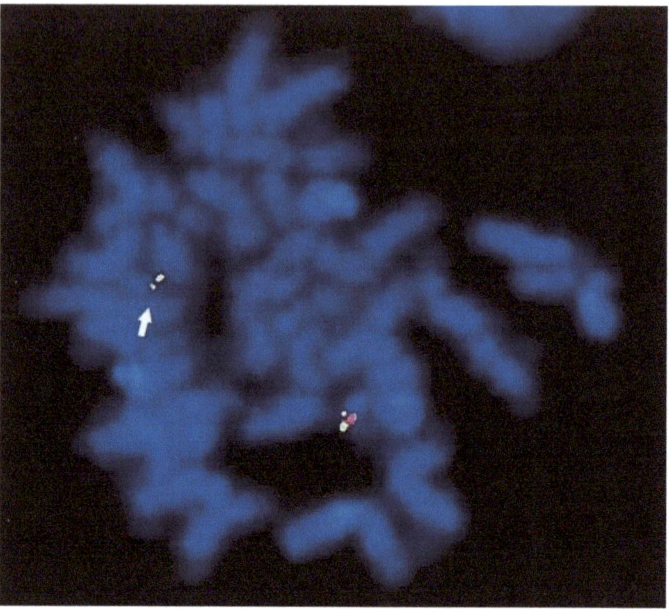

Fig. (4). FISH for 22q11.2. The red signal indicates the 22q11.2 region and the green signal is the control region. The arrow indicates the deleted chromosome 22, showing the presence of the control region only.

Heart defects are present in 85% of cases, and the most common are VSD (62%), right aortic arch (52%) and tetralogy of Fallot (21%).

DiGeorge and velo-cardio-facial syndromes were considered separate entities, but it is now known that both are different aspects of the same condition. The DiGeorge phenotype is evident in the neonatal period, with cardiopathy, hypocalcemia, absence of thymic tissue and immunodeficiency. In velo-cardio-facial syndrome, the diagnosis is usually made later, and a cleft palate or an insufficiency of the palatine veil are frequent. It is important to note whether one parent has a submucosal cleft or a nasal voice, which may be the only symptoms in some cases [3].

Williams Syndrome

Williams syndrome phenotype has been described in 1961 and includes typical faces with thick lips, epicanthus, periorbital edema, clear irises with star patterns, intellectual deficiency with verbal functioning far superior to other cognitive functions, hypersensitivity to sounds and a friendly personality. The etiology was clarified in 1993 as a deletion in the long arm of chromosome 7 - 7q11.23, including approximately 17 genes, one of them being elastin, responsible for cardiovascular alterations. The diagnosis is made by FISH with a probe specific for the region.

Cardiovascular defects include supravalvar aortic stenosis (the malformation described in the original Williams patients), peripheral pulmonary artery stenosis, ASD, VSD, renal artery stenosis with hypertension, aortic hypoplasia, and other arterial abnormalities. Other frequent anomalies are renal malformations and hypercalcemia [3].

Monogenic Diseases

Noonan Syndrome and Other RASopathies

Noonan syndrome was described in 1963 and includes epicanthal folds, ptosis, ocular hypertelorism, downslanting palpebral fissures, a short or webbed neck, a low posterior hairline, cubitus valgus, cryptorchidism, lymphedema, coagulation disorders, ocular disorders, deafness and heart disease. There may be short stature and intellectual impairment, and feeding difficulties are very frequent in infants. Other conditions, such as Costello's syndrome and cardio-facial-cutaneous syndrome, present similar phenotypes with overlapping characteristics since all are caused by mutations in genes involved in the same pathway (RAS-mitoge--activated protein kinase), which is known as RASopathies. The genes involved in the pathway are *PTPN11* (40-50% of Noonan cases are due to mutations in this gene), *SOS1, RAF1, KRAS, BRAF, MEK1* and *NRAS*. RASopathies have an autosomal dominant inheritance, usually due to a new mutation, and a relation with advanced paternal age. In at least 30% of the cases, one of the parents is affected, and because it is a condition with variable expressiveness, it is important to carefully evaluate the parents in search of signs of the syndrome. In cases where one parent is affected, the risk of recurrence is 50%.

In the intrauterine period, there may be increased nuchal translucency measurement, hygroma and hydrops, and in the female fetus, a differential diagnosis with Turner syndrome should be made. The frequent cardiovascular alterations are pulmonary stenosis secondary to a dysplastic or thickened valve, hypertrophic cardiomyopathy, ASD, tetralogy of Fallot, coarctation of the aorta, and abnormalities of the mitral valve and atrioventricular canal [3].

Type II Glycogenosis or Pompe Disease

Infantile-onset Pompe disease is rare, with an estimated prevalence of 1:138,000, but taking this diagnosis into consideration is very important because there is a specific treatment. The disease involves an innate error in the metabolism of the group of lysosomal storage diseases, is of autosomal recessive inheritance, and is caused by the deficiency of the alpha-1,4-glucosidase enzyme. The risk of recurrence to the offspring of parents with an affected child is 25%. The diagnosis is made by enzymatic dosing in blood.

The major changes in the infantile form occur in the skeletal muscles and myocardium, beginning before 12 months of life (usually at approximately 4 months, but may be in the neonatal period). Infants present with severe hypotonia, eating difficulty, dyspnea and hypertrophic cardiomyopathy with an early death. The late form, beginning after 12 months, mainly affects the skeletal muscles.

Recombinant alpha-glucosidase enzyme replacement therapy is indicated once the diagnosis is confirmed and it significantly changes the course of the disease [11, 12].

Teratogenic Syndromes

Fetal Alcohol Syndrome/Fetal Alcohol Spectrum

Intrauterine exposure to alcohol leads to multiple abnormalities, the most significant being neurological disorders, such as intellectual disability, behavioral disorders and central nervous system (CNS) malformations. It is considered the most frequent environmental cause of intellectual disability and is avoidable in 100% of cases. The diagnosis is clinical through physical examination, the history of alcohol ingestion during pregnancy, and the exclusion of other causes. It is considered that there is no safe limit for the consumption of alcohol during pregnancy, and every report of its use should be valued. It is often difficult to obtain this information, either because the mother denies having consumed any alcohol or because many of the children are not raised by their biological families.

Physical characteristics include low weight, microcephaly, short palpebral fissures, smooth upper lip filters, abnormal joints and abnormal palm creases. In milder forms, there may be no physical changes, only cognitive and behavioral changes. The most frequent malformations are cardiovascular, usually VSD and ASD, and there may be coarctation of the aorta and tetralogy of Fallot. There may also be malformations of the skeletal and CNS [3, 13, 14].

Retinoic Acid Embryopathy

Isotretinoin was recognized as a teratogen in 1985, and its defect spectrum was described. A risk of malformation of 35% is considered in the offspring of women who become pregnant while using the medication and maintains medication use after the 15th postconceptional day.

The spectrum of malformations includes craniofacial (facial asymmetry, microtia/anotia, facial paralysis, micrognathia) and CNS (hydrocephalus, microcephaly, neuronal migration defects, cerebellar abnormalities) malformations. Cardiac malformations are severe, occurring in more than half of patients and include conotruncal defects (tetralogy of Fallot, transposition of the great vessels, truncus arteriosus, double outlet of right ventricle), interrupted and hypoplastic aortic arch and heart left hypoplastic syndrome [3, 15, 16].

Congenital Rubella Syndrome

Rubella is an infectious disease caused by a virus of the rubivirus genus. Its symptoms are mild and may be asymptomatic. However, when contracted during pregnancy, it can cause serious problems in the fetus. The likelihood of problems occurring, and their severity depends on gestational age: when the disease occurs in women less than 12 weeks pregnant, approximately 80% of those exposed are affected and when it occurs between 12 and 16 weeks, 50% are affected. After 16 weeks of gestation, congenital abnormalities and growth restriction are rare.

The classical triad includes deafness, ocular abnormalities such as cataracts, retinopathy and microphthalmia, and cardiovascular anomalies, mainly PDA and pulmonary artery stenosis. Congenital rubella syndrome is preventable through vaccination [17, 18].

Diabetic Embryopathy

Maternal hyperglycemia is a known teratogenic agent, with mechanisms not yet well established. The incidence of congenital anomalies is related to maternal levels of glycated hemoglobin, and the risk is the same for type 1 and type 2 diabetes mellitus. The critical effect of hyperglycemia occurs between 2- and 6- weeks post conception, which makes glycemic control fundamental not only during pregnancy but also during the preconception period.

Frequent cardiac defects include defects of laterality and rotation (or heterotaxia), abnormalities of the axis, atrioventricular defect and membranous VSD. Exposure to hyperglycemia in the last months of pregnancy increases the risk of hypertrophic cardiomyopathy.

Caudal regression (agenesis/vertebral hypoplasia with lower limb hypoplasia) is the congenital defect most strongly related to maternal diabetes. Member defects (hypoplasia and defects of reduction), neural tube defects and VATER/VACTERL are also frequent [5, 19, 20].

LABORATORY INVESTIGATION

In the investigation of a child with a congenital heart defect of possible genetic etiology, we can use several complementary exams. The choice of the exams depends on the probable etiology and availability of the baby's biological material, as summarized below:

Cytogenetic Analysis (Karyotype)

Karyotype is the set of metaphasic chromosomes organized by size and morphology. Its analysis allows the evaluation of the number and presence of structural changes, such as translocations, deletions and duplications. In general, the cells used are peripheral blood lymphocytes, but other cell types, such as skin fibroblasts and bone marrow cells, may be used. For prenatal diagnosis, samples of chorionic villi, amniotic fluid or blood from the umbilical cord are used. There is a need for cell culture to perform the test.

The main limitations of the technique are the chromosomal anomalies that are below the limit of detection (chromosomal microaberrations), the presence of low degree mosaicism, and marking chromosomes and the complex structural rearrangements. The latter two cases can be detected by the karyotype, but there is a need for other techniques for better characterization.

Indications for karyotype in children include the following:

- Specific chromosome syndrome suspected;

- Dysmorphisms, possibly associated with intellectual disability, malformations and/or short stature;

- Presence of two or more malformations;

- Developmental delay/intellectual disability and one or more malformations;

- Small for gestational age and one or more malformations;

- Stillborns or neonatal death;

- Females with short stature even in the absence of dysmorphic features/malformations;

- Ambiguous genitalia.

Comparative Genomic Hybridization (CGH Array)

Comparative genomic hybridization (CGH array) is a technique based on the cohybridization of DNA to be analyzed with reference DNA, both labeled with different colored fluorochromes in a slide containing thousands of rows of DNA sequences. It allows the detection of microdeletions and microduplications that are not visible cytogenetically.

The material to be studied is DNA, usually extracted from peripheral blood cells or saliva, but any tissue can be used. The limitations of the test are microaberrations below the technique's limit of detection and structural chromosomal anomalies without loss or gain of material (balanced translocations).

Indications for CGH array:

- Suspected known microdeletion/microduplication syndrome;

- Investigation of chromosomal microaberrations in cases where the karyotype is normal;

- Better definition of visible structural anomalies in the karyotype;

-When there is no material available to perform cytogenetics. This may be necessary in abortion material, stillbirths, and patients who have died before blood could be collected for karyotype (in these cases, a skin biopsy can be made or blood that was stored for other tests can be used);

- When the test is easily available and relatively inexpensive, the CGH array can be the first screening test instead of the karyotype.

In Situ Hybridization with Fluorescence (FISH)

In situ hybridization with fluorescence (FISH) is based on the hybridization of the chromosomal DNA with fluorescence-labeled probes, using the specific segment of DNA to be studied. The FISH technique can be used in both metaphase chromosomes and interphase nuclei. For this reason, there is no need for cell culture, allowing rapid results and use in buccal smear samples and fixed histological sections. The main limitation of the technique is the need for clinical suspicion since the probes are specific to each region of the DNA.

Indications for FISH:

- Investigation of numerical chromosomal abnormalities when there is a need for rapid or fixed tissue diagnosis;

- Suspected known microdeletion syndrome;

- Better definition of anomalies that were seen in the karyotype;

- Investigation of translocations not detectable cytogenetically (in parents of patients with structural chromosome abnormalities).

DNA Sequencing and Detection of Specific Mutations

The purpose of these tests is to determine variations in the base pair sequence of the subject's DNA by screening for mutations in known genes. DNA extraction can be performed from any available tissue. The techniques used vary according to the purpose but are generally based on the amplification of available DNA through the polymerase chain reaction (PCR) technique.

Screening for specific mutations is used in suspected cases from families with known mutations and in diseases and/or population groups where there are single or few frequent mutations. The complete sequencing of a gene is the determination of the sequence of base pairs that compose it. The result is then compared to a standard sequence, looking for variants which will later be classified according to the probability of being pathogenic. The individual sequencing of a gene is indicated in the investigation of conditions caused by a single gene (or few genes). In cases where mutations in several genes can cause similar phenotypes, the use of panels (where many genes are sequenced together) is more cost-effective.

Complete exome sequencing is a test where the entire coding part of the genome (the exons) is sequenced and, with the aid of bioinformatics, the genes of interest are screened for variants. It can be used in the same way as the gene panels and in cases of probable monogenic etiology, when there is not a specific suspicion [3, 21, 22].

EVALUATION OF INFANTS WITH CONGENITAL HEART DISEASE

In most genetic syndromes, congenital heart disease is one of the most common defects. Therefore, an infant with a detected congenital heart disease should be carefully examined for dysmorphic features, for example, small, nonfamiliar variations in the morphology or size of the eyes, ears or hands. The presence of dysmorphia in a patient with heart disease suggests that it is not an isolated malformation but rather a part of a malformative syndrome. Often, the pattern of dysmorphia may lead to a clinically recognizable diagnosis, such as Down syndrome [3].

A brief neurological evaluation is also important, mainly looking for changes in tone and difficulty of suction, which are frequent in malformative syndromes in the neonatal period.

During a physical examination, other associated congenital defects should also be taken into consideration. The objective is not only therapeutic but also to help in the etiological diagnosis since some conditions have typical patterns of malformation. It is important to order some basic complementary exams, such as abdominal and transfontanellar ultrasonography, to look for occult anomalies, even in babies with an apparently normal physical examination. Other imaging tests may be ordered according to physical examination and diagnostic suspicion.

A geneticist evaluation should be requested for infants with congenital heart disease in the following cases:

• Suspicion of specific genetic syndrome;

• Presence of facial or limb dysmorphia;

• Presence of at least one other malformation;

• In infants who are small or large for their gestational age without a definite cause.

When a patient with a birth defect is a stillbirth or has a high risk of neonatal death, the case should be documented as best as possible. The family should be informed of the importance of the investigation and permission for the following procedures must be requested:

• Photograph;

• Perform the imaging tests that are possible;

• Collect blood for karyotype (heparin tube - green cap or heparinized syringe) and for DNA extraction (EDTA tube - purple cap) and store in the refrigerator (it cannot be frozen; blood can be collected through umbilical cord puncture in the delivery room or soon after death by intracardiac puncture);

• Request necropsy;

• Give the family a summary of the hospitalization with requested exams, the results of exams that already exist and photos;

• Refer the family to genetic counseling.

GENETIC COUNSELING

The primary objective of genetic counseling is to provide information to the family in a nondirective way. It consists of confirming the diagnosis (whenever possible), obtaining the family history and establishing recurrence risks. The information provided should include the etiology, prognosis, therapeutic possibilities, risk of recurrence, possibilities for prevention and prenatal screening.

The risks of recurrence for the parents of a baby with a congenital defect depend on the etiology of the disease in question and can be summarized as follows:

• Isolated malformations and associations: empirical risk of 3-5%;
• Free trisomy: 1% risk + maternal age risk;
• Inherited translocations: must be calculated individually, as they depend on the type of translocation and the gender of the carrier;
• Chromosomal microaberrations: low risk when a cryptic translocation in one of the parents is ruled out. If one parent has the same microaberrations, the risk to their offspring is 50%;
• Monogenic autosomal dominant diseases: if a parent is a carrier, the risk to their offspring is 50%. When both parents are normal, the risk is 2-3% (possibility of gonadal cell mosaicism);
• Monogenic autosomal recessive diseases: 25% risk for the parents;
• X-linked monogenic diseases: female carriers transmit the gene to 50% of their offspring, and the manifestation depends on the sex of the child and the disease (some X-linked conditions may manifest in female carriers) [3, 4, 23].

SOME USEFUL SITES

• OMIM - Online Mendelian Inheritance in Man. www.omim.org — catalog of Mendelian human diseases, allows consultations by diagnosis and by clinical characteristics.

• Genereviews. https://www.ncbi.nlm.nih.gov/books/NBK1116/ — information on genetic conditions including diagnosis, clinical follow-up and genetic counseling.

CONSENT FOR PUBLICATION

Not applicable.

CONFLICT OF INTEREST

The authors confirm that the contents of this chapter have no conflict of interest.

ACKNOWLEDGEMENTS

Declare none.

REFERENCES

[1]   Turnpenny P, Ellard S. Emery's Elements of Medical Genetics. 15th ed., Philadelphia, PA: Elsevier 2017.

[2]   França EB, Lansky S, Rego MAS, *et al.* Leading causes of child mortality in Brazil, in 1990 and 2015: estimates from the Global Burden of Disease. Rev Bras Epidemiol 2017; 20(20) (Suppl. 01): 46-60.
[http://dx.doi.org/10.1590/1980-5497201700050005] [PMID: 28658372]

[3]   Jones KL, Jones MC, del Campo M. Smith's Recognizable Patterns of Human Malformation. 7th ed., Philadephia, PA: Elsevier Sauders 2013.

[4]   Hamosh A, Scott AF, Amberger J, Valle D, McKusick VA. Online Mendelian Inheritance in Man (OMIM). Hum Mutat 2000; 15(1): 57-61.
[http://dx.doi.org/10.1002/(SICI)1098-1004(200001)15:1<57::AID-HUMU12>3.0.CO;2-G] [PMID: 10612823]

[5]   Basu M, Garg V. Maternal hyperglycemia and fetal cardiac development: Clinical impact and underlying mechanisms. Birth Defects Res 2018; 110(20): 1504-16.
[http://dx.doi.org/10.1002/bdr2.1435] [PMID: 30576094]

[6]   Asim A, Kumar A, Muthuswamy S, Jain S, Agarwal S. "Down syndrome: an insight of the disease". J Biomed Sci 2015; 22: 41.
[http://dx.doi.org/10.1186/s12929-015-0138-y] [PMID: 26062604]

[7]   Lo NS, Leung PM, Lau KC, Yeung CY. Congenital cardiovascular malformations in Chinese children with Down's syndrome. Chin Med J (Engl) 1989; 102(5): 382-6.
[PMID: 2530065]

[8]   de Rubens Figueroa J, del Pozzo Magaña B, Pablos Hach JL, Calderón Jiménez C, Castrejón Urbina R. [Heart malformations in children with Down syndrome]. Rev Esp Cardiol 2003; 56(9): 894-9.
[http://dx.doi.org/10.1016/S0300-8932(03)76978-4] [PMID: 14519277]

[9]   Bermudez BE, Medeiros SL, Bermudez MB, Novadzki IM, Magdalena NI. Down syndrome: Prevalence and distribution of congenital heart disease in Brazil. Sao Paulo Med J 2015; 133(6): 521-4.
[http://dx.doi.org/10.1590/1516-3180.2015.00710108] [PMID: 26648279]

[10]   Gonsalez CH. Síndrome de Turner 2019.www.ghente.org/ciencia/genetica/turner.htm

[11]   Dasouki M, Jawdat O, Almadhoun O, *et al.* Pompe disease: literature review and case series. Neurol Clin 2014; 32(3): 751-776, ix.
[http://dx.doi.org/10.1016/j.ncl.2014.04.010] [PMID: 25037089]

[12]   Chan J, Desai AK, Kazi ZB, *et al.* The emerging phenotype of late-onset Pompe disease: A systematic literature review. Mol Genet Metab 2017; 120(3): 163-72.
[http://dx.doi.org/10.1016/j.ymgme.2016.12.004] [PMID: 28185884]

[13]   Caputo C, Wood E, Jabbour L. Impact of fetal alcohol exposure on body systems: A systematic review. Birth Defects Res C Embryo Today 2016; 108(2): 174-80.
[http://dx.doi.org/10.1002/bdrc.21129] [PMID: 27297122]

[14]   Gupta KK, Gupta VK, Shirasaka T. An update on fetal alcohol syndrome-pathogenesis, risks, and treatment. Alcohol Clin Exp Res 2016; 40(8): 1594-602.
[http://dx.doi.org/10.1111/acer.13135] [PMID: 27375266]

[15]   Lammer EJ, Chen DT, Hoar RM, *et al.* Retinoic acid embryopathy. N Engl J Med 1985; 313(14): 837-41.
[http://dx.doi.org/10.1056/NEJM198510033131401] [PMID: 3162101]

[16]   Mondal D, R Shenoy S, Mishra S. Retinoic acid embryopathy. Int J Appl Basic Med Res 2017; 7(4): 264-5.
[http://dx.doi.org/10.4103/ijabmr.IJABMR_469_16] [PMID: 29308367]

[17]   Masresha B, Shibeshi M, Kaiser R, Luce R, Katsande R, Mihigo R. Congenital rubella syndrome in the african region - data from sentinel surveillance. J Immunol Sci 2018; (Suppl.)146-50.
[http://dx.doi.org/10.29245/2578-3009/2018/si.1122] [PMID: 30957103]

[18]   Pilania RK, Verma S, Kumar P, Sachdeva RK, Jayashree M, Singh M. Congenital rubella syndrome at tertiary care hospital in North India: Results from a retrospective assessment. J Trop Pediatr 2019; 65(3): 297-300.
[http://dx.doi.org/10.1093/tropej/fmy045] [PMID: 31158287]

[19]   Eriksson UJ, Wentzel P. The status of diabetic embryopathy. Ups J Med Sci 2016; 121(2): 96-112.
[http://dx.doi.org/10.3109/03009734.2016.1165317] [PMID: 27117607]

[20]   Nasri HZ, Houde Ng K, Westgate MN, Hunt AT, Holmes LB. Malformations among infants of mothers with insulin-dependent diabetes: Is there a recognizable pattern of abnormalities? Birth Defects Res 2018; 110(2): 108-13.
[http://dx.doi.org/10.1002/bdr2.1155] [PMID: 29377640]

[21]   Hehir-Kwa JY, Pfundt R, Veltman JA. Exome sequencing and whole genome sequencing for the detection of copy number variation. Expert Rev Mol Diagn 2015; 15(8): 1023-32.
[http://dx.doi.org/10.1586/14737159.2015.1053467] [PMID: 26088785]

[22]   LaDuca H, Farwell KD, Vuong H, *et al.* Exome sequencing covers >98% of mutations identified on targeted next generation sequencing panels. PLoS One 2017; 12(2)e0170843
[http://dx.doi.org/10.1371/journal.pone.0170843] [PMID: 28152038]

[23]   Borgulova I, Putzova M, Soldatova I, *et al.* Preimplantation genetic diagnosis of X-linked diseases examined by indirect linkage analysis. Bratisl Lek Listy 2015; 116(9): 542-6.
[http://dx.doi.org/10.4149/BLL_2015_103] [PMID: 26435019]

CHAPTER 9

Environmental Factors Associated with Congenital Heart Diseases

Ana Luisa Neves[*]

Department of Pediatric Cardiology, University Hospital Center of S. João; Faculty of Medicine, University of Porto, Porto, Portugal

Abstract: Congenital heart diseases (CHD) are common, of largely unknown etiology, with high mortality. This chapter presents the available information on environmental factors that may alter the risk for CHD. Information regarding parental characteristics and conditions, maternal therapeutic drug exposures, parental nontherapeutic drug exposures, and environmental exposures are presented. Aside from some cardiac teratogens and prenatal maternal conditions or exposures associated with an increased risk for CHD, such as thalidomide, and retinoids, smoking, maternal rubella infection, phenylketonuria, hypertension, and diabetes, studies investigating most of environmental risk factors have yielded conflicting results. Associations were found for febrile illness, *in vitro* fertilization, stressful life events, hyperhomocysteinemia, obesity, hypertension, antihypertensives, bronchodilators, anticonvulsant drugs, non-therapeutic drugs, alcohol, air pollution, disinfectant products, pesticides, solvents, metals and landfill/hazardous waste sites. Some principles for prevention can be useful, as preconception and prenatal care with specific attention to the intake of folic acid, vaccination for rubella, detection and effective management of phenylketonuria, hypertension, and diabetes, discussion of any medicine use, avoidance of infections and chemical exposures, alcohol, smoking, and non-therapeutic drugs. Women receiving therapeutic drugs should be regularly monitored. In addition, screening for CHD should be performed when environmental risk factors are present. Further investigations for the development of prevention and intervention are needed.

Keywords: Air pollution, Alcohol, Chemical exposure, Congenital heart disease, Diabetes, Disinfectant by-products, Drug exposures, Environmental risk factors, Etiology, Febrile illness, Folic acid, Hazardous waste sites, Hypertension, Infection, Obesity, Rubella, Smoking, Solvents, Teratogens, Vitamin A congeners/retinoids.

---

[*] **Address Correspondence Ana Luisa Neves:** Department of Pediatric Cardiology, Centro Hospitalar Universitário de S. João, E.P.E., Alameda Prof. Hernâni Monteiro, 4200-319, Porto, Portugal; E-mail: alneves1@med.up.pt

INTRODUCTION

The incidence of moderate and severe forms of congenital heart disease (CHD) is about 6/1,000 live births [1]. Scarce information is available regarding the adverse effect of environmental risk factors in CHD [2]. More than 66% of congenital defects relate to unknown, most likely multifactorial causes, including environmental risk factors [3]. Environmental exposure refers to any factor that is not genetic, and more specifically to the fetal-placental-maternal environment [3]. Increased knowledge about environmental factors could allow preventive strategies to reduce CHD [2]. Environmental risk factors are divided into four categories: parental demographics or conditions, maternal therapeutic drug exposures, parental nontherapeutic drug exposures, and parental environmental exposures [4].

ENVIRONMENTAL FACTORS ASSOCIATED WITH CONGENITAL HEART DISEASES

Demographic and Conditions

Demographics

Maternal age is associated with CHD [5 - 10]. In the Baltimore-Washington Infant Study (BWIS), advanced maternal age was found to be associated with an increased risk of Ebstein's anomaly and d-transposition of the great arteries (d-TGA). Younger age was associated with tricuspid atresia [11]. The Metropolitan Atlanta Congenital Defects Program, identified older mothers as more likely to have a child with an atrial septal defect (ASD), coarctation of the aorta (CoA), or d-TGA [5]. In the USA, a detailed analysis of the National Birth Defects Prevention Study (NBDPS) database, advanced maternal age was associated with ASD, tetralogy of Fallot (TOF), and ventricular septal defects (VSD), whereas younger maternal age was associated with total anomalous pulmonary venous return and tricuspid atresia. Paternal age was found to be [12] associated with CHD [8, 9]. A matched case-control study identified an association between advanced paternal age and VSD [9].

Diabetes

Pregestational diabetes has an absolute risk of CHD of 3–5% live births, relative risk or likelihood ratio ≈5% live births; level of evidence (LOE) I/A [13]. Pregestational diabetes has been associated with multiple types of CHD including ASD, atrioventricular septal defect, CoA, double-outlet right ventricle, pulmonary atresia, total anomalous pulmonary venous return, d-TGA, TOF, truncus arteriosus, and VSD [11, 14 - 16]. Diabetes is associated with a higher relative risk of certain specific cardiac defects, including 6.22 for heterotaxy, 4.72 for truncus arteriosus, 2.85 for TGA and 18.24 for single ventricle defects [13, 17, 18]. Garne *et al.* showed an association with ASD, VSD, d-TGA and CoA [15]. The increased risk of ASD, VSD, and d-TGA has been described by Correa *et al.* [14]. The strongest associations with overt maternal diabetes were found with double outlet right ventricle, and truncus arteriosus in a study based on the BWIS database [19]. The spectrum of maternal diabetes mellitus-related CHD includes, particularly TGA, double outlet right ventricle, and common truncus [16, 19]. Additionally, maternal pre-gestational diabetes may be an independent risk factor for mortality among infants with CHD [16]. Hypertrophic cardiomyopathy showed a strong association with maternal diabetes [20, 21]. Hyperglycemia plays a critical role [14], so metabolic control is important in diabetic women preconception and during pregnancy.

In pregestational diabetes, fetal echocardiography should be performed at 18–22 weeks [13]. Gestational diabetes mellitus with HbA1c <6% has a low absolute risk (<1%); LOE III/B [13]. If HbA1c >6%, fetal echocardiography in the third trimester may be considered to assess for ventricular hypertrophy [13].

Phenylketonuria

Phenylketonuria has an absolute risk of 12–14 (% live births), OR of 10–15% and LOE I/A [22, 23]. Preconception metabolic control may affect risk [13]. Fetal echocardiography should be performed if periconception phenylalanine level >10 mg/dL [13].

Maternal Lupus or Sjögrens

The association of maternal lupus and other connective tissue diseases with congenital complete heart block (CHB) is well known. Lupus or Sjögrens if SSA/SSB autoantibody positive [13, 24 - 26] has an absolute risk of 1-5% live births [13]. High SSA values (≥50 U/mL) may correlate with increased fetal risk [13, 26]. In addition, women with both autoantibodies and hypothyroidism are at a 9-fold increased risk of having an affected fetus or neonate compared with those with SSA or SSB alone [25]. Fetal echocardiography should be performed at 16 weeks, then weekly or every other week to 28 weeks. Concern for late myocardial involvement [26] may justify additional assessments in the third trimester [13].

Maternal Febrile Illness and Infections

Certain infections, specifically maternal rubella, have been associated with a higher incidence of specific cardiac malformations [27] such as patency of the ductus arteriosus (PDA) and VSD. Febrile illness was positively associated with the occurrence of CHD in offspring [27]. In a study in Finland, maternal upper respiratory infection was twice as common among the hypoplastic left heart syndrome (HLHS) group [28]. There were associations between fever and influenza and specific CHD, namely right-sided obstructive and atrioventricular septal defects in infants with Down syndrome. Maternal antipyretic use in the setting of fever or influenza tended to decrease these associations [29]. Parvovirus, coxsackie virus, adenovirus, and cytomegalovirus may cause fetal myocarditis [13]. Referral for fetal cardiac evaluation is indicated for first-trimester rubella (*Class I; Level of Evidence C*), or an infection with suspicion of fetal myocarditis (*Class I; Level of Evidence C*). No consistent associations have been identified between CHD and infections in a review [2].

Hyperhomocysteinemia

Folate is a key factor in cardiovascular development. A compromised folate or vitamin B12 status results in hyperhomocysteinemia. Three studies demonstrated increased risk of CHD in infants born to mothers with high homocysteine levels. However, these studies had small sample sizes, again suggesting that further investigation is warranted [30 - 32].

Hypertension

Hypertension is common in pregnancy. Multiple studies have identified an approximate two-fold increased risk of CHD among infants born to mothers with hypertension during pregnancy [28, 33, 34]. When the databases were stratified by defect, no significant associations remained. Further research must be performed [34, 35].

Overweight and Obesity

Findings have demonstrated each category of increased weight to be significantly associated with the development of CHD [36 - 41]. Mothers with a body mass index (BMI) greater than 30 kg/m^2 were identified as more likely to have an infant with ASD [38, 42], VSD [42], aortic valve stenosis [38], HLHS [37, 38], pulmonary valve stenosis [38], or truncus arteriosus [43], whereas infants born to mothers with a BMI greater than 40 kg/m^2 were more likely to have a double-outlet right ventricle [37, 38, 42, 43].

Assisted Reproduction Technology

There are conflicting reports on the direct association of the use of assisted reproduction technology and CHD malformations in offspring. Recent reports suggest that the increased incidence of CHD in these pregnancies may be attributable to the increased risk specifically for multiple pregnancies [44, 45], advanced maternal age and the unknown effect of the underlying reason for subfertility [46 - 49]. Nevertheless, the overall risk of CHD in infants conceived through *in vitro* fertilization seems to be slightly higher than that for reference populations with a risk of 1.1% to 3.3% [44, 46, 47, 50]. When stratified by defect, ASD, aortic valve stenosis, CoA, TOF, and VSD demonstrated an association [11, 49, 51, 52]. Referral for fetal cardiac evaluation is reasonable if the pregnancy is a result of assisted reproduction technology (*Class IIa; Level of Evidence A*) [13].

Socioeconomic Status

Socioeconomic status has been investigated as a potential risk factor in the development of CHD. In an investigation in Denmark, low maternal and paternal socio-occupational status was associated with infant CHD [53]. A small case-control study in Lithuania showed a 3.4-fold elevation in risk for an infant with a CHD born to mothers with low socioeconomic status [54]. In the USA, household socioeconomic status was associated with the risk of CHD [55].

Stress

The relationship between maternal stress and birth defects has been evaluated [56]. In China, a case-control study identified a threefold greater risk for infants with CHD born to mothers who reported stressful life events during the periconceptional period [57]. In the California Birth Defects Monitoring Program, an association of CHD with d-TGA was identified [58]. Further investigation with larger studies is needed [2]. Table **1** summarizes the literature regarding the environmental risk factors – Demographics and conditions significantly associated with CHD.

ENVIRONMENTAL FACTORS ASSOCIATED WITH CONGENITAL HEART DISEASES – THERAPEUTIC DRUG EXPOSURES

Antihypertensive Drugs

Studies investigating the maternal use of antihypertensive medications and CHD development have conflicting results. Li *et al.* [34] and Banhidy *et al.* [62], have not reported significant associations with antihypertensive medications. Angiotensin-converting enzyme (ACE) inhibitors exposure in the first trimester was associated with increased risk for CHD in a large control population [63], mainly ASD or PDA. Analyses of the Swedish Medical Birth Register [64] and the NBDPS [33] databases identified a two- to three-fold increase in the risk for CHD as a group [33, 64]. Previous NBDPS findings from 1997 to 2003 suggested that maternal antihypertensive use was associated with CHD. Fisher *et al.* re-examined associations between specific antihypertensive medication classes and specific CHD with additional NBDPS data from 2004 to 2011 and observed increased risk of CoA, pulmonary valve stenosis, perimembranous VSD, and secundum ASD. The associations for these phenotypes were statistically significant for mothers who reported β-blocker use or renin–angiotensin system blocker use; estimates for other antihypertensive medication classes were generally based on fewer exposed cases and were less stable but remained elevated, suggesting that antihypertensive medication use may be associated with increased risk of specific CHD, although they could not completely rule out confounding by underlying disease characteristics [35]. Li *et al.* found that ACE inhibitors in the first trimester had a risk profile similar to the use of other antihypertensives regarding malformations in live born offspring and associated the increased risk of malformations to the underlying hypertension rather than the drugs [34]. Referral for fetal cardiac evaluation is reasonable for maternal therapeutic drugs including ACE inhibitors (*Class IIa; Level of Evidence B*) between 18-22 weeks [13].

Table 1. Environmental factors associated with congenital heart diseases – Demographics and conditions.

Exposure	Reference	Database	CHD Cases (n)	Controls (n)	OR or RR (95% CI)
Demographics					
Advanced maternal age	Miller *et al.*2011 [5]	MACDP (1968–2005)	739	1,301,143	1.2 (1.1–1.3)
	Hollier *et al.*2000 [6]	PHHS (1988–1994)	3,757	102,728	4.0 (1.7–9.2)
	Kidd *et al.*1993 [7]	NSW/ACT (1981–1984)	1,479	343,521	1.3 (1.1–1.4)
	Ferencz *et al.*1993 [10]	BWIS (1981–1989)	3,377	3,572	1.3 (1.1–1.5)
Advanced paternal age	Yang *et al.*2007 [8]	NCHS (1999–2000)	9,767	77,514	1.2 (1.1–1.4)
	Bassili *et al.*2000 [9]	EHS (1995–1997)	894	894	1.5 (1.2–2.0)
Young paternal age	Yang *et al.*2007 [8]	Bei/Heb provinces (1988)	497	6,222	2.3 (1.9–2.8)
Pre-gestational diabetes	Garne *et al.*2012 [15]	EUROCAT (1990–2005)	323	92,976	2.2 (1.9–2.6)

(Table 1) cont.....

Exposure	Reference	Database	CHD Cases (n)	Controls (n)	OR or RR (95% CI)
Diabetes mellitus type 1	Banhidy *et al.*2010 [59]	HCCSCA (1980–1996)	4,480	38,151	2.5 (1.6–3.9)
Pre-gestational diabetes	Correa *et al.*2008 [14]	NBDPS (1997–2003)	3,519	4,689	4.6 (2.9–7.5)
Pre-gestational diabetes	Loffredo *et al.*2001 [16]	BWIS (1981–1989)	3,377	3,572	3.0 (1.9–4.8)
Febrile illness	Acs *et al.* 2005 [60]	HCCSCA (1980–1996)	4,480	38,151	2.6 (1.2–5.4)
	Liu *et al.* 2009 [57]	Shan province (2004–2005)	164	328	5.9 (2.7–13.1)
	Botto *et al.* 2001 [27]	ABDCCS (1968–1980)	829	3,029	1.8 (1.4–2.4)
	Tikkanen *et al.* [28]	FRCM (1982–1983)	583	756	1.5 (1.1–2.1)
Influenza	Acs *et al.* 2005 [61]	HCCSCA (1980–1996)	4,480	38,151	1.7 (1.3–2.3)
Hypertension	Li *et al.* 2011 [34]	KPNCa (1995–2008)	6,873	453,078	1.4 (1.3–1.5)
	Cato *et al.* 2009 [33]	NBDPS (1997–2003)	5,021	4,796	1.8 (1.1–2.7)
	Tikkanen *et al.* 1990 [28]	FRCM (1982–1983)	583	756	2.6 (1.1–5.2)
Hyperhomocysteinemia	Hobbs *et al.* 2011 [30]	ARHMS (1998–2008)	417	250	1.5 (1.2–1.8)
	Verkleij-Haboort *et al.* 2006 [31]	HAVEN (2003–2005)	151	183	2.9 (1.4–6.0)
	Wenstrom *et al.* 2001 [32]	APGC (1988–1998)	26	116	3.5 (1.2–10.2)
Pre-pregnancy weight					
Overweight (BMI 25–30 kg/m²)	Watkins *et al.* 2003 [39]	ABDRFSS (1993–1997)	195	330	2.0 (1.2–3.1)
Obese (BMI >30 kg/m²)	Madsen *et al.* 2013 [37]	WCHARS (1992–2007)	14,412	141,420	1.2 (1.2–1.3)
	Mills *et al.* 2010 [38]	NYSCMR (1993–2003)	7,392	56,304	1.2 (1.1–1.2)
	Blomberg *et al.* 2010 [36]	SMBR (1995–2007)	11,163	1,235,877	1.2 (1.1–1.2)
	Watkins *et al.* 2003 [39]	ABDRFSS (1993–1997)	195	330	2.0 (1.2–3.4)

(Table 1) cont.....

Exposure	Reference	Database	CHD Cases (n)	Controls (n)	OR or RR (95% CI)
Severely obese (BMI >40 kg/m^2)	Blomberg *et al.*2010 [36]	SMBR (1995–2007)	11,163	1,235,877	1.5 (1.2–1.8)
Reproductive history Infertility/ART	Tararbit *et al.* 1990 [49]	PaRCM (1987–2006)	5,493	3,104	1.4 (1.1–1.7)
Socioeconomic status (low)	Kuciene *et al.* 2009 [54]	Kaunas (1999–2005)	187	643	3.4 (1.5–7.6)
	Varela *et al.* 2009 [53]	DNBC (1997–2002)	659	81,453	1.6 (1.3–2.0)
Stress	Liu *et al.* 2009 [57]	Shan province (2004–2005)	164	328	2.7 (1.5–4.8)

ART: assisted reproduction technology; CHD: congenital heart defects; OR: odds ratio; RR: relative risk; CI: confidence interval; BMI: body mass index.

Bronchodilators

A New York State population-based study suggests that both maternal asthma status and asthma medication use, particularly bronchodilators, may play a role in cardiac malformations in offspring [65].

Anticonvulsant Drugs

Large epidemiological studies of the offspring of epileptic women have been published, however is not clear whether the malformations found are due to the epilepsy or the anticonvulsant therapy [66]. There are characteristic anomalies associated with some of the anticonvulsants as fetal hydantoin syndrome. Phenytoin and valproic acid are Food and Drug Administration (FDA) category D (Studies show fetal risk in human beings; use of drug may be acceptable even with risks, such as in life-threatening illnesses or where safer drugs are ineffective) [66]. In a meta-analysis including a group of untreated epileptic women as control subjects, the incidence of malformations in the unmedicated epileptic control subjects was similar to that for the normal population. Cardiac malformations were found in 1.8% of 1208 carbamazepine-exposed fetuses [67]. Fetal echocardiogram may be considered, although its usefulness has not been established if exposure occurs (*Class IIb; Level of Evidence A*) [13].

Lithium

Lithium use during pregnancy has been associated with Ebstein's anomaly [66, 68]. However, more recent studies and literature analyses have suggested that the risk is not as high as initially thought [69]. Fetal echocardiogram may be considered, although its usefulness has not been established if exposure occurs

(*Class IIb; Level of Evidence B*) [13].

Antidepressant Drugs

Maternal use of any antidepressants during the periconceptional period is associated with CHD [10]. Fluoxetine use was associated with an increased risk of isolated VSD [70]. Use of tricyclic antidepressants was associated with a higher risk than other antidepressants [71, 72]. Paroxetine exposure was associated with increased risk of CHD, specifically with right ventricular outflow tract defects [70, 73]. On the other hand, other studies have not identified a significant association between maternal antidepressant use and CHD [74, 75]. Referral for fetal cardiac evaluation may be considered for paroxetine (*Class IIb; Level of Evidence A*) [13].

Vitamin K Antagonists

Vitamin K antagonists as warfarin used in the first trimester of pregnancy have been reported to be teratogenic. A recent multicenter, prospective study suggests that there was no increased risk of CHD despite an increased risk of other birth defects [76]. A detailed anatomy scan should be performed [13].

Anti-infection Drugs

Antibiotics and antifungals are commonly prescribed during the periconceptional period of pregnancy. Erythromycins, and cephalosporins, although used commonly by pregnant women, were not associated with many birth defects [77]. Sulfonamides were associated with HLHS and CoA. Nitrofurantoins were associated with HLHS and ASD. These increased risks were reduced if the mother concomitantly took folic acid supplementation [78, 79]. The BWIS identified a significant association between metronidazole use and the development of CHD [10]. Two metanalyses showed no increased risk of CHD, associated with maternal use of metronidazole [80, 81].

Retinoic Acid

Retinoic acid, a vitamin A analog, is contraindicated in pregnancy (FDA category X); however, inadvertent use may occur. Conotruncal defects and aortic arch anomalies were reported in association with its use [82]. Fetal echocardiogram is recommended if exposure occurs (*Class I; Level of Evidence B*) [13].

Thalidomide

Thalidomide is a cardiac teratogen and therefore contraindicated during pregnancy and among women planning a pregnancy (FDA category X).

Thalidomide is associated with VSD, ASD and conotruncal defects [83]. No safe dose of thalidomide treatment during fetal development has been established.

Nonsteroidal Anti-inflammatory Drugs

The use of nonsteroidal anti-inflammatory drugs (NSAIDs) in early gestation has been associated with a small increased risk for CHD [84]. Maternal use of aspirin is reported to be associated with interrupted aortic arch [85] and pulmonary valve stenosis [86]. Ibuprofen has been associated with an increased risk of CHD [10] namely atrioventricular septal defect, double-outlet right ventricle and d-TGA [11]. A more recent large study using a Norwegian Cohort did not confirm this association [87]. An association between maternal use of naproxen and CHD overall has been demonstrated using the Swedish Medical Birth Register [88]. NSAIDs are sometimes used for tocolysis in the late second- and third- trimester fetus and may cause ductal constriction [89]. Doppler ductal constriction is evident in 25% to 50% of indomethacin exposed fetuses, but it is usually mild and resolves with drug discontinuation [90]. Fetal cardiac evaluation may be considered for maternal use of NSAIDs in the first or second trimester (*Class IIb; Level of Evidence B*) and NSAIDs used in the third trimester (*Class I; Level of Evidence A*) [13]. Table **2** summarizes the literature regarding the environmental risk factors – Therapeutic drug exposure significantly associated with CHD.

Protective Effect of Folic Acid

Multivitamin supplements containing folic acid may reduce the risk for some types of CHD [27, 92, 93]. Using the Atlanta Birth Defects Case-Control Study [94], approximately one in four major cardiac defects could be prevented by periconceptional multivitamin use. With the EUROCAT [95] database, use of periconceptional folic acid supplements was related to approximately 20% reduction in the prevalence of any CHD. In the Hungarian cohort-controlled trial of periconceptional multivitamin supplementation, the occurrence of CHD was reduced in the supplemented cohort [96]. Among the subtypes, d-TGA and VSD exhibited significant risk reduction [97]. Reduction in risk was present when the multivitamin supplementation was used at about the time of conception or early in the first month of pregnancy [3, 94, 96, 98, 99]. World Health Organization recommends that all women trying to conceive until 12 weeks of gestation, should take a folic acid supplement (400 µg folic acid daily). High-dose folic acid supplementation (4 mg per day starting one month prior to conception) should be considered with following pregnancies after one child with CHD [100].

Table 2. Environmental factors associated with congenital heart diseases – therapeutic drug exposures.

Therapeutic Drug	Reference	Database	CHD Cases (n)	Controls (n)	OR or RR (95% CI)
Antihypertensives					
β-blockers Pulmonary valve stenosis and secundum ASD	Caton *et al.* [33]	NBDPS (1997-2003)	5021	4796	2.6 (1.2–5.3)
ACE inhibitors	Cooper *et al.* [63]	TN Medicaid (1985–2000)	209	29,096	3.7 (1.9–7.3)
Early pregnancy antihypertensive	Fisher *et al.* [35]	NBDPS (2004 to 2011)	10625	11137	
CoA					2.50 (1.52–4.11)
Pulmonary valve stenosis					2.19 (1.44–3.34)
Perimembranous VSD					1.90 (1.09–3.31)
Secundum ASD					1.94 (1.36–2.79)
Bronchodilators	Lin *et al.* [65]	NYSCMR (1988–1991)	502	1,066	2.2 (1.1–4.6)
Anticonvulsants	Hernandez-Diaz *et al.* 2000 [78]	SEUBDS (1976–1988)	3,870	8,387	2.2 (1.4–3.5)
Antidepressants (any)	Ferencz *et al.*1993 [10]	BWIS (1981–1989)	3,377	3,572	3.0 (1.2–7.6)
SSRI	Malm *et al.* 2011 [70]	FRCM (1996–2003)	8,253	635,583	1.3 (1.1–1.6)
Fluoxetine VSD	Malm *et al.* 2011 [70]				2.03, 95% (CI 1.28-3.21)
Paroxetine Right ventricular outflow tract defects	Malm *et al.* 2011 [70]				4.68, 95% (CI 1.48-14.74).
Paroxetine	Bar-Oz *et al.* [73]	Meta-analysis			1.72 (CI 1.22–2.42)
Paroxetine	Reis *et al.* [72]	SMBR (1995–2007)	1,208	1,062,190	1.7 (1.1–2.5)
SNRI **Venlafaxine**	Polen *et al.* [71]	NBDPS (1997–2007)	8,069	8,002	2.7 (1.5–5.0)
Anti-infection					

(Table 2) cont.....

Therapeutic Drug	Reference	Database	CHD Cases (n)	Controls (n)	OR or RR (95% CI)
Sulfonamides	Czeizel *et al.* [79]	HCCSCA (1980–1996	4,467	38,151	2.1 (1.4–3.3)
	Hernandez-Diaz *et al.* [78]	SEUBDS (1976–1988)	3,870	8,387	3.4 (1.8–6.4)
Sulfonamides	Crider *et al.* [77]	Population-based, multisite	5269	4941	
			HLHS		3.2 (1.3-7.6)
			CoA		2.7 (1.3-5.6)
Nitrofurantoin	Crider *et al.* [77]	Population-based, multisite	HLHS		4.2 (1.9-9.1)
		Population-based, multisite	ASD		1.9 (1.1-3.4)
Antifungals Metronidazole	Ferencz *et al.* [91]	BWIS (1981–1989)	3,377	3,572	2.5 (1.1–5.8)
Ibuprofen	Ferencz *et al.* [91]	BWIS (1981–1989)	3,377	3,572	1.4 (1.1–1.8)
Naproxen	Kallen *et al.* [88]	SMBR (1995–2001)	5,565	577,730	1.7 (1.1–2.5)

CHD: congenital heart defects; OR: odds ratio; RR: relative risk; CI: confidence interval; ASD: atrial septal defect; HLHS: hypoplastic left heart syndrome; CoA: coarctation of the aorta; SSRI: Selective serotonin-reuptake inhibitors; SNRI: serotonin-norepinephrine reuptake inhibitors; VSD: ventricular septal defect; ACE: angiotensin-converting enzyme.

Vitamin D

Deficient vitamin D status was associated with CHD in offspring [101]. Improvement of the periconceptional maternal vitamin D status is recommended with emphasis in safe sunlight exposure, a higher dietary intake of fish and seafood, and the use of a low dose vitamin D supplement [102]. The Endocrine Society suggests that pregnant and lactating women require at least 600 IU/day of vitamin D and recognizes that in order to maintain a serum concentration >75 nmol/l, 1500–2000 IU/day of vitamin D may be needed [103].

Environmental Factors Associated with Congenital Heart Diseases – Nontherapeutic Drug Exposures

Alcohol

Studies have documented the wide-ranging teratogenic effects of alcohol consumption during pregnancy on birth outcomes, including CHD [104]. A case-control study that examined the risk of congenital anomalies with different sporadic and daily doses of alcohol consumption in Spain reported an increased risk of CHD as a group only with the highest level of maternal consumption of alcohol per day (>92 g/d) [105]. A case-control study using the Pregnancy Risk Assessment Monitoring System database also reported a threefold risk for CHD among mothers who reported periconceptional alcohol use [106]. When study databases were stratified by defect, increased risks were observed for ASD [28], d-TGA, and VSD [107 - 109]. Pregnancy Risk Assessment Monitoring Survey shown that multiple episodes of maternal binge drinking in early pregnancy may increase the odds of CHD, and this relationship was more dramatic when combined with maternal smoking [106]. One case-control study of conotruncal defects in Atlanta showed no association with maternal reports of alcohol consumption or "binge" drinking [104].

Caffeine

Concern that maternal ingestion of caffeine may lead to birth defects prompted the FDA to caution pregnant women to limit their caffeine intake [66]. However, no evidence for a teratogenic effect of caffeine was identified on the NBDPS [10, 110].

Cigarette Smoking

There is an association between maternal exposure to cigarette smoking and CHD [111, 112]. Two recent metanalyses demonstrated a modest association of cigarette use and CHD [113, 114]. Maternal smoking during pregnancy was associated with septal and right-sided obstructive defects [115]. In addition, passive smoke exposure demonstrated a significant association between maternal passive smoke exposure and atrioventricular septal defects [116] and secundum ASD [117]. A study demonstrated an increased risk of CHD among fathers who reported smoking [118-120].

Other Drugs

A review performed at Boston City Hospital showed an increased risk of CHD for infants born to mothers who used cocaine prenatally [121]. Maternal marijuana use was associated with VSD [107] and paternal marijuana use was associated with CHD [10]. Table **3** summarizes the literature regarding the environmental risk factors – Nontherapeutic drug exposure significantly associated with CHD.

Air Pollution

Maternal exposure to environmental air pollution has been associated with CHD [122]. Were observed associations between CO and TOF, particulate matter <10 μm (PM <10 μm) with ASD [14] and PDA [123], and SO_2 with VSD [124]. Moderate association of NO_2 with CoA was found, as well as between SO_2, PM10

[125] and PM2.5 with CHD [112, 126]. A meta-analysis [127] found that NO_2 was significantly associated with CoAo. Vrijheid *et al.* found associations between NO_2 and SO_2 exposures and CoA and TOF, and PM $\leq$10 μm exposure and ASD [128]. Other studies have shown little or no association with CHD development [129, 130]. The epidemiological evidence for a causal association between air pollutants exposure and the risk of CHD is still to be considered limited [111, 129]. Maternal exposure to cyanide or heavy metals was associated with CHD [131, 132]. Agricultural chemicals [104] and insecticides have been associated with an increased risk of conotruncal defects. Maternal reports of potential exposure to herbicides and rodenticides were associated with an increased risk of d-TGA [133] and of potential exposure to pesticides with total anomalous pulmonary venous return, membranous VSD [11], PDA [134], TOF, HLHS, CoA, pulmonary valve stenosis and ASD and VSD [135].

Table 3. Environmental factors associated with congenital heart diseases – nontherapeutic drug exposures.

Nontherapeutic drug	Reference	Database	CHD cases (n)	Controls (n)	OR or RR (95% CI)
Alcohol Maternal use Binge drinking	Mateja *et al.* 2012 [106]	PRAMS (1996–2005)	237	948	3.0 (1.2–7.5)
Maternal use Binge drinking+ cigarette smoking	Mateja *et al.* 2012 [106]	PRAMS (1996–2005)	237	948	9.45, 95% CI 2.53-35.31
Cigarette smoking Maternal use	Karataza *et al.* 2011 [119]	Patras (2006–2009)	157	208	2.8 (1.8–4.6)
Cigarette smoking Maternal use	Hackshaw *et al.*2011 [113]	Systematic review	-	-	1.09 (1.02-1.17)
	Lee *et al.*2013 [114]	Meta-analysis	-	-	1.1 (1.02-1.21))
	Zhang *et al.* 2017 [120]	Meta-analysis	-	-	1.1 (1.04-1.18)
Cigarette smoking Paternal use	Cresci *et al.* 2011 [118]	Italy (2008–2010)	360	360	1.7 (1.1–2.6)
Cocaine Maternal use	Ferencz *et al.*1993 [91]	BWIS (1981–1989)	3,377	3,572	1.6 (1.1–2.3)
	Lipshultz *et al.*1991 [121]	Boston City (1988–1990)	49	505	3.7 (1.4–9.4)
Cocaine Paternal use	Ferencz *et al.*1993 [91]	BWIS (1981–1989)	3,377	3,572	1.7 (1.3–2.2)

Nontherapeutic drug	Reference	Database	CHD cases (n)	Controls (n)	OR or RR (95% CI)
Marijuana Paternal use	Ferencz *et al.*1993 [91]	BWIS (1981–1989)	3,377	3,572	1.2 (1.1–1.4)

CHD: congenital heart defects; OR: odds ratio; RR: relative risk; CI: confidence interval.

Chemical Exposures/Organic Solvents

Exposure to chemicals may lead to CHD. Organic solvents exposure was associated with CoA, HLHS, d-TGA [11] and VSD [136]. Maternal occupational exposure to phthalates and alkylphenolic compounds were associated with CHD [137] and specifically with VSD, ASD, PDA and pulmonary valve stenosis. Paternal exposure to phthalates and polychlorinated compounds was associated with VSD, while exposure to alkylphenolic compounds was associated with CoA [138, 139]. Paternal exposure to phthalates or alkylphenolic compounds was a risk factor for VSD and pulmonary valve stenosis [140]. Parental exposure to hair dye was also found to be a risk factor [141]. Maternal exposure to dyes, lacquers or paints was associated with CHD [142].

Water Contamination

Multiple studies have examined the relationship between maternal exposure to contaminated water and CHD. Exposure to ground water contamination with trichloroethylene [143 - 148] and dichloroethylene was associated with CHD [145]. Two large reviews have reported no association between maternal exposure to trichloroethylene contaminated water and CHD [146, 147]. A meta-analysis of drinking water trihalomethane and chlorination by-product exposure found a modest association for all CHD, with greater correlation for septal defects [149]; a study of exposure through bathing and showering found an association with bromodichloromethanes [112]. An drinking water study had found an association of arsenic with CoA but not with any other CHD and no association for lead or mercury [150]. When metal concentrations were measured in hair, it was found that arsenic levels were significantly higher in almost every CHD sub-type and were dose-dependent [151]. Hair cadmium was also associated with a 2.81-fold increase in the incidence of conotruncal defects for levels in the highest group and there was an additive effect of the presence of both cadmium and arsenic [151]. Hair lead was also found to be dose dependently associated with the presence of certain sub-types of CHD in a case control study [152]. One study found that high blood lead was associated with total CHD, conotruncal defects, septal defects and right ventricular outflow tract obstruction [153]. An area of Italy polluted with lead from ceramic factories was found to have a higher incidence of CHD [154], while an investigation of paternal employment found that lead exposure was associated with increased risk of VSD [155]. Hair aluminum was associated with total CHD and particularly septal and conotruncal defects and right ventricular outflow tract obstruction [156]. Recent studies investigated cord blood and found that presence of aluminum and barium were associated with higher incidence of CHD that presence of aluminum was associated with higher incidence of CHD [157, 158]. Selenium may be protective [150, 153].

Hazardous Waste Sites

Large population-based studies have evaluated the risk of CHD in communities located close to hazardous waste sites with limited results. One study found an increased risk of all CHD as a group [159]. Two studies found no associations with CHD [160, 161]. A case control study found that living within a mile of any waste site was associated with truncus arteriosus [162]. A five-country EUROHAZCON study found that maternal residence within 3 km of a landfill site was associated with increased risk of CHD [130]. Recent studies tend to show an association with CHD and exposure to solvents, a range of metals, landfill sites or hazardous waste sites [112].

Other Environmental Exposures

Evaluations of possible associations of heart defects with maternal exposure to ionizing radiation have been limited. The BWIS examined possible associations of CHD with maternal reports of exposure to ionizing radiation in occupational settings or as part of medical or dental evaluations and found few reports of such exposures and no evidence of any associations [11]. A study considered paternal occupational exposure in the six months prior to conception and found an association between ionizing radiation and endocardial cushion defect without Down syndrome [163]. Table **4** summarizes the literature regarding the environmental exposures.

Table 4. Environmental factors associated with congenital heart diseases – Environmental exposures.

Environmental Exposures	Reference	Database	CHD Cases (n)	Controls (n)	OR or RR (95% CI)
Air pollution	Ren *et al*. 2018 [125]	Population based study	321	30,990	PM10 exposure of $\geq$92 µg m^{-3} 1.16 (1.06–1.28)
	Liu *et al*. 2017 [126]	Hospital-based case control study	700	110,720	PM10 exposure 1.28 (1.03–1.61)

(Table 3) cont.....

Environmental Exposures	Reference	Database	CHD Cases (n)	Controls (n)	OR or RR (95% CI)
Pesticides	Rappazzo *et al.* 2016 [134]	Case control study	6358	298,548	ASD: 1.70 (1.34– 2.14) PDA: OR 1.50 (1.22– 1.85)
Any pesticides	Loffredo *et al.*2001 [133]	Population based study	TGA		2.0 (1.2–3.3)
Herbicides			TGA		2.8 (1.3–7.2)
Rodenticides			TGA		4.7 (1.4–12.1)
Neonicotinoids	Carmichael *et al.*2014 [135]	Case control study	TOF		2.4 (1.1–5.1)
Strobin			HLHS		2.9 (1.2–7.0)
Triazine			HLHS		2.2 (1.0–5.1)
Pyridazinone			CoA		2.9 (1.1–7.5)
Avermectin			VSD		2.8 (1.2–6.2)
Dichlorophenoxy acid			ASD		2.3(1.2–4.5)
Chemical exposures/ Organic solvents					
Maternal cyanide exposure	Shaw *et al.*1992 [131]	San Francisco (1983–1985)	5,046	20,882	2.2 (1.3–3.9)
Maternal heavy metal exposure	Shaw *et al.*1992 [131]	San Francisco (1983–1985)	5,046	20,882	1.5 (1.1–2.3)
Paternal phthalate exposure	Snijder *et al.*2012 [138]	Case control study HAVEN (2003–2010)	424 All CHD	480	2.08 (1.27–3.40)
			VSD		2.84 (1.37–5.92)
Paternal alkylphenolic compound exposure	Snijder *et al.*2012 [138]	HAVEN (2003–2010)	424	480	1.8 (1.1–3.0)
			CoA		3.85 (1.17–12.67)
Paternal phthalate exposure	Wijnands *et al.*2014 [139]	Case control study	VSD		1.93 (1.05–3.54).
Phthalates	Wang *et al.*2013 [137]	Case control study	357 All CHD	270	1.6 (1.0–2.6)
Alkylphenolic compounds	Wang *et al.*2013 [137]	Case control study	357 All CHD	270	1.8 (1.1–3.0)

(Table 3) cont.....

Environmental Exposures	Reference	Database	CHD Cases (n)	Controls (n)	OR or RR (95% CI)
Maternal occupational phthalate exposure	Wang *et al.*2015 [140]	Hospital based case control study	707	593	
			VSD		3.7 (1.7–8.0)
			PDA		3.8 (1.6–8.9)
			ASD		3.5 (1.4–8.7)
			PVS		4.2 (1.1–16.0)
Maternal alkylphenolic compound exposure:	Wang *et al.*2015 [140]	Hospital based case control study	VSD		2.2 (1.3–3.6)
			PDA		2.0 (1.1–3.5)
			PVS		3.8 (1.5–9.4)
Maternal heavy metal exposure	Wang *et al.*2015 [140]	Hospital based case control study	VSD		7.3 (2.0–27.6);
			ASD		6.5 (1.1–36.7)
Paternal occupational phthalate exposure	Wang *et al.*2015 [140]	Hospital based case control study	VSD		1.6 (1.0–2.4)
			PVS		2.4 (1.1–5.2)
Paternal alkylphenolic compound exposure	Wang *et al.*2015 [140]	Hospital based case control study	VSD		1.5 (1.0–2.2)
Maternal exposure to any housing renovations	Liu *et al.*2013 [142]	Hospital based case control study	560 All CHD	472	1.89 (1.29–2.77)
Moved into a new house within one month after decoration at 3 months before pregnancy	Liu *et al.*2013 [142]	Hospital based case control study	All CHD		2.38 (1.03–5.48)
Moved into a new house within one month after decoration during first trimester	Liu *et al.*2013 [142]	Hospital based case control study	All CHD		4.00 (1.62–9.86)
Drinking water contaminants Dichloroethylene	Bove *et al.* 1995 [145]	New Jersey (1985–1988)	108	52,334	2.8 (1.3–5.9)* * 90% CI
Trichloroethylene	Yauck *et al.*2004 [144]	Milwaukee (1997–1999)	245	3,780	6.2 (2.6–14.5)
Bromodichloromethane exposure during first month of gestation	Grazuleviciene *et al.*2013 [164]	Cohort study	57 All CHD	2,903	2.16 (1.05–4.46)
Hazardous waste site	Malik *et al.*2004 [165]	Dallas County (1979–1984)	1,283	2,292	1.2 (1.1–1.4)

(Table 3) cont.....

Environmental Exposures	Reference	Database	CHD Cases (n)	Controls (n)	OR or RR (95% CI)
Any waste site	Langlois *et al.*2009 [162] Truncus arteriosus	Case control study	101	4,368	2.80 (1.19–6.54)
Hazardous waste sites	Langlois *et al.*2009 [162] Truncus arteriosus	Case control study	101	4,368	4.99 (1.26–14.51)
Proximity to hazardous waste sites and release of chemicals into the air	Kuehl *et al.*2003 [141] TGA	Case control study	36	3,495	13.4 (95% CI: 4.7–37.8)
Residence within 3 km of hazardous industrial waste site	Dolk *et al.*1998 [130]	Population-based register study	248 Septal defects	2366	1.49 (1.09–2.04)
	Dolk *et al.*1998 [130]		63 Arterial or venous anomalies	2366	1.81 (1.02–3.20)

CHD: congenital heart defects; OR: odds ratio; RR: relative risk; CI: confidence interval; HLHS: hypoplastic left heart syndrome; TAPVR: total anomalous pulmonary venous return; AVSD: atrioventricular septal defect; VSD: ventricular septal defect; CoA: coarctation of the aorta; PDA: persistent ductus arteriosus; PVS: pulmonary vein stenosis.

CONCLUSION

Studies investigating most of the environmental risk factors have limited results due to small samples, difficulty to perform precise measurements of exposures, recall and confounding bias. Thalidomide, retinoids, maternal rubella infection, phenylketonuria, hypertension, diabetes, alcohol, organic solvents, smoking and air pollution have been associated with CHD. Prevention should be provided, with preconception care. Previous conditions such as diabetes, hypertension and phenylketonuria should be detected and properly managed. The vaccination plan should be updated. Balanced nutrition as well as the use of a multivitamin containing folic acid should be provided. Exposures such as infections, organic solvents, alcohol, smoking, and non-therapeutic drugs should be avoided. Pregnancy follow-up should be provided with screening for CHD if risk factors are present. Additional investigations about environmental risk factors are needed to improve prevention strategies.

CONSENT FOR PUBLICATION

Not applicable.

CONFLICT OF INTEREST

The authors confirm that the contents of this chapter have no conflict of interest.

ACKNOWLEDGEMENTS

Declare none.

REFERENCES

[1]　Hoffman JI, Kaplan S. The incidence of congenital heart disease. J Am Coll Cardiol 2002; 39(12): 1890-900.
[http://dx.doi.org/10.1016/S0735-1097(02)01886-7] [PMID: 12084585]

[2]　Patel SS, Burns TL. Nongenetic risk factors and congenital heart defects. Pediatr Cardiol 2013; 34(7): 1535-55.
[http://dx.doi.org/10.1007/s00246-013-0775-4] [PMID: 23963188]

[3]　Huhta J, Linask KK. Environmental origins of congenital heart disease: the heart-placenta connection. Semin Fetal Neonatal Med 2013; 18(5): 245-50.
[http://dx.doi.org/10.1016/j.siny.2013.05.003] [PMID: 23751925]

[4]　Wilson PD, Loffredo CA, Correa-Villaseñor A, Ferencz C. Attributable fraction for cardiac malformations. Am J Epidemiol 1998; 148(5): 414-23.
[http://dx.doi.org/10.1093/oxfordjournals.aje.a009666] [PMID: 9737553]

[5]　Miller A, Riehle-Colarusso T, Siffel C, Frías JL, Correa A. Maternal age and prevalence of isolated congenital heart defects in an urban area of the United States. Am J Med Genet A 2011; 155A(9): 2137-45.
[http://dx.doi.org/10.1002/ajmg.a.34130] [PMID: 21815253]

[6]　Hollier LM, Leveno KJ, Kelly MA, MCIntire DD, Cunningham FG. Maternal age and malformations in singleton births. Obstet Gynecol 2000; 96(5 Pt 1): 701-6.
[PMID: 11042304]

[7]　Kidd SA, Lancaster PA, McCredie RM. The incidence of congenital heart defects in the first year of life. J Paediatr Child Health 1993; 29(5): 344-9.
[http://dx.doi.org/10.1111/j.1440-1754.1993.tb00531.x] [PMID: 8240861]

[8]　Yang Q, Wen SW, Leader A, Chen XK, Lipson J, Walker M. Paternal age and birth defects: how strong is the association? Hum Reprod 2007; 22(3): 696-701.
[http://dx.doi.org/10.1093/humrep/del453] [PMID: 17164268]

[9]　Bassili A, Mokhtar SA, Dabous NI, Zaher SR, Mokhtar MM, Zaki A. Risk factors for congenital heart diseases in Alexandria, Egypt. Eur J Epidemiol 2000; 16(9): 805-14.
[http://dx.doi.org/10.1023/A:1007601919164] [PMID: 11297222]

[10]　Ferencz C, Rubin JD, Loffredo CA, Magee CA. Epidemiology of congenital heart disease: the Baltimore-Washington Infant Study: 1981–1989. Mount Kisco, NY: Futura Publishing Co 1993.

[11]　Ferencz C, Loffredo CA, Corea-Villasenor A, Wilson PD. Genetic and environmental risk factors of major cardiovascular malformations: the Baltimore-Washington Infant Study: 1981–1989. Armonk, NY: Futura Publishing Co 1997; p. 463.

[12]　Kazaura M, Lie RT, Skjaerven R. Paternal age and the risk of birth defects in Norway. Ann Epidemiol 2004; 14(8): 566-70.
[http://dx.doi.org/10.1016/j.annepidem.2003.10.003] [PMID: 15350956]

[13]　Donofrio MT, Moon-Grady AJ, Hornberger LK, *et al.* American Heart Association Adults With Congenital Heart Disease Joint Committee of the Council on Cardiovascular Disease in the Young and

Council on Clinical Cardiology, Council on Cardiovascular Surgery and Anesthesia, and Council on Cardiovascular and Stroke Nursing. Diagnosis and treatment of fetal cardiac disease: a scientific statement from the American Heart Association. Circulation 2014; 129(21): 2183-242.
[http://dx.doi.org/10.1161/01.cir.0000437597.44550.5d] [PMID: 24763516]

[14]   Correa A, Gilboa SM, Besser LM, Botto LD, Moore CA, Hobbs CA, *et al.* Diabetes mellitus and birth defects. Am J Obstet Gynecol 2008; 199:237: e1-9.
[http://dx.doi.org/10.1016/j.ajog.2008.06.028]

[15]   Garne E, Loane M, Dolk H, *et al.* Spectrum of congenital anomalies in pregnancies with pregestational diabetes. Birth Defects Res A Clin Mol Teratol 2012; 94(3): 134-40.
[http://dx.doi.org/10.1002/bdra.22886] [PMID: 22371321]

[16]   Loffredo CA, Wilson PD, Ferencz C. Maternal diabetes: an independent risk factor for major cardiovascular malformations with increased mortality of affected infants. Teratology 2001; 64(2): 98-106.
[http://dx.doi.org/10.1002/tera.1051] [PMID: 11460261]

[17]   Ray JG, O'Brien TE, Chan WS. Preconception care and the risk of congenital anomalies in the offspring of women with diabetes mellitus: a meta-analysis. QJM 2001; 94(8): 435-44.
[http://dx.doi.org/10.1093/qjmed/94.8.435] [PMID: 11493721]

[18]   Lisowski LA, Verheijen PM, Copel JA, *et al.* Congenital heart disease in pregnancies complicated by maternal diabetes mellitus. An international clinical collaboration, literature review, and meta-analysis. Herz 2010; 35(1): 19-26.
[http://dx.doi.org/10.1007/s00059-010-3244-3] [PMID: 20140785]

[19]   Ferencz C, Rubin JD, McCarter RJ, Clark EB. Maternal diabetes and cardiovascular malformations: predominance of double outlet right ventricle and truncus arteriosus. Teratology 1990; 41(3): 319-26.
[http://dx.doi.org/10.1002/tera.1420410309] [PMID: 2326756]

[20]   Ferencz C, Neill CA. Cardiomyopathy in infancy: observations in an epidemiologic study. Pediatr Cardiol 1992; 13(2): 65-71.
[http://dx.doi.org/10.1007/BF00798206] [PMID: 1614921]

[21]   Dervisoglu P, Kosecik M, Kumbasar S. Effects of gestational and pregestational diabetes mellitus on the foetal heart: a cross-sectional study. J Obstet Gynaecol 2018; 38(3): 408-12.
[http://dx.doi.org/10.1080/01443615.2017.1410536] [PMID: 29355062]

[22]   Costedoat-Chalumeau N, Amoura Z, Lupoglazoff JM, *et al.* Outcome of pregnancies in patients with anti-SSA/Ro antibodies: a study of 165 pregnancies, with special focus on electrocardiographic variations in the children and comparison with a control group. Arthritis Rheum 2004; 50(10): 3187-94.
[http://dx.doi.org/10.1002/art.20554] [PMID: 15476223]

[23]   Friedman DM, Kim MY, Copel JA, *et al.* PRIDE Investigators. Utility of cardiac monitoring in fetuses at risk for congenital heart block: the PR Interval and Dexamethasone Evaluation (PRIDE) prospective study. Circulation 2008; 117(4): 485-93.
[http://dx.doi.org/10.1161/CIRCULATIONAHA.107.707661] [PMID: 18195175]

[24]   Jaeggi E, Laskin C, Hamilton R, Kingdom J, Silverman E. The importance of the level of maternal anti-Ro/SSA antibodies as a prognostic marker of the development of cardiac neonatal lupus erythematosus a prospective study of 186 antibody-exposed fetuses and infants. J Am Coll Cardiol 2010; 55(24): 2778-84.
[http://dx.doi.org/10.1016/j.jacc.2010.02.042] [PMID: 20538173]

[25]   Spence D, Hornberger L, Hamilton R, Silverman ED. Increased risk of complete congenital heart block in infants born to women with hypothyroidism and anti-Ro and/or anti-La antibodies. J Rheumatol 2006; 33(1): 167-70.
[PMID: 16292791]

[26]   Saleeb S, Copel J, Friedman D, Buyon JP. Comparison of treatment with fluorinated glucocorticoids to

the natural history of autoantibody-associated congenital heart block: retrospective review of the research registry for neonatal lupus. Arthritis Rheum 1999; 42(11): 2335-45.
[http://dx.doi.org/10.1002/1529-0131(199911)42:11<2335::AID-ANR12>3.0.CO;2-3]　　[PMID: 10555029]

[27] Botto LD, Lynberg MC, Erickson JD. Congenital heart defects, maternal febrile illness, and multivitamin use: a population-based study. Epidemiology 2001; 12(5): 485-90.
[http://dx.doi.org/10.1097/00001648-200109000-00004] [PMID: 11505164]

[28] Tikkanen J, Heinonen OP. Risk factors for cardiovascular malformations in Finland. Eur J Epidemiol 1990; 6(4): 348-56.
[http://dx.doi.org/10.1007/BF00151707] [PMID: 2091934]

[29] Oster ME, Riehle-Colarusso T, Alverson CJ, Correa A. Associations between maternal fever and influenza and congenital heart defects. J Pediatr 2011; 158(6): 990-5.
[http://dx.doi.org/10.1016/j.jpeds.2010.11.058] [PMID: 21256509]

[30] Hobbs CA, MacLeod SL, Jill James S, Cleves MA. Congenital heart defects and maternal genetic, metabolic, and lifestyle factors. Birth Defects Res A Clin Mol Teratol 2011; 91(4): 195-203.
[http://dx.doi.org/10.1002/bdra.20784] [PMID: 21384532]

[31] Verkleij-Hagoort AC, Verlinde M, Ursem NT, *et al.* Maternal hyperhomocysteinaemia is a risk factor for congenital heart disease. BJOG 2006; 113(12): 1412-8.
[http://dx.doi.org/10.1111/j.1471-0528.2006.01109.x] [PMID: 17081182]

[32] Wenstrom KD, Johanning GL, Johnston KE, DuBard M. Association of the C677T methylenetetrahydrofolate reductase mutation and elevated homocysteine levels with congenital cardiac malformations. Am J Obstet Gynecol 2001; 184(5): 806-12.
[http://dx.doi.org/10.1067/mob.2001.113845] [PMID: 11303187]

[33] Caton AR, Bell EM, Druschel CM, *et al.* National Birth Defects Prevention Study. Antihypertensive medication use during pregnancy and the risk of cardiovascular malformations. Hypertension 2009; 54(1): 63-70.
[http://dx.doi.org/10.1161/HYPERTENSIONAHA.109.129098] [PMID: 19433779]

[34] Li DK, Yang C, Andrade S, Tavares V, Ferber JR. Maternal exposure to angiotensin converting enzyme inhibitors in the first trimester and risk of malformations in offspring: a retrospective cohort study. BMJ 2011; 343: d5931.
[http://dx.doi.org/10.1136/bmj.d5931] [PMID: 22010128]

[35] Fisher SC, Van Zutphen AR, Werler MM, *et al.* National Birth Defects Prevention Study. Maternal Antihypertensive Medication Use and Congenital Heart Defects: Updated Results From the National Birth Defects Prevention Study. Hypertension 2017; 69(5): 798-805.
[http://dx.doi.org/10.1161/HYPERTENSIONAHA.116.08773] [PMID: 28373593]

[36] Blomberg MI, Källén B. Maternal obesity and morbid obesity: the risk for birth defects in the offspring. Birth Defects Res A Clin Mol Teratol 2010; 88(1): 35-40.
[PMID: 19711433]

[37] Madsen NL, Schwartz SM, Lewin MB, Mueller BA. Prepregnancy body mass index and congenital heart defects among offspring: a population-based study. Congenit Heart Dis 2013; 8(2): 131-41.
[http://dx.doi.org/10.1111/j.1747-0803.2012.00714.x] [PMID: 22967199]

[38] Mills JL, Troendle J, Conley MR, Carter T, Druschel CM. Maternal obesity and congenital heart defects: a population-based study. Am J Clin Nutr 2010; 91(6): 1543-9.
[http://dx.doi.org/10.3945/ajcn.2009.28865] [PMID: 20375192]

[39] Watkins ML, Rasmussen SA, Honein MA, Botto LD, Moore CA. Maternal obesity and risk for birth defects. Pediatrics 2003; 111(5 Pt 2): 1152-8.
[PMID: 12728129]

[40] Watkins ML, Botto LD. Maternal prepregnancy weight and congenital heart defects in offspring.

Epidemiology 2001; 12(4): 439-46.
[http://dx.doi.org/10.1097/00001648-200107000-00014] [PMID: 11428386]

[41]   Simeone RM, Tinker SC, Gilboa SM, *et al.* National Birth Defects Prevention Study. Proportion of selected congenital heart defects attributable to recognized risk factors. Ann Epidemiol 2016; 26(12): 838-45.
[http://dx.doi.org/10.1016/j.annepidem.2016.10.003] [PMID: 27894567]

[42]   Cedergren MI, Källén BA. Maternal obesity and infant heart defects. Obes Res 2003; 11(9): 1065-71.
[http://dx.doi.org/10.1038/oby.2003.146] [PMID: 12972676]

[43]   Queisser-Luft A, Kieninger-Baum D, Menger H, Stolz G, Schlaefer K, Merz E. [Does maternal obesity increase the risk of fetal abnormalities? Analysis of 20,248 newborn infants of the Mainz Birth Register for detecting congenital abnormalities]. Ultraschall Med 1998; 19(1): 40-4.
[PMID: 9577892]

[44]   Bahtiyar MO, Campbell K, Dulay AT, *et al.* Is the rate of congenital heart defects detected by fetal echocardiography among pregnancies conceived by *in vitro* fertilization really increased?: a case-historical control study. J Ultrasound Med 2010; 29(6): 917-22.
[http://dx.doi.org/10.7863/jum.2010.29.6.917] [PMID: 20498466]

[45]   Schofield SJ, Doughty VL, van Stiphout N, *et al.* Assisted conception and the risk of CHD: a case-control study. Cardiol Young 2017; 27(3): 473-9.
[http://dx.doi.org/10.1017/S1047951116000743] [PMID: 27226023]

[46]   Katalinic A, Rösch C, Ludwig M. German ICSI Follow-Up Study Group. Pregnancy course and outcome after intracytoplasmic sperm injection: a controlled, prospective cohort study. Fertil Steril 2004; 81(6): 1604-16.
[http://dx.doi.org/10.1016/j.fertnstert.2003.10.053] [PMID: 15193484]

[47]   Rimm AA, Katayama AC, Diaz M, Katayama KP. A meta-analysis of controlled studies comparing major malformation rates in IVF and ICSI infants with naturally conceived children. J Assist Reprod Genet 2004; 21(12): 437-43.
[http://dx.doi.org/10.1007/s10815-004-8760-8] [PMID: 15704519]

[48]   Rimm AA, Katayama AC, Katayama KP. A meta-analysis of the impact of IVF and ICSI on major malformations after adjusting for the effect of subfertility. J Assist Reprod Genet 2011; 28(8): 699-705.
[http://dx.doi.org/10.1007/s10815-011-9583-z] [PMID: 21625967]

[49]   Tararbit K, Houyel L, Bonnet D, *et al.* Risk of congenital heart defects associated with assisted reproductive technologies: a population-based evaluation. Eur Heart J 2011; 32(4): 500-8.
[http://dx.doi.org/10.1093/eurheartj/ehq440] [PMID: 21138932]

[50]   Lie RT, Lyngstadaas A, Ørstavik KH, Bakketeig LS, Jacobsen G, Tanbo T. Birth defects in children conceived by ICSI compared with children conceived by other IVF-methods; a meta-analysis. Int J Epidemiol 2005; 34(3): 696-701.
[http://dx.doi.org/10.1093/ije/dyh363] [PMID: 15561745]

[51]   Reefhuis J, Honein MA, Schieve LA, Correa A, Hobbs CA, Rasmussen SA. National Birth Defects Prevention Study. Assisted reproductive technology and major structural birth defects in the United States. Hum Reprod 2009; 24(2): 360-6.
[http://dx.doi.org/10.1093/humrep/den387] [PMID: 19010807]

[52]   Reefhuis J, Honein MA, Schieve LA, Rasmussen SA. National Birth Defects Prevention Study. Use of clomiphene citrate and birth defects, National Birth Defects Prevention Study, 1997-2005. Hum Reprod 2011; 26(2): 451-7.
[http://dx.doi.org/10.1093/humrep/deq313] [PMID: 21112952]

[53]   Varela MM, Nohr EA, Llopis-González A, Andersen AM, Olsen J. Socio-occupational status and congenital anomalies. Eur J Public Health 2009; 19(2): 161-7.
[http://dx.doi.org/10.1093/eurpub/ckp003] [PMID: 19221022]

[54]	Kuciene R, Dulskiene V. Maternal socioeconomic and lifestyle factors during pregnancy and the risk of congenital heart defects. Medicina (Kaunas) 2009; 45(11): 904-9.
[http://dx.doi.org/10.3390/medicina45110116] [PMID: 20051723]

[55]	Yang J, Carmichael SL, Canfield M, Song J, Shaw GM. National Birth Defects Prevention Study. Socioeconomic status in relation to selected birth defects in a large multicentered US case-control study. Am J Epidemiol 2008; 167(2): 145-54.
[http://dx.doi.org/10.1093/aje/kwm283] [PMID: 17947220]

[56]	Carmichael SL, Shaw GM, Yang W, Abrams B, Lammer EJ. Maternal stressful life events and risks of birth defects. Epidemiology 2007; 18(3): 356-61.
[http://dx.doi.org/10.1097/01.ede.0000259986.85239.87] [PMID: 17435445]

[57]	Liu S, Liu J, Tang J, Ji J, Chen J, Liu C. Environmental risk factors for congenital heart disease in the Shandong Peninsula, China: a hospital-based case-control study. J Epidemiol 2009; 19(3): 122-30.
[http://dx.doi.org/10.2188/jea.JE20080039] [PMID: 19398851]

[58]	Carmichael SL, Shaw GM. Maternal life event stress and congenital anomalies. Epidemiology 2000; 11(1): 30-5.
[http://dx.doi.org/10.1097/00001648-200001000-00008] [PMID: 10615840]

[59]	Bánhidy F, Acs N, Puhó EH, Czeizel AE. Congenital abnormalities in the offspring of pregnant women with type 1, type 2 and gestational diabetes mellitus: a population-based case-control study. Congenit Anom (Kyoto) 2010; 50(2): 115-21.
[http://dx.doi.org/10.1111/j.1741-4520.2010.00275.x] [PMID: 20184644]

[60]	Acs N, Bánhidy F, Puhó EH, Czeizel AE. Possible association between acute pelvic inflammatory disease in pregnant women and congenital abnormalities in their offspring: a population-based case-control study. Birth Defects Res A Clin Mol Teratol 2008; 82(8): 563-70.
[http://dx.doi.org/10.1002/bdra.20480] [PMID: 18553461]

[61]	Acs N, Bánhidy F, Puhó E, Czeizel AE. Maternal influenza during pregnancy and risk of congenital abnormalities in offspring. Birth Defects Res A Clin Mol Teratol 2005; 73(12): 989-96.
[http://dx.doi.org/10.1002/bdra.20195] [PMID: 16323157]

[62]	Bánhidy F, Acs N, Puhó EH, Czeizel AE. Chronic hypertension with related drug treatment of pregnant women and congenital abnormalities in their offspring: a population-based study. Hypertens Res 2011; 34(2): 257-63.
[http://dx.doi.org/10.1038/hr.2010.227] [PMID: 21107325]

[63]	Cooper WO, Hernandez-Diaz S, Arbogast PG, *et al.* Major congenital malformations after first-trimester exposure to ACE inhibitors. N Engl J Med 2006; 354(23): 2443-51.
[http://dx.doi.org/10.1056/NEJMoa055202] [PMID: 16760444]

[64]	Lennestål R, Otterblad Olausson P, Källén B. Maternal use of antihypertensive drugs in early pregnancy and delivery outcome, notably the presence of congenital heart defects in the infants. Eur J Clin Pharmacol 2009; 65(6): 615-25.
[http://dx.doi.org/10.1007/s00228-009-0620-0] [PMID: 19198819]

[65]	Lin S, Herdt-Losavio M, Gensburg L, Marshall E, Druschel C. Maternal asthma, asthma medication use, and the risk of congenital heart defects. Birth Defects Res A Clin Mol Teratol 2009; 85(2): 161-8.
[http://dx.doi.org/10.1002/bdra.20523] [PMID: 19067406]

[66]	Jenkins KJ, Correa A, Feinstein JA, *et al.* American Heart Association Council on Cardiovascular Disease in the Young. Noninherited risk factors and congenital cardiovascular defects: current knowledge: a scientific statement from the American Heart Association Council on Cardiovascular Disease in the Young: endorsed by the American Academy of Pediatrics. Circulation 2007; 115(23): 2995-3014.
[http://dx.doi.org/10.1161/CIRCULATIONAHA.106.183216] [PMID: 17519397]

[67]	Matalon S, Schechtman S, Goldzweig G, Ornoy A. The teratogenic effect of carbamazepine: a meta-

analysis of 1255 exposures. Reprod Toxicol 2002; 16(1): 9-17.
[http://dx.doi.org/10.1016/S0890-6238(01)00199-X] [PMID: 11934528]

[68]   Nora JJ, Nora AH, Toews WH. Letter: Lithium, Ebstein's anomaly, and other congenital heart defects. Lancet 1974; 2(7880): 594-5.
[http://dx.doi.org/10.1016/S0140-6736(74)91918-7] [PMID: 4140306]

[69]   Jacobson SJ, Jones K, Johnson K, *et al.* Prospective multicentre study of pregnancy outcome after lithium exposure during first trimester. Lancet 1992; 339(8792): 530-3.
[http://dx.doi.org/10.1016/0140-6736(92)90346-5] [PMID: 1346886]

[70]   Malm H, Artama M, Gissler M, Ritvanen A. Selective serotonin reuptake inhibitors and risk for major congenital anomalies. Obstet Gynecol 2011; 118(1): 111-20.
[http://dx.doi.org/10.1097/AOG.0b013e318220edcc] [PMID: 21646927]

[71]   Polen KN, Rasmussen SA, Riehle-Colarusso T, Reefhuis J. National Birth Defects Prevention Study. Association between reported venlafaxine use in early pregnancy and birth defects, national birth defects prevention study, 1997-2007. Birth Defects Res A Clin Mol Teratol 2013; 97(1): 28-35.
[http://dx.doi.org/10.1002/bdra.23096] [PMID: 23281074]

[72]   Reis M, Källén B. Delivery outcome after maternal use of antidepressant drugs in pregnancy: an update using Swedish data. Psychol Med 2010; 40(10): 1723-33.
[http://dx.doi.org/10.1017/S0033291709992194] [PMID: 20047705]

[73]   Bar-Oz B, Einarson T, Einarson A, *et al.* Paroxetine and congenital malformations: meta-Analysis and consideration of potential confounding factors. Clin Ther 2007; 29(5): 918-26.
[http://dx.doi.org/10.1016/j.clinthera.2007.05.003] [PMID: 17697910]

[74]   Alwan S, Reefhuis J, Rasmussen SA, Olney RS, Friedman JM. National Birth Defects Prevention Study. Use of selective serotonin-reuptake inhibitors in pregnancy and the risk of birth defects. N Engl J Med 2007; 356(26): 2684-92.
[http://dx.doi.org/10.1056/NEJMoa066584] [PMID: 17596602]

[75]   Lattimore KA, Donn SM, Kaciroti N, Kemper AR, Neal CR Jr, Vazquez DM. Selective serotonin reuptake inhibitor (SSRI) use during pregnancy and effects on the fetus and newborn: a meta-analysis. J Perinatol 2005; 25(9): 595-604.
[http://dx.doi.org/10.1038/sj.jp.7211352] [PMID: 16015372]

[76]   Schaefer C, Hannemann D, Meister R, *et al.* Vitamin K antagonists and pregnancy outcome. A multi-centre prospective study. Thromb Haemost 2006; 95(6): 949-57.
[http://dx.doi.org/10.1160/TH06-02-0108] [PMID: 16732373]

[77]   Crider KS, Cleves MA, Reefhuis J, Berry RJ, Hobbs CA, Hu DJ. Antibacterial medication use during pregnancy and risk of birth defects: National Birth Defects Prevention Study. Arch Pediatr Adolesc Med 2009; 163(11): 978-85.
[http://dx.doi.org/10.1001/archpediatrics.2009.188] [PMID: 19884587]

[78]   Hernández-Díaz S, Werler MM, Walker AM, Mitchell AA. Folic acid antagonists during pregnancy and the risk of birth defects. N Engl J Med 2000; 343(22): 1608-14.
[http://dx.doi.org/10.1056/NEJM200011303432204] [PMID: 11096168]

[79]   Czeizel AE, Rockenbauer M, Sørensen HT, Olsen J. The teratogenic risk of trimethoprim-sulfonamides: a population based case-control study. Reprod Toxicol 2001; 15(6): 637-46.
[http://dx.doi.org/10.1016/S0890-6238(01)00178-2] [PMID: 11738517]

[80]   Caro-Patón T, Carvajal A, Martin de Diego I, Martin-Arias LH, Alvarez Requejo A, Rodríguez Pinilla E. Is metronidazole teratogenic? A meta-analysis. Br J Clin Pharmacol 1997; 44(2): 179-82.
[http://dx.doi.org/10.1046/j.1365-2125.1997.00660.x] [PMID: 9278206]

[81]   Burtin P, Taddio A, Ariburnu O, Einarson TR, Koren G. Safety of metronidazole in pregnancy: a meta-analysis. Am J Obstet Gynecol 1995; 172(2 Pt 1): 525-9.
[http://dx.doi.org/10.1016/0002-9378(95)90567-7] [PMID: 7856680]

[82]   Lammer EJ, Chen DT, Hoar RM, *et al.* Retinoic acid embryopathy. N Engl J Med 1985; 313(14): 837-41.
[http://dx.doi.org/10.1056/NEJM198510033131401] [PMID: 3162101]

[83]   Smithells RW, Newman CG. Recognition of thalidomide defects. J Med Genet 1992; 29(10): 716-23.
[http://dx.doi.org/10.1136/jmg.29.10.716] [PMID: 1433232]

[84]   Ericson A, Källén BA. Nonsteroidal anti-inflammatory drugs in early pregnancy. Reprod Toxicol 2001; 15(4): 371-5.
[http://dx.doi.org/10.1016/S0890-6238(01)00137-X] [PMID: 11489592]

[85]   Loffredo CA, Ferencz C, Wilson PD, Lurie IW. Interrupted aortic arch: an epidemiologic study. Teratology 2000; 61(5): 368-75.
[http://dx.doi.org/10.1002/(SICI)1096-9926(200005)61:5<368::AID-TERA8>3.0.CO;2-N]   [PMID: 10777832]

[86]   Hernandez RK, Werler MM, Romitti P, Sun L, Anderka M. National Birth Defects Prevention S. Nonsteroidal antiinflammatory drug use among women and the risk of birth defects. Am J Obstet Gynecol 2012; 206:228: e1-8.

[87]   van Gelder MM, Roeleveld N, Nordeng H. Exposure to non-steroidal anti-inflammatory drugs during pregnancy and the risk of selected birth defects: a prospective cohort study. PLoS One 2011; 6(7)e22174
[http://dx.doi.org/10.1371/journal.pone.0022174] [PMID: 21789231]

[88]   Källén BA, Otterblad Olausson P. Maternal drug use in early pregnancy and infant cardiovascular defect. Reprod Toxicol 2003; 17(3): 255-61.
[http://dx.doi.org/10.1016/S0890-6238(03)00012-1] [PMID: 12759093]

[89]   Koren G, Florescu A, Costei AM, Boskovic R, Moretti ME. Nonsteroidal antiinflammatory drugs during third trimester and the risk of premature closure of the ductus arteriosus: a meta-analysis. Ann Pharmacother 2006; 40(5): 824-9.
[http://dx.doi.org/10.1345/aph.1G428] [PMID: 16638921]

[90]   Huhta JC, Moise KJ, Fisher DJ, Sharif DS, Wasserstrum N, Martin C. Detection and quantitation of constriction of the fetal ductus arteriosus by Doppler echocardiography. Circulation 1987; 75(2): 406-12.
[http://dx.doi.org/10.1161/01.CIR.75.2.406] [PMID: 3802445]

[91]   Ferencz C, Boughman JA. Congenital heart disease in adolescents and adults. Teratology, genetics, and recurrence risks. Cardiol Clin 1993; 11(4): 557-67.
[http://dx.doi.org/10.1016/S0733-8651(18)30138-3] [PMID: 8252559]

[92]   Czeizel AE. Periconceptional folic acid containing multivitamin supplementation. Eur J Obstet Gynecol Reprod Biol 1998; 78(2): 151-61.
[http://dx.doi.org/10.1016/S0301-2115(98)00061-X] [PMID: 9622312]

[93]   Botto LD, Mulinare J, Erickson JD. Do multivitamin or folic acid supplements reduce the risk for congenital heart defects? Evidence and gaps. Am J Med Genet A 2003; 121A(2): 95-101.
[http://dx.doi.org/10.1002/ajmg.a.20132] [PMID: 12910485]

[94]   Botto LD, Mulinare J, Erickson JD. Occurrence of congenital heart defects in relation to maternal multivitamin use. Am J Epidemiol 2000; 151(9): 878-84.
[http://dx.doi.org/10.1093/oxfordjournals.aje.a010291] [PMID: 10791560]

[95]   van Beynum IM, Kapusta L, Bakker MK, den Heijer M, Blom HJ, de Walle HE. Protective effect of periconceptional folic acid supplements on the risk of congenital heart defects: a registry-based case-control study in the northern Netherlands. Eur Heart J 2010; 31(4): 464-71.
[http://dx.doi.org/10.1093/eurheartj/ehp479] [PMID: 19952004]

[96]   Czeizel AE, Dobó M, Vargha P. Hungarian cohort-controlled trial of periconceptional multivitamin supplementation shows a reduction in certain congenital abnormalities. Birth Defects Res A Clin Mol

Teratol 2004; 70(11): 853-61.
[http://dx.doi.org/10.1002/bdra.20086] [PMID: 15523663]

[97]   Botto LD, Khoury MJ, Mulinare J, Erickson JD. Periconceptional multivitamin use and the occurrence of conotruncal heart defects: results from a population-based, case-control study. Pediatrics 1996; 98(5): 911-7.
[PMID: 8909485]

[98]   Werler MM, Hayes C, Louik C, Shapiro S, Mitchell AA. Multivitamin supplementation and risk of birth defects. Am J Epidemiol 1999; 150(7): 675-82.
[http://dx.doi.org/10.1093/oxfordjournals.aje.a010070] [PMID: 10512421]

[99]   Han M, Neves AL, Serrano M, Brinez P, Huhta JC, Acharya G, *et al.* Effects of alcohol, lithium, and homocysteine on nonmuscle myosin-II in the mouse placenta and human trophoblasts. Am J Obstet Gynecol 2012; 207:104: e7-19.
[http://dx.doi.org/10.1016/j.ajog.2012.05.007]

[100]   Huhta JC, Linask K. When should we prescribe high-dose folic acid to prevent congenital heart defects? Curr Opin Cardiol 2015; 30(1): 125-31.
[http://dx.doi.org/10.1097/HCO.0000000000000124] [PMID: 25389654]

[101]   Koster MPH, van Duijn L, Krul-Poel YHM, *et al.* A compromised maternal vitamin D status is associated with congenital heart defects in offspring. Early Hum Dev 2018; 117: 50-6.
[http://dx.doi.org/10.1016/j.earlhumdev.2017.12.011] [PMID: 29287191]

[102]   Obermann-Borst SA, Vujkovic M, de Vries JH, *et al.* A maternal dietary pattern characterised by fish and seafood in association with the risk of congenital heart defects in the offspring. BJOG 2011; 118(10): 1205-15.
[http://dx.doi.org/10.1111/j.1471-0528.2011.02984.x] [PMID: 21585642]

[103]   Holick MF, Binkley NC, Bischoff-Ferrari HA, *et al.* Endocrine Society. Evaluation, treatment, and prevention of vitamin D deficiency: an Endocrine Society clinical practice guideline. J Clin Endocrinol Metab 2011; 96(7): 1911-30.
[http://dx.doi.org/10.1210/jc.2011-0385] [PMID: 21646368]

[104]   Sun J, Chen X, Chen H, *et al.* Maternal Alcohol Consumption Before and During Pregnancy and the Risks of Congenital Heart Defects in Offspring: A Systematic Review and Meta-analysis. Congenit Heart Dis 2015; 10(5): E216-24.
[http://dx.doi.org/10.1111/chd.12271] [PMID: 26032942]

[105]   Martínez-Frías ML, Bermejo E, Rodríguez-Pinilla E, Frías JL. Risk for congenital anomalies associated with different sporadic and daily doses of alcohol consumption during pregnancy: a case-control study. Birth Defects Res A Clin Mol Teratol 2004; 70(4): 194-200.
[http://dx.doi.org/10.1002/bdra.20017] [PMID: 15108246]

[106]   Mateja WA, Nelson DB, Kroelinger CD, Ruzek S, Segal J. The association between maternal alcohol use and smoking in early pregnancy and congenital cardiac defects. J Womens Health (Larchmt) 2012; 21(1): 26-34.
[http://dx.doi.org/10.1089/jwh.2010.2582] [PMID: 21895513]

[107]   Williams LJ, Correa A, Rasmussen S. Maternal lifestyle factors and risk for ventricular septal defects. Birth Defects Res A Clin Mol Teratol 2004; 70(2): 59-64.
[http://dx.doi.org/10.1002/bdra.10145] [PMID: 14991912]

[108]   Tikkanen J, Heinonen OP. Risk factors for atrial septal defect. Eur J Epidemiol 1992; 8(4): 509-15.
[http://dx.doi.org/10.1007/BF00146368] [PMID: 1397217]

[109]   Grewal J, Carmichael SL, Ma C, Lammer EJ, Shaw GM. Maternal periconceptional smoking and alcohol consumption and risk for select congenital anomalies. Birth Defects Res A Clin Mol Teratol 2008; 82(7): 519-26.
[http://dx.doi.org/10.1002/bdra.20461] [PMID: 18481814]

[110]   Browne ML, Hoyt AT, Feldkamp ML, *et al.* Maternal caffeine intake and risk of selected birth defects

in the National Birth Defects Prevention Study. Birth Defects Res A Clin Mol Teratol 2011; 91(2): 93-101.
[http://dx.doi.org/10.1002/bdra.20752] [PMID: 21254365]

[111] Baldacci S, Gorini F, Santoro M, Pierini A, Minichilli F, Bianchi F. Environmental and individual exposure and the risk of congenital anomalies: a review of recent epidemiological evidence Epidemiol Prev 2018; 42 (3-4 Suppl 1): 1-34.

[112] Nicoll R. Environmental contaminants and congenital heart defects: a re-evaluation of the evidence. Int J Environ Res Public Health 2018; 15(10): E2096.
[http://dx.doi.org/10.3390/ijerph15102096] [PMID: 30257432]

[113] Hackshaw A, Rodeck C, Boniface S. Maternal smoking in pregnancy and birth defects: a systematic review based on 173 687 malformed cases and 11.7 million controls. Hum Reprod Update 2011; 17(5): 589-604.
[http://dx.doi.org/10.1093/humupd/dmr022] [PMID: 21747128]

[114] Lee LJ, Lupo PJ. Maternal smoking during pregnancy and the risk of congenital heart defects in offspring: a systematic review and metaanalysis. Pediatr Cardiol 2013; 34(2): 398-407.
[http://dx.doi.org/10.1007/s00246-012-0470-x] [PMID: 22886364]

[115] Malik S, Cleves MA, Honein MA, *et al.* National Birth Defects Prevention Study. Maternal smoking and congenital heart defects. Pediatrics 2008; 121(4): e810-6.
[http://dx.doi.org/10.1542/peds.2007-1519] [PMID: 18381510]

[116] Patel SS, Burns TL, Botto LD, *et al.* National Birth Defects Prevention Study. Analysis of selected maternal exposures and non-syndromic atrioventricular septal defects in the National Birth Defects Prevention Study, 1997-2005. Am J Med Genet A 2012; 158A(10): 2447-55.
[http://dx.doi.org/10.1002/ajmg.a.35555] [PMID: 22903798]

[117] Hoyt AT, Canfield MA, Romitti PA, Botto LD, Anderka MT, Krikov SV, *et al.* Associations between maternal periconceptional exposure to secondhand tobacco smoke and major birth defects. Am J Obstet Gynecol 2016; 215:613: e1-e11.
[http://dx.doi.org/10.1016/j.ajog.2016.07.022]

[118] Cresci M, Foffa I, Ait-Ali L, *et al.* Maternal and paternal environmental risk factors, metabolizing GSTM1 and GSTT1 polymorphisms, and congenital heart disease. Am J Cardiol 2011; 108(11): 1625-31.
[http://dx.doi.org/10.1016/j.amjcard.2011.07.022] [PMID: 21890078]

[119] Karatza AA, Giannakopoulos I, Dassios TG, Belavgenis G, Mantagos SP, Varvarigou AA. Periconceptional tobacco smoking and isolated congenital heart defects in the neonatal period. Int J Cardiol 2011; 148(3): 295-9.
[http://dx.doi.org/10.1016/j.ijcard.2009.11.008] [PMID: 19951824]

[120] Zhang D, Cui H, Zhang L, Huang Y, Zhu J, Li X. Is maternal smoking during pregnancy associated with an increased risk of congenital heart defects among offspring? A systematic review and meta-analysis of observational studies. J Matern Fetal Neonatal Med 2017; 30(6): 645-57.
[http://dx.doi.org/10.1080/14767058.2016.1183640] [PMID: 27126055]

[121] Lipshultz SE, Frassica JJ, Orav EJ. Cardiovascular abnormalities in infants prenatally exposed to cocaine. J Pediatr 1991; 118(1): 44-51.
[http://dx.doi.org/10.1016/S0022-3476(05)81842-6] [PMID: 1986097]

[122] Ritz B, Yu F, Fruin S, Chapa G, Shaw GM, Harris JA. Ambient air pollution and risk of birth defects in Southern California. Am J Epidemiol 2002; 155(1): 17-25.
[http://dx.doi.org/10.1093/aje/155.1.17] [PMID: 11772780]

[123] Strickland MJ, Klein M, Correa A, *et al.* Ambient air pollution and cardiovascular malformations in Atlanta, Georgia, 1986-2003. Am J Epidemiol 2009; 169(8): 1004-14.
[http://dx.doi.org/10.1093/aje/kwp011] [PMID: 19258486]

[124]   Gilboa SM, Mendola P, Olshan AF, *et al.* Relation between ambient air quality and selected birth defects, seven county study, Texas, 1997-2000. Am J Epidemiol 2005; 162(3): 238-52.
[http://dx.doi.org/10.1093/aje/kwi189] [PMID: 15987727]

[125]   Ren Z, Zhu J, Gao Y, *et al.* Maternal exposure to ambient PM_{10} during pregnancy increases the risk of congenital heart defects: Evidence from machine learning models. Sci Total Environ 2018; 630: 1-10.
[http://dx.doi.org/10.1016/j.scitotenv.2018.02.181] [PMID: 29471186]

[126]   Liu CB, Hong XR, Shi M, *et al.* Effects of Prenatal PM_{10} Exposure on Fetal Cardiovascular Malformations in Fuzhou, China: A Retrospective Case-Control Study. Environ Health Perspect 2017; 125(5)057001
[http://dx.doi.org/10.1289/EHP289] [PMID: 28557713]

[127]   Chen EK, Zmirou-Navier D, Padilla C, Deguen S. Effects of air pollution on the risk of congenital anomalies: a systematic review and meta-analysis. Int J Environ Res Public Health 2014; 11(8): 7642-68.
[http://dx.doi.org/10.3390/ijerph110807642] [PMID: 25089772]

[128]   Vrijheid M, Martinez D, Manzanares S, *et al.* Ambient air pollution and risk of congenital anomalies: a systematic review and meta-analysis. Environ Health Perspect 2011; 119(5): 598-606.
[http://dx.doi.org/10.1289/ehp.1002946] [PMID: 21131253]

[129]   Hansen CA, Barnett AG, Jalaludin BB, Morgan GG. Ambient air pollution and birth defects in brisbane, australia. PLoS One 2009; 4(4)e5408
[http://dx.doi.org/10.1371/journal.pone.0005408] [PMID: 19404385]

[130]   Dolk H, Armstrong B, Lachowycz K, *et al.* Ambient air pollution and risk of congenital anomalies in England, 1991-1999. Occup Environ Med 2010; 67(4): 223-7.
[http://dx.doi.org/10.1136/oem.2009.045997] [PMID: 19819865]

[131]   Shaw GM, Schulman J, Frisch JD, Cummins SK, Harris JA. Congenital malformations and birthweight in areas with potential environmental contamination. Arch Environ Health 1992; 47(2): 147-54.
[http://dx.doi.org/10.1080/00039896.1992.10118769] [PMID: 1567240]

[132]   Shaw GM, Nelson V, Iovannisci DM, Finnell RH, Lammer EJ. Maternal occupational chemical exposures and biotransformation genotypes as risk factors for selected congenital anomalies. Am J Epidemiol 2003; 157(6): 475-84.
[http://dx.doi.org/10.1093/aje/kwg013] [PMID: 12631536]

[133]   Loffredo CA, Silbergeld EK, Ferencz C, Zhang J. Association of transposition of the great arteries in infants with maternal exposures to herbicides and rodenticides. Am J Epidemiol 2001; 153(6): 529-36.
[http://dx.doi.org/10.1093/aje/153.6.529] [PMID: 11257060]

[134]   Rappazzo KM, Warren JL, Meyer RE, *et al.* Maternal residential exposure to agricultural pesticides and birth defects in a 2003 to 2005 North Carolina birth cohort. Birth Defects Res A Clin Mol Teratol 2016; 106(4): 240-9.
[http://dx.doi.org/10.1002/bdra.23479] [PMID: 26970546]

[135]   Carmichael SL, Yang W, Roberts E, *et al.* Residential agricultural pesticide exposures and risk of selected congenital heart defects among offspring in the San Joaquin Valley of California. Environ Res 2014; 135: 133-8.
[http://dx.doi.org/10.1016/j.envres.2014.08.030] [PMID: 25262086]

[136]   Tikkanen J, Heinonen OP. Risk factors for ventricular septal defect in Finland. Public Health 1991; 105(2): 99-112.
[http://dx.doi.org/10.1016/S0033-3506(05)80283-5] [PMID: 2068244]

[137]   Wang C, Xie L, Zhou K, *et al.* Increased risk for congenital heart defects in children carrying the ABCB1 Gene C3435T polymorphism and maternal periconceptional toxicants exposure. PLoS One 2013; 8(7): e68807.

[http://dx.doi.org/10.1371/journal.pone.0068807] [PMID: 23874772]

[138] Snijder CA, Vlot IJ, Burdorf A, *et al.* Congenital heart defects and parental occupational exposure to chemicals. Hum Reprod 2012; 27(5): 1510-7.
[http://dx.doi.org/10.1093/humrep/des043] [PMID: 22357765]

[139] Wijnands KP, Zeilmaker GA, Meijer WM, Helbing WA, Steegers-Theunissen RP. Periconceptional parental conditions and perimembranous ventricular septal defects in the offspring. Birth Defects Res A Clin Mol Teratol 2014; 100(12): 944-50.
[http://dx.doi.org/10.1002/bdra.23265] [PMID: 25196200]

[140] Wang C, Zhan Y, Wang F, *et al.* Parental occupational exposures to endocrine disruptors and the risk of simple isolated congenital heart defects. Pediatr Cardiol 2015; 36(5): 1024-37.
[http://dx.doi.org/10.1007/s00246-015-1116-6] [PMID: 25628158]

[141] Kuehl KS, Loffredo CA. Population-based study of l-transposition of the great arteries: possible associations with environmental factors. Birth Defects Res A Clin Mol Teratol 2003; 67(3): 162-7.
[http://dx.doi.org/10.1002/bdra.10015] [PMID: 12797457]

[142] Liu Z, Li X, Li N, *et al.* Association between maternal exposure to housing renovation and offspring with congenital heart disease: a multi-hospital case-control study. Environ Health 2013; 12: 25.
[http://dx.doi.org/10.1186/1476-069X-12-25] [PMID: 23522351]

[143] Watson RE, Jacobson CF, Williams AL, Howard WB, DeSesso JM. Trichloroethylene-contaminated drinking water and congenital heart defects: a critical analysis of the literature. Reprod Toxicol 2006; 21(2): 117-47.
[http://dx.doi.org/10.1016/j.reprotox.2005.07.013] [PMID: 16181768]

[144] Yauck JS, Malloy ME, Blair K, Simpson PM, McCarver DG. Proximity of residence to trichloroethylene-emitting sites and increased risk of offspring congenital heart defects among older women. Birth Defects Res A Clin Mol Teratol 2004; 70(10): 808-14.
[http://dx.doi.org/10.1002/bdra.20060] [PMID: 15390315]

[145] Bove FJ, Fulcomer MC, Klotz JB, Esmart J, Dufficy EM, Savrin JE. Public drinking water contamination and birth outcomes. Am J Epidemiol 1995; 141(9): 850-62.
[http://dx.doi.org/10.1093/oxfordjournals.aje.a117521] [PMID: 7717362]

[146] Goldberg SJ, Lebowitz MD, Graver EJ, Hicks S. An association of human congenital cardiac malformations and drinking water contaminants. J Am Coll Cardiol 1990; 16(1): 155-64.
[http://dx.doi.org/10.1016/0735-1097(90)90473-3] [PMID: 2358589]

[147] Shaw GM, Swan SH, Harris JA, Malcoe LH. Maternal water consumption during pregnancy and congenital cardiac anomalies. Epidemiology 1990; 1(3): 206-11.
[http://dx.doi.org/10.1097/00001648-199005000-00005] [PMID: 2081254]

[148] Hardin BD, Kelman BJ, Brent RL. Trichloroethylene and dichloroethylene: a critical review of teratogenicity. Birth Defects Res A Clin Mol Teratol 2005; 73(12): 931-55.
[http://dx.doi.org/10.1002/bdra.20192] [PMID: 16342278]

[149] Nieuwenhuijsen MJ, Martinez D, Grellier J, *et al.* Chlorination disinfection by-products in drinking water and congenital anomalies: review and meta-analyses. Environ Health Perspect 2009; 117(10): 1486-93.
[http://dx.doi.org/10.1289/ehp.0900677] [PMID: 20019896]

[150] Zierler S, Theodore M, Cohen A, Rothman KJ. Chemical quality of maternal drinking water and congenital heart disease. Int J Epidemiol 1988; 17(3): 589-94.
[http://dx.doi.org/10.1093/ije/17.3.589] [PMID: 3209340]

[151] Jin X, Tian X, Liu Z, *et al.* Maternal exposure to arsenic and cadmium and the risk of congenital heart defects in offspring. Reprod Toxicol 2016; 59: 109-16.
[http://dx.doi.org/10.1016/j.reprotox.2015.12.007] [PMID: 26743994]

[152] Liu Z, Yu Y, Li X, *et al.* Maternal lead exposure and risk of congenital heart defects occurrence in

offspring. Reprod Toxicol 2015; 51: 1-6.
[http://dx.doi.org/10.1016/j.reprotox.2014.11.002] [PMID: 25462788]

[153] Ou Y, Bloom MS, Nie Z, *et al.* Associations between toxic and essential trace elements in maternal blood and fetal congenital heart defects. Environ Int 2017; 106: 127-34.
[http://dx.doi.org/10.1016/j.envint.2017.05.017] [PMID: 28645012]

[154] Vinceti M, Rovesti S, Bergomi M, *et al.* Risk of birth defects in a population exposed to environmental lead pollution. Sci Total Environ 2001; 278(1-3): 23-30.
[http://dx.doi.org/10.1016/S0048-9697(00)00885-8] [PMID: 11669270]

[155] Silver SR, Pinkerton LE, Rocheleau CM, Deddens JA, Michalski AM, Van Zutphen AR. Birth defects in infants born to employees of a microelectronics and business machine manufacturing facility. Birth Defects Res A Clin Mol Teratol 2016; 106(8): 696-707.
[http://dx.doi.org/10.1002/bdra.23520] [PMID: 27224896]

[156] Liu Z, Lin Y, Tian X, *et al.* Association between maternal aluminum exposure and the risk of congenital heart defects in offspring. Birth Defects Res A Clin Mol Teratol 2016; 106(2): 95-103.
[http://dx.doi.org/10.1002/bdra.23464] [PMID: 26707789]

[157] Liu Z, He C, Chen M, *et al.* The effects of lead and aluminum exposure on congenital heart disease and the mechanism of oxidative stress. Reprod Toxicol 2018; 81: 93-8.
[http://dx.doi.org/10.1016/j.reprotox.2018.07.081] [PMID: 30031113]

[158] Zhang N, Liu Z, Tian X, *et al.* Barium exposure increases the risk of congenital heart defects occurrence in offspring. Clin Toxicol (Phila) 2018; 56(2): 132-9.
[http://dx.doi.org/10.1080/15563650.2017.1343479] [PMID: 28705031]

[159] Croen LA, Shaw GM, Sanbonmatsu L, Selvin S, Buffler PA. Maternal residential proximity to hazardous waste sites and risk for selected congenital malformations. Epidemiology 1997; 8(4): 347-54.
[http://dx.doi.org/10.1097/00001648-199707000-00001] [PMID: 9209846]

[160] Orr M, Bove F, Kaye W, Stone M. Elevated birth defects in racial or ethnic minority children of women living near hazardous waste sites. Int J Hyg Environ Health 2002; 205(1-2): 19-27.
[http://dx.doi.org/10.1078/1438-4639-00126] [PMID: 12018013]

[161] Dummer TJ, Dickinson HO, Parker L. Adverse pregnancy outcomes near landfill sites in Cumbria, northwest England, 1950--1993. Arch Environ Health 2003; 58(11): 692-8.
[http://dx.doi.org/10.3200/AEOH.58.11.692-698] [PMID: 15702893]

[162] Langlois PH, Brender JD, Suarez L, *et al.* Maternal residential proximity to waste sites and industrial facilities and conotruncal heart defects in offspring. Paediatr Perinat Epidemiol 2009; 23(4): 321-31.
[http://dx.doi.org/10.1111/j.1365-3016.2009.01045.x] [PMID: 19523079]

[163] Correa-Villaseñor A, Ferencz C, Loffredo C, Magee C. The Baltimore-Washington Infant Study Group. Paternal exposures and cardiovascular malformations. J Expo Anal Environ Epidemiol 1993; 3 (Suppl. 1): 173-85.
[PMID: 9857303]

[164] Grazuleviciene R, Kapustinskiene V, Vencloviene J, Buinauskiene J, Nieuwenhuijsen MJ. Risk of congenital anomalies in relation to the uptake of trihalomethane from drinking water during pregnancy. Occup Environ Med 2013; 70(4): 274-82.
[http://dx.doi.org/10.1136/oemed-2012-101093] [PMID: 23404756]

[165] Malik S, Schecter A, Caughy M, Fixler DE. Effect of proximity to hazardous waste sites on the development of congenital heart disease. Arch Environ Health 2004; 59(4): 177-81.
[http://dx.doi.org/10.3200/AEOH.59.4.177-181] [PMID: 16189989]

CHAPTER 10

Labor Management of Pregnant Women with Fetuses with Congenital Heart Diseases

Edward Araujo Júnior[1,2,*], Christiane Simioni[1], Milene Carvalho Carrilho[1] and Luciano Marcondes Machado Nardozza[1]

[1] *Discipline of Fetal Medicine, Department of Obstetrics, Paulista School of Medicine, Federal University of São Paulo (EPM-UNIFESP), São Paulo-SP, Brazil*

[2] *Medical course, Municipal University of São Caetano do Sul (USCS), Bela Vista Campus, São Paulo-SP, Brazil*

Abstract: Congenital heart defects (CHDs) are the most common defects at birth. Thus, their prenatal diagnosis is extremely important, since early intervention, when required, dramatically reduces newborn mortality. CHDs, that occur both at the intrauterine phase and during the first hours of life, are well tolerated and do not require specialized care during delivery. However, some severe CHDs have an increased risk of hemodynamic instability and may require maintenance of fetal shunts after birth. In these cases, planning the time of delivery and selecting a tertiary hospital are necessary. In some cases, there may be maternal or fetal indications to anticipate delivery, including a variety of obstetric ones. Thus, the birth of a newborn with CHD is a multidisciplinary event, involving obstetricians, neonatologists, and cardiologists.

Keywords: Congenital heart defects, Neonatal care, Prenatal diagnosis, Type of delivery.

INTRODUCTION

Congenital heart defects (CHDs) have an occurrence rate of 4 to 13/1,000 live births [1, 2] and are the most common defects at birth [3 - 5]. It is also estimated that 10% of all gestational losses are due to severe forms of CHDs [6]. Of those born with CHD, about 50% require surgical intervention or evolve with permanent sequelae [4]. According to data from the World Health Organization (WHO), during the years 1950 and 1994, 42% of newborn deaths were due to a CHD [1].

---

* **Address Correspondence Edward Araujo Júnior:** Discipline of Fetal Medicine, Department of Obstetrics, Paulista School of Medicine, Federal University of São Paulo (EPM-UNIFESP), São Paulo-SP, Brazil; Tel: +55-11-37965944; E-mail: araujojred@terra.com.br

There is considerable evidence supporting the heritability of CHDs, indicating a strong correlation with both genetic and environmental factors, however, most CHDs cases are attributed to multifactorial causes involving multiple risk factors that are the result of genetic, epigenetic and environmental ones [6]. Recently, after the outbreak of the Zika virus (ZIKV) infection in Brazil, minor cardiac defects (atrial septal defect, ventricular septal defect, and patent ductus arteriosus) have been reported in fetuses of mothers who have been infected with the ZIKV (positive PCR for the ZIKV), with a higher prevalence in pregnant women presenting cutaneous rashes in the second trimester and/or fetuses with alterations in the central nervous system [7].

Prenatal diagnosis of cardiac defects reduces mortality rate after birth, as it allows early intervention when needed. Other benefits of prenatal diagnosis include parental counseling, screening for other correlated pathologies, planning of the time of delivery, and selection of a tertiary hospital with the ability to provide the necessary care to the newborn with CHD [1, 4, 5].

Most CHDs are well tolerated *in utero*, do not present a risk of hemodynamic instability at birth or in the first days of life, and do not require specialized care during delivery. However, some severe CHDs have an increased risk of hemodynamic instability after delivery and may require maintenance of fetal shunts (*e.g.*, to maintain the permeability of the ductus arteriosus) and/or immediate postnatal interventions [8]. To identify the fetuses with CHD at risk of hemodynamic instability at birth, it is important to understand the physiology of fetal circulation and the transition to the extrauterine one [8].

PRENATAL DIAGNOSIS OF HEART DEFECTS

During ultrasound examinations, it is easier to identify major cardiac defects, thus cardiac malformations diagnosed during the prenatal period lead often to severe and complex pathologies. This is also the main reason for the referral of pregnant women for fetal echocardiography. The association with extracardiac malformations and chromosomal aberrations is also responsible for the diagnosis of most fetal heart defects upon referral for echocardiography due to fetal morphological alterations or due to a positive first and second trimester screening. The inverse may also occur since the identification of a cardiac structural defects may raise the suspicion of other fetal alterations and/or associated syndromes.

Congenital Heart Defects without the Risk of Hemodynamic Instability at Birth

This group includes left-to-right shunt lesions, such as ventricular septal defects (VSDs), atrial septal defects (ASDs), atrioventricular septal defects (AVSDs), and mild valve anomalies. Left-to-right shunt lesions usually become hemodynamically unstable weeks after birth, when a decreased pulmonary vascular resistance causes a significant left-to-right shunt and associated pulmonary overcirculation [8]. Similarly, cardiac function is generally stable after birth in newborns diagnosed during the prenatal period with a mild isolated valve abnormality [9]. These conditions do not require specialized care in the delivery room, childbirth can frequently occur in primary and secondary hospitals and the newborns can be evaluated both in the nursery and in the outpatient clinic [10 - 12].

Congenital Heart Defects with a Minimal Risk of Hemodynamic Instability at Birth

This group mainly includes CHDs that depend on the permeability of ductus arteriosus for the maintenance of the systemic or pulmonary circulation after birth. The ductus arteriosus usually closes 12 to 72 hours after birth [9] and, therefore, these newborns should not be compromised in the delivery room or in the immediate perinatal period [13, 14]. In these cases, prostaglandin E1 therapy may be used to maintain ductal patency. After initial stabilization, the newborn should be sent to the cardiac tertiary care center for an early intervention and/or surgery [8].

Congenital Heart Defects with a High Risk of Hemodynamic Instability at Birth

This group includes cardiac defects that require immediate stabilization after birth with intervention in the immediate perinatal period. Newborns with these conditions should be born in a hospital with pediatric neonatology and cardiology units available on-site, with rapid access to an interventional cardiac catheterization service and cardiac surgery. Examples of CHDs in this category include hypoplastic left heart syndrome (HLHS) with restrictive or closed foramen ovale, transposition of the great arteries (TGA), arrhythmias that are hard to control, complete heart block, tetralogy of Fallot (TOF) with absent pulmonary valve and concern with airway obstruction or with hydrops, severe Ebstein's anomaly with hydrops, and total anomalous pulmonary venous connection obstruction [8].

TYPE OF BIRTH IN CONGENITAL HEART DISEASES DIAGNOSED IN THE PRENATAL PERIOD

Interatrial Septal Anomalies

Interatrial communications (IACs) are classified according to their embryogenesis, location in relation to the oval fossa, and size. Four types are classified in order of frequency: ostium secundum (80% of the cases, usually occurs alone), ostium primum, venous sinus, and coronary sinus. Isolated IACs with no other associated anomalies have a good prognosis.

Intrauterine, the blood usually flows from the right to the left atrium by foramen ovale and therefore the normal physiology is not drastically affected. At birth, newborns are asymptomatic, and the obstetric approach should not be modified.

In cases of restrictive foramen ovale with progressive heart failure, the resolution of the gestation should be also considered, even if prematurely, to prevent worsening of fetal hydrops, which should disappear in the postnatal period due to an establishment of the circulation in series [15].

Ventricular Septal Defects

Most ventricular septal defects (VSDs) appears in isolation, but 40% occur as part of another or more structural cardiac anomalies [16]. Isolated VSDs are the most commonly recognized cardiac defect, accounting for 9.7% of the defects in fetuses and 30% in newborns. They can vary in size and can be single or multiple.

Most isolated VSDs evolve to spontaneous closure before birth (74%). Of those that do not close before birth, 76% will close in the first year of life. The size and the location of the defect influence the spontaneous closure index. In general, apical, perimembranous, and large defects remain permeable, and smaller muscular defects present a greater tendency to close [16]. In these cases, prenatal care should be followed normally, but, immediately after birth, a careful physical evaluation of the newborn should be performed. Newborns with larger defects may need treatment that includes drugs and/or surgery. Surgical intervention is usually necessary when there is pulmonary hypertension, congestive heart failure or hypoxia.

Large inlet defects, which are the most common ones in fetuses, are indicative of a specific fetal karyotype, since they have a high association with trisomy. VSDs associated with chromosomal disorders affect the prognosis and the obstetric approach. The delivery planning of a fetus with a genetic syndrome should be discussed individually with the medical team and the parents, depending on the viability of the fetus and postnatal survival.

Atrioventricular Septal Defects

Atrioventricular septal defects (AVSDs) refer to various cardiac malformations that include abnormalities in the development of the interatrial septum, interventricular septum, and atrioventricular (mitral and tricuspid) valves. Also called atrioventricular canal defects or endocardial cushion defects, the AVSD has an incidence of approximately 2.9% among all congenital heart defects and has been associated with a variety of syndromes and chromosomal abnormalities, accounting for 40% of all cardiac malformations in individuals with Down syndrome [16]. The incidence of CHDs in children of mothers with AVSD is 14%, much higher than most CHDs.

In the complete form of AVSD, the symptoms usually occur early as a result of the large increase in pulmonary blood flow associated with increased pulmonary artery pressure and common atrioventricular valve insufficiency. These newborns usually present together with heart failure, recurrent respiratory infections, and developmental delay. Complete AVSD should be surgically repaired before one year of age to avoid a potentially irreversible pulmonary vascular obstructive disease [16].

The type of delivery of a fetus with septal anomalies should be discussed individually with the medical team and the parents, and a vaginal delivery can be considered in most cases.

Hypoplastic Left Heart Syndrome

Hypoplastic left heart syndrome (HLHS) is the most severe left heart obstructive lesion. To varying degrees, it consists of a small left ventricle and is associated with aortic atresia, hypoplastic ascending aorta, atresia or hypoplasia of the mitral valve and small left atrium. It is the most common cause of death due to CHDs in the initial neonatal period, accounting for 25% of all cardiac deaths [16].

At birth, a newborn with HLHS may appear normal, but starts to develop cyanosis within a few hours due to the mix of arterial and venous blood. Survival depends on the blood flowing from the right ventricle through the ductus arteriosus to the descending aorta. Administration of prostaglandin E1 is recommended to keep the ductus arteriosus permeable.

Without a surgical intervention, newborns with HLHS will die soon after birth. The surgical procedures are aimed at separating the pulmonary and systemic circulations and reducing pulmonary vascular resistance and ventricular pressure overload. The existing surgical technique for HLHS is the Norwood procedure, performed in three stages: stage 1 in the first days of life, stage 2 around 3-4 months of age and stage 3 around 1-2 years of age. Cardiac transplantation for these newborns can be considered. The association of HLHS with cardiovascular anomalies is high. The most common malformations are the coarctation of the aorta and atresia of the mitral valve [16].

Pregnant women with HLHS fetuses can deliver vaginally, but the time of delivery must be planned due to the requirement of a surgical intervention immediately postpartum. Thus, delivery should occur in a tertiary hospital with a readily available surgical team to assist the newborn. Therefore, vaginal delivery or cesarean section should be chosen, both at term, according to the appropriate obstetric standards for each patient.

Right Ventricle Hypoplasia (Pulmonary Atresia with Intact Ventricular Septum/Tricuspid Atresia)

Hypoplasia of the right ventricle rarely occurs as an isolated event. Most commonly, it results from pulmonary atresia with an intact ventricular septum and corresponds to about 1 to 3% of CHDs. It occurs in 0.1 to 0.4 in every 10,000 live births. The classification includes the bipartite ventricle with input, trabecular and output components, bipartite with input and output components, and unipartite with input components. These classifications are useful to determine the surgical treatment that will be used and the prognosis [16]. Tricuspid atresia also results in a hypoplastic right ventricle and is defined as the complete agenesis of the tricuspid valve, resulting in lack of communication in the right side of the heart, between the right atrium and the right ventricle.

Prostaglandin E1 is administered to newborns with pulmonary atresia with an intact ventricular septum at birth to maintain the permeability of the ductus arteriosus until surgery is performed. The type of surgery required depends on the type of associated cardiovascular anomalies [16]. The delivery planning for these pregnant women should be discussed individually with the medical team and the parents.

Univentricular Heart

The univentricular heart disease is a condition in which there are two atrioventricular valves, or one atrioventricular valve associated with a single functional ventricle. It is a rare cardiac anomaly that occurs in 2.5% of live births with congenital heart defects.

The existence of a single ventricle alone does not usually lead to significant hemodynamic changes. Nevertheless, a serial ultrasonographic examination is required to investigate signs of congestive heart failure. If this is not detected, there is no indication to change the type of delivery, but childbirth should occur in a tertiary reference center [15].

After birth, the hemodynamics of the univentricular heart greatly depends on other associated anomalies. The newborns are usually submitted to palliative procedures with early pulmonary artery banding to avoid pulmonary over circulation and heart failure and wait a few months for the Glenn or hemi-Fontan cavopulmonary correction (deviation of blood from the superior vena cava to the right pulmonary artery). After a variable period, on average of two years, the Fontan surgery is completed by directing the flow of the inferior vena cava to the pulmonary artery [15].

Aortic Stenosis and Pulmonary Stenosis

Aortic stenosis can be caused by a variety of lesions that obstruct the outflow of the left ventricle. It occurs in about 3 to 6% of newborns with CHDs. Associated cardiac malformations are observed in about 30% of all cases. Valve stenosis is the most common type of aortic stenosis, occurring in 60-70% of patients with aortic stenosis.

The prognosis and conduct depend on the severity of the lesion, the gestational age at which the diagnosis was made, and the presence of associated anomalies. While advising the parents, it is important to clarify that a severe aortic stenosis diagnosed at 20 to 24 weeks may not present left ventricular enlargement during the gestation, having a typical appearance of an HLHS at 36 weeks, which will prevent biventricular surgical correction, not infrequently leading to fetal hydrops and death. In these situations, the Norwood surgery would be indicated, and all the three steps would be required to complete the correction [15].

Intrauterine balloon valvuloplasty has been reported to improve left ventricular function in cases of critical aortic stenosis. This procedure involves the passage of a 5 mm catheter through the apex of the left ventricle and through the aortic valve. A balloon is then inflated inside the aortic ring.

Without a surgical intervention, the symptomatic newborn with severe aortic stenosis will not survive. Prostaglandin E1 should be administered at birth to maintain the permeability of the ductus arteriosus, thus relieving pulmonary hypertension and maintaining systemic perfusion. The surgical intervention usually consists of transventricular valvotomy, along with open techniques. Critical aortic stenosis requires replacement of the valve.

The obstetric conduct should include ultrasonographic examinations and serial fetal echocardiography to rule out early signs of congestive heart failure and hemodynamic decompensation. The anticipation of delivery in these cases should be avoided since it further increases the mortality rate. Elective cesarean section after pulmonary maturity (after 37 weeks of gestation) is advised in a tertiary center with a cardiovascular surgical team prepared to follow the case in the postnatal period [15].

Congenital pulmonary artery stenosis is defined as the obstruction of the right ventricular outflow tract, either due to an abnormal pulmonary valve or narrowing of the infundibulum. It represents 7.4% of the structural cardiac anomalies of all live births. The obstruction most commonly occurs due to a pulmonary valve anomaly (bicuspid or quadricuspid), with varying degrees of fusion of the leaflets of the valve. Dysplastic pulmonary valves are frequently found in patients with Noonan syndrome [15]. Isolated pulmonary stenosis leads to obstruction of the right ventricular outflow tract and, depending on the degree of stenosis, can lead to congestive heart failure in the fetus.

As with aortic stenosis, the prognosis and conduct depend on the severity of the lesion, the gestational age at which the diagnosis was made, and the presence of associated anomalies. In this case, it is also important to inform the parents that a severe pulmonary stenosis diagnosed at 20 to 24 weeks may not show growth of the right ventricle during the gestation, presenting a typical hypoplastic right heart syndrome at 36 weeks, which will prevent the biventricular surgical correction [15].

Expansion of the pulmonary valve with a balloon catheter has been a good postnatal treatment option for cases with a good size right ventricle.

The obstetric conduct should include serial fetal echocardiography to follow-up the growth and function of both right heart ventricle and pulmonary valve.

Elective cesarean section is advisable after reaching pulmonary maturity (after 37 weeks of gestation) in a tertiary center with a cardiovascular surgical team prepared to follow the case in the postnatal period.

Coarctation of the Aorta

The coarctation of the aorta is the narrowing of the aortic lumen resulting in an obstruction to the blood flow. In 98% of cases, the narrowing is located between the origin of the left subclavian artery and the ductus arteriosus. It is the fifth most common malformation among CHDs. In 32% of cases, coarctation is an isolated anomaly [16]. The coarctation of the aorta causes obstruction of the left ventricular outflow tract and, depending on the severity of the lesion, may lead to left ventricle failure and to hypoperfusion in important organs as well as in the lower limbs.

The prognosis and conduct depend on the severity of the lesion and the gestational age at which the diagnosis was made. Serial ultrasonographic follow-up during prenatal care is recommended to accompany the aggravation or failure of the growth of the aortic arch.

The obstetric conduct should consider the delivery in a tertiary center at around 38 weeks. A hemodynamics and/or cardiovascular surgery team should be prepared to follow the case of the newborn.

Ebstein's Anomaly

The Ebstein's anomaly is defined as the apical displacement of the leaflets of the tricuspid valve (usually the posterior leaflet) from their normal location at the atrioventricular junction inside the right ventricle. This results in a reduction of the functional right ventricle caused by the atrialization of the right ventricular inlet [16]. It occurs at a frequency of 3 to 7% of all fetal heart defects and in 1 to 20,000 live births. The Ebstein's anomaly has been linked to maternal ingestion of lithium carbonate, a drug that is used to treat manic-depressive psychosis, suggesting that lithium is a specific teratogen.

When the Ebstein's anomaly is diagnosed intrauterus, the fetus should be closely monitored to follow the progression of the cardiac dysfunction with resulting cardiomegaly, increased tricuspid insufficiency, tachyarrhythmia, and onset of fetal hydrops. The early cardiomegaly may compromise the prognosis as it impairs the normal development of the lungs. Early neonatal death due to ventilatory impairments is not rare.

The worsening of the intrauterine conditions may be an indication for the delivery, although it is known in advance that the prognosis is poor. An elective full-term cesarean section is recommended in a tertiary hospital under the care of a pediatric cardiology and intensive care team.

Tetralogy of Fallot

The tetralogy of Fallot is the most common cyanotic congenital heart defect and occurs in 7 to 10% of children with CHDs, with a prevalence of around 2-2.5/10,000 live births [17]. As the name suggests, the tetralogy of Fallot consists of four classic features: ventricular septal defect (VSD), aortic cavity (biventricular origin of the aortic valve), infundibulum-valvular pulmonary stenosis, and right ventricle hypertrophy.

Fetuses with the classic form of the tetralogy of Fallot tend to evolve well in the postnatal period, getting stabilized around the first week of life, and being discharged and receiving outpatient follow-up care while waiting for the best time for the surgical intervention. Surgeries are usually palliative, of the pulmonary systemic anastomosis type, although there are already quite encouraging results with the early corrective surgery.

The dependent ductus arteriosus and the required prostaglandin therapy are usually factors associated with pulmonary atresia or more severe obstruction of the right ventricular outflow tract. These tend to represent a more severe type of the disease, progressing with congestive heart failure. The hospital mortality rate is usually high, over 50%.

Pregnant women whose fetuses are carriers of the tetralogy of Fallot should be referred for full-term delivery at a tertiary reference center, with an available pediatric cardiologist and a cardiac surgery team.

Transposition of the Great Arteries

The transposition of the great arteries (TGA) is a frequent cyanotic heart defect, characterized by an altered exit of the great arteries from the ventricles, that is, the aorta arises from the right ventricle and the pulmonary artery from the left ventricle. It occurs in 5 to 7% of all cases of CHDs in childhood and has a prevalence of around 2-3/10,000 live births.

The TGA is rarely associated with chromosomal or extracardiac anomalies. Therefore, counseling will depend on the type of cardiac defect detected. Echocardiographic monitoring should be repeated monthly to investigate the development of other late-onset lesions.

There is a strict indication for delivery to occur in a tertiary reference center, with an available pediatric cardiologist and a cardiac surgery team. The delivery must occur in the hospital that will then follow the cardiac condition of the new delivery to avoid any transfer.

Double Outlet Right Ventricle

The double outlet right ventricle (DORV) refers to cardiac lesions with an abnormal ventriculoarterial connection. The DORV is more commonly defined as a disease in which more than 50% of the aortic root and pulmonary artery originate from the ventricle that has the morphological characteristics of a right one, regardless of whether this ventricle is located to the right. The incidence in newborns is around 0.03-0.07 per 1,000 live births.

The prognosis will depend on the type of DORV, by the complexity of the associated lesions and by the presence of chromosomal anomalies, such as trisomy of chromosomes 13 and 18. A serial echocardiographic follow-up is mandatory to investigate the development of late-onset lesions. It is advisable that childbirth occurs in a tertiary reference center, with an available pediatric cardiologist and cardiac surgery team.

PLANNING THE BIRTH OF FETUSES DIAGNOSED WITH CONGENITAL HEART DISEASES

The delivery planning should consider three main factors: the risk of hemodynamic instability at birth, the resources of the region, the presence of obstetric complications.

Selecting the Hospital and the Transfer of the Newborn

Most newborns with CHDs do not require specialized perinatal care and it is recommended that they are born at the local hospital and followed up as outpatients [18]. However, if a specialized pediatric cardiology and intensive care team are required after delivery, the selected birth location must take into account these special needs [8].

Gestational Age at Delivery

Recent studies have shown that delivery in fetuses diagnosed with severe CHDs tends to occur sooner than in those with a CHD diagnosis made after birth [19]. This is a concerning finding since healthy newborns born at 37 or 38 weeks of gestation are at a higher risk of worse outcomes as compared to those born later, at 39 or 40 weeks [8, 20]. Study has shown that newborns with CHDs stay in intensive care units for longer periods and present higher mortality when born before 39 weeks [20]. Therefore, if there are no fetal or maternal indications for prematurity, the potential advantages of elective preterm delivery of fetuses with CHDs should be carefully considered [8].

In addition to increased mortality, there is increasing evidence that the decision on the time of delivery of fetuses with CHDs should also consider the potential effect of the gestational age at birth on the neurological outcome and, therefore, the full-term delivery of these newborns, or the closest possible to full-term, may improve brain development and decrease susceptibility to postnatal lesions [8].

Type of Delivery

Most experts agree that, in the absence of cardiac failure, hemodynamic decompensation, fetal hydrops, or sustained fetal arrhythmia, elective preterm delivery does not confer an advantage [8]. It is often stated that vaginal delivery should be the preferred option in fetuses with CHD [8], leaving cesarean sections for obstetric indications. Data from retrospective studies show that prenatal diagnosis of severe CHD, such as HLHS, TGA, DORV or TOF, increases the likelihood of cesarean sections. In fetuses with CHDs, the mode of delivery has not been shown to affect the Apgar score, pre- and post-operative morbidity, including the risk of hemodynamic instability, metabolic acidosis and end-organ dysfunction, duration of hospitalization, or survival for surgery or hospital discharge [21]. Two retrospective studies have concluded that vaginal delivery is safe for fetuses with CHDs in most cases [8, 21], but the impact on functional outcomes and long-term brain development are largely unknown [8].

Fetal Vitality During Labor

The decision to perform a vaginal delivery in women with a prenatal diagnosis of fetal CHD opens a debate on how to monitor these fetuses during labor in order to identify and act on those with risk of hypoxemia, to minimize the risk of hypoxic-ischemic encephalopathy and adverse long-term neurological outcome.

Retrospective study evaluated the use of cardiotocography during labor of fetuses with CHDs and shown that these fetuses present higher percentage of non-reassuring traces, but no characteristic fetal heart rate pattern has been related to specific cardiac pathologies [22]. As in normal fetuses, the use of continuous cardiotocography during labor of fetuses with CHDs has been associated with an increased rate of emergency cesarean sections [22].

CONCLUSION

The detection of intrauterine CHD allows for better prenatal counseling and delivery planning, especially when urgent postnatal intervention is required, which can be anticipated based on available predictive models. Perinatal management should be tailored to the specific needs of the mother and fetus and should include decisions about location and time and mode of delivery. In selected cases, there may be maternal or fetal indications supporting the anticipation of delivery, including a variety of obstetric indications, such as preterm birth, maternal comorbidities, complications during pregnancy, or non-reassuring fetal vitality test results. Collaboration between specialized obstetric and pediatric services and a careful perinatal management and delivery planning after a prenatal CHD diagnosis can improve the perinatal status of newborns, possibly improving both survival and long-term outcomes.

CONSENT FOR PUBLICATION

Not applicable.

CONFLICT OF INTEREST

The authors confirm that the contents of this chapter have no conflict of interest.

ACKNOWLEDGEMENTS

Declare none.

REFERENCES

[1]   Carvalho JS, Allan LD, Chaoui R, *et al.* International Society of Ultrasound in Obstetrics and Gynecology. ISUOG Practice Guidelines (updated): sonographic screening examination of the fetal heart. Ultrasound Obstet Gynecol 2013; 41(3): 348-59.
[http://dx.doi.org/10.1002/uog.12403] [PMID: 23460196]

[2]   Carvalho JS, Mavrides E, Shinebourne EA, Campbell S, Thilaganathan B. Improving the effectiveness of routine prenatal screening for major congenital heart defects. Heart 2002; 88(4): 387-91.
[http://dx.doi.org/10.1136/heart.88.4.387] [PMID: 12231598]

[3]   Foy PM, Wheller JJ, Samuels P, Evans KD. Evaluation of the fetal heart at 14 to 18 weeks' gestation in fetuses with a screening nuchal translucency greater than or equal to the 95th percentile. J Ultrasound Med 2013; 32(10): 1713-9.
[http://dx.doi.org/10.7863/ultra.32.10.1713] [PMID: 24065251]

[4]   Lai CW, Chau AK, Lee CP. Comparing the accuracy of obstetric sonography and fetal echocardiography during pediatric cardiology consultation in the prenatal diagnosis of congenital heart disease. J Obstet Gynaecol Res 2016; 42(2): 166-71.
[http://dx.doi.org/10.1111/jog.12870] [PMID: 26555867]

[5]   McBrien A, Sands A, Craig B, Dornan J, Casey F. Impact of a regional training program in fetal echocardiography for sonographers on the antenatal detection of major congenital heart disease. Ultrasound Obstet Gynecol 2010; 36(3): 279-84.
[http://dx.doi.org/10.1002/uog.7616] [PMID: 20205153]

[6]   Maslen CL. Recent advances in placenta-heart interactions. Front Physiol 2018; 9: 735.
[http://dx.doi.org/10.3389/fphys.2018.00735] [PMID: 29962966]

[7]   Orofino DHG, Passos SRL, de Oliveira RVC, *et al.* Cardiac findings in infants with *in utero* exposure to Zika virus- a cross sectional study. PLoS Negl Trop Dis 2018; 12(3):e0006362.
[http://dx.doi.org/10.1371/journal.pntd.0006362] [PMID: 29579059]

[8]   Sanapo L, Moon-Grady AJ, Donofrio MT. Perinatal and delivery management of infants with congenital heart disease. Clin Perinatol 2016; 43(1): 55-71.
[http://dx.doi.org/10.1016/j.clp.2015.11.004] [PMID: 26876121]

[9]   Lim MK, Hanretty K, Houston AB, Lilley S, Murtagh EP. Intermittent ductal patency in healthy newborn infants: demonstration by colour Doppler flow mapping. Arch Dis Child 1992; 67(10 Spec No): 1217-8.
[http://dx.doi.org/10.1136/adc.67.10_Spec_No.1217] [PMID: 1444565]

[10]   Friedman AH, Fahey JT. The transition from fetal to neonatal circulation: normal responses and implications for infants with heart disease. Semin Perinatol 1993; 17(2): 106-21.
[PMID: 8327901]

[11]   Donofrio MT, Duplessis AJ, Limperopoulos C. Impact of congenital heart disease on fetal brain development and injury. Curr Opin Pediatr 2011; 23(5): 502-11.
[http://dx.doi.org/10.1097/MOP.0b013e32834aa583] [PMID: 21881507]

[12]   Rosenthal GL. Patterns of prenatal growth among infants with cardiovascular malformations: possible fetal hemodynamic effects. Am J Epidemiol 1996; 143(5): 505-13.
[http://dx.doi.org/10.1093/oxfordjournals.aje.a008771] [PMID: 8610666]

[13]   Johnson BA, Ades A. Delivery room and early postnatal management of neonates who have prenatally diagnosed congenital heart disease. Clin Perinatol 2005; 32(4): 921-946, ix.
[http://dx.doi.org/10.1016/j.clp.2005.09.014] [PMID: 16325670]

[14]   Donofrio MT, Skurow-Todd K, Berger JT, *et al.* Risk-stratified postnatal care of newborns with congenital heart disease determined by fetal echocardiography. J Am Soc Echocardiogr 2015; 28(11): 1339-49.
[http://dx.doi.org/10.1016/j.echo.2015.07.005] [PMID: 26298099]

[15]   McElhinney DB, Marshall AC, Wilkins-Haug LE, *et al.* Predictors of technical success and postnatal biventricular outcome after *in utero* aortic valvuloplasty for aortic stenosis with evolving hypoplastic left heart syndrome. Circulation 2009; 120(15): 1482-90.
[http://dx.doi.org/10.1161/CIRCULATIONAHA.109.848994] [PMID: 19786635]

[16]   Słodki M, Rizzo G, Augustyniak A, *et al.* Retrospective cohort study of prenatally and postnatally diagnosed coarctation of the aorta (CoA): prenatal diagnosis improve neonatal outcome in severe CoA. J Matern Fetal Neonatal Med 2018; 5: 1-5. Epub ahead of print
[http://dx.doi.org/10.1080/14767058.2018.1510913] [PMID: 30185080]

[17]   Allan L, Hornberger L, Sharland SG. Textbook of Fetal Cardiolgy. London: Oxford University Press 2005.

[18]   Donofrio MT, Moon-Grady AJ, Hornberger LK, *et al.* American Heart Association Adults With Congenital Heart Disease Joint Committee of the Council on Cardiovascular Disease in the Young and Council on Clinical Cardiology, Council on Cardiovascular Surgery and Anesthesia, and Council on Cardiovascular and Stroke Nursing. Diagnosis and treatment of fetal cardiac disease: a scientific statement from the American Heart Association. Circulation 2014; 129(21): 2183-242.
[http://dx.doi.org/10.1161/01.cir.0000437597.44550.5d] [PMID: 24763516]

[19]   Levey A, Glickstein JS, Kleinman CS, *et al.* The impact of prenatal diagnosis of complex congenital heart disease on neonatal outcomes. Pediatr Cardiol 2010; 31(5): 587-97.
[http://dx.doi.org/10.1007/s00246-010-9648-2] [PMID: 20165844]

[20]   Costello JM, Polito A, Brown DW, *et al.* Birth before 39 weeks' gestation is associated with worse outcomes in neonates with heart disease. Pediatrics 2010; 126(2): 277-84.
[http://dx.doi.org/10.1542/peds.2009-3640] [PMID: 20603261]

[21]   Walsh CA, MacTiernan A, Farrell S, *et al.* Mode of delivery in pregnancies complicated by major fetal congenital heart disease: a retrospective cohort study. J Perinatol 2014; 34(12): 901-5.
[http://dx.doi.org/10.1038/jp.2014.104] [PMID: 24875409]

[22]   Ueda K, Ikeda T, Iwanaga N, *et al.* Intrapartum fetal heart rate monitoring in cases of congenital heart disease. Am J Obstet Gynecol 2009; 201(1): 64.e1-6.
[http://dx.doi.org/10.1016/j.ajog.2009.03.015] [PMID: 19481721]

CHAPTER 11

Fetal Cardiac Intervention

Pablo Marantz[1,*], **Sofía Grinenco**[1] and **Lucas Otãno**[2]

[1] *Department of Pediatric Cardiology, Hospital Italiano de Buenos Aires, Buenos Aires, Argentina*

[2] *Department of Obstetrics and Gynecology, Fetal Medicine Unit, Hospital Italiano de Buenos Aires, Buenos Aires, Argentina*

Abstract: Fetal heart interventions have been developed for select cardiac defects in order to alter the natural history of disease and improve patients' outcomes. Intervention rationale and patient selection criteria, as well as associated risks and procedural technical considerations have been reviewed. Fetal aortic valvuloplasty is performed in fetuses with severe aortic stenosis with evolving hypoplastic left heart syndrome, with improving rates of biventricular outcome and early survival; and in rare cases of fetuses with aortic stenosis with severe mitral insufficiency and restrictive foramen ovale. Fetal atrial septoplasty with atrial septal stent placement in patients with hypoplastic left heart syndrome with intact or highly restrictive atrial septum has not yet demonstrated a decrease in the disease's associated mortality. There is limited data regarding the results of fetal pulmonary valvuloplasty in fetuses with pulmonary atresia with intact ventricular septum with evolving hypoplastic right ventricle. Pericardiocentesis for severe pericardial effusion secondary to heart tumors or a cardiac diverticulum or aneurysm continues to be a rare procedure in an exceptional condition. Key aspects regarding selection criteria for intervention and technical and clinical results, require further study in a multicenter collaborative approach.

Keywords: Aortic valve stenosis, Catheterization, Congenital heart defects, Critical aortic stenosis, Diverticulum, Fetal cardiac intervention, Fetal cardiology, Fetal echocardiography, Fetal heart, Fetal pulmonary valvuloplasty, Fetal therapies, Hydrops fetalis, Hypoplastic left heart syndrome, Intrauterine valvuloplasty, Mitral valve insufficiency, Pericardial effusion, Prenatal diagnosis, Pulmonary atresia with intact ventricular septum, Stent, Ultrasonography.

INTRODUCTION

Fetal cardiac interventions have been performed during the last decades in at least 35 specialized centers across the world. They are technically challenging procedures, performed by multidisciplinary teams in highly selected cases. The

---

* **Address Correspondence Pablo Marantz:** Department of Pediatric Cardiology, Hospital Italiano de Buenos Aires, Tte. Gral. Juan Domingo Perón 4190,C.A.B.A., Buenos Aires, Argentina C1199ABB; Tel: (54 11) 4959-0200; E-mail: pablo.marantz@hospitalitaliano.org.ar

Edward Araujo Júnior, Nathalie Jeanne M. Bravo-Valenzuela and Alberto Borges Peixoto (Eds.)

accumulated experience and expertise, enhanced since 2011 by the creation of a multicenter International Fetal Cardiac Intervention Registry (IFCIR; www.ifcir.com), has allowed general consensus in terms of indication and patient selection criteria for fetal cardiac interventions, and in procedural technique aspects [1]. Information regarding these patients´ clinical outcomes, and optimal postnatal therapeutic strategies will require further international collaboration in research focused on the evaluation of mid and long-term follow-up.

INTERVENTION RATIONALE AND PATIENT SELECTION CRITERIA

The aim of fetal heart interventions is to modify the natural history of certain congenital heart defects (CHD) and thus improve patients´ prognosis in terms of survival and quality of life after birth. These CHD can evolve during gestation with heart failure, hydrops and fetal demise; or they can progress with damage and hypoplasia of heart valves, chambers and/or vessels, and with severe myocardial and/or pulmonary vasculature damage [2 - 4] (Table 1). There are specific fetal echocardiographic criteria, concerning both structural and functional aspects of these CHD, that are considered when selecting patients for these procedures [5 - 9].

Table 1. Types of congenital heart defects amenable to fetal cardiac interventions, and type of procedures performed.

Congenital Heart Defect	Fetal Cardiac Intervention
Aortic stenosis with echocardiographic criteria of progression to HLHS	Fetal aortic valvuloplasty
Aortic stenosis with severe mitral insufficiency, restrictive FO and severely dilated left atrium	Fetal aortic valvuloplasty and/or fetal atrial septoplasty with atrial septal stent placement
HLHS with severely restrictive FO or intact atrial septum	Fetal atrial septoplasty with atrial septal stent placement
Pulmonary atresia with intact ventricular septum and echocardiographic criteria of progression to hypoplastic right ventricle and single-ventricle circulation	Fetal pulmonary valvuloplasty
Severe pericardial effusion, generally secondary to heart tumors or cardiac diverticulum	Fetal Pericardiocentesis (serial pericardiocentesis or placement of a pericardiac amniotic shunt in cases with recurrence of pericardial effusion)

HLHS: hypoplastic left heart syndrome; FO: foramen ovale.

Fetal cardiac procedures can be performed during the second trimester or the first weeks of the third trimester. Intervening in this stage of gestation has the potential of avoiding the development of severe and irreversible heart and pulmonary damage. Moreover, the cannulas and stylet needles and the coronary balloon catheters available for these procedures are most suitable for fetuses in this stage of gestation. Chromosomal abnormalities and major anomalies in other organs should always be ruled out before selecting a patient for intervention.

In our series, at Hospital Italiano de Buenos Aires, among 54 patients selected during a 13-year-period for fetal heart intervention based on fetal echocardiographic findings, three were excluded for intervention at detecting major fetal extracardiac anomalies or chromosomal defects (Fig. **1**).

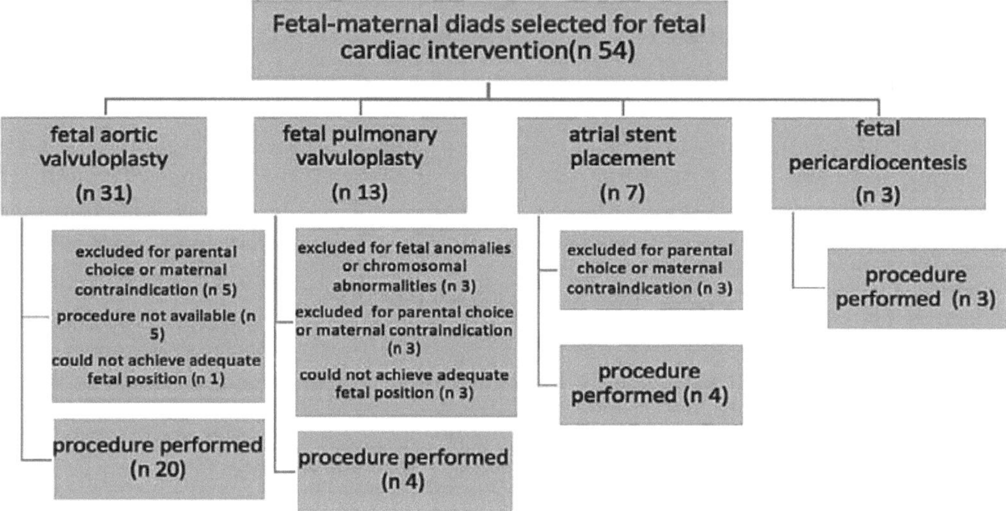

Fig. (1). Patients selected for fetal heart intervention at Hospital Italiano de Buenos Aires.

PATIENTS´ RISKS AND TECHNICAL CONSIDERATIONS

Fetal interventions should be safe for the mother. No significant maternal adverse outcomes related to fetal heart interventions have been reported to date [10].

Maternal laparotomy, that was initially used in order to aid fetal positioning maneuvers, has been currently abandoned as a practice, not actually having demonstrated benefits [1]. Achieving appropriate fetal position, which varies according to the type of fetal cardiac procedure performed is crucial for procedural technical success. If the fetus is not spontaneously in the proper position, fetal external version maneuvers are required.

The procedures are usually performed under maternal regional anesthesia, spinal or epidural, and fetal analgesia and neuromuscular blockade (which involves a combination of fentanyl, vecuronium or pancuronium, and atropine). Fetal medication is administered by intramuscular or umbilical cord puncture, under permanent ultrasonographic guidance. A cannula (12 cm, 18 or 19-gauge, for most interventions) and stylet needle are introduced through the maternal abdomen, uterine wall, amniotic cavity, fetal chest wall and into the heart or into the pericardium cavity. According to the fetal procedure required, pericardial fluid can be extracted, a coronary angioplasty balloon catheter progressed across the aortic or pulmonary valves for valvuloplasty, or a pre-mounted stent can be delivered and placed across the atrial septum.

Fetal cardiac procedures pose significant risks for the fetuses. The most frequent associated complications are: hemopericardium, bradycardia with hemodynamic instability, and tachyarrhythmias. Intraprocedural resuscitation maneuvers include pericardiocentesis or pericardial drainage for significant effusion ($\geq$ 3 mm), intracardiac and/or intramuscular administration of epinephrine or atropine for persistent fetal bradycardia ($\leq$ 110 bpm for $\geq$ 60 seconds), or, less frequently, administration of digoxin for persistent supraventricular tachycardia [11]. Overall procedural related fetal death was 7% in our center, and 11% in the initial report of the IFCIR [1]. The number of procedures required to ensure a center's learning curve and ongoing proficiency, and the team-based skill sets required for these maternal-fetal complex interventions, are still under scrutiny. A systematic review, with a metanalysis, of perinatal outcomes and intrauterine complications following fetal heart interventions for CHD by Araujo Júnior *et al.* has brought out the current difficulties and limitations in data analysis due to the absence of randomized controlled trials [12].

FETAL AORTIC VALVULOPLASTY FOR FETAL AORTIC STENOSIS EVOLVING TO HYPOPLASTIC LEFT HEART SYNDROME

Fetuses with severe valvar aortic stenosis in the mid-second or beginning of the third trimester of gestation, undergo myocardial damage due to subendocardial ischemia and abnormal coronary blood flow; and impeded left-sided heart structures' growth, with progression to a hypoplastic left heart syndrome (HLHS).

A fetal aortic valvuloplasty has the potential of modifying the disease's natural history by allowing an increase in antegrade aortic flow, and thus improving left ventricular function and growth, and aortic and mitral valves' growth [13].

There are specific fetal echocardiographic criteria for selecting the patients for intervention, including a threshold scoring system proposed to identify those cases with a higher likeliness for achieving a biventricular pathway after a fetal aortic valvuloplasty [5] (Table **2**) (Fig. **2**). In recent studies, other factors, such as left ventricle (LV) pressure, size of the ascending aorta and diastolic function have been associated likelihood of biventricular circulation after fetal aortic valvuloplasty [14, 15].

Table 2. Criteria for patient selection for fetal aortic valvuloplasty.

1. Severe valvar AoV stenosis (decreased valve leaflets mobility with antegrade Doppler color flow jet across AoV smaller than valve annulus diameter, and with none or minimal sub valvar outflow obstruction)
2. LV with qualitatively depressed function, but generating at least 10 mmHg pressure gradient across AoV or 15 mmHg mitral regurgitation jet gradient
3. LV long-axis Z score ≥ -2 and MV annulus diameter Z score > -3
4. Retrograde or bidirectional flow in the transverse aortic arch; OR 2 of the following: monophasic mitral inflow Doppler pattern, left-to-right flow across the atrial septum or an intact atrial septum, and bidirectional flow in pulmonary veins
5. Threshold scoring system, fulfilling at least 4 of the following criteria:
a. LV long-axis Z score > 0
b. LV short-axis Z score > 0
c. AoV annulus Z score > -3.5
d. MV annulus Z score > -2
e. MV regurgitation or AoV stenosis maximum systolic gradient ≥ 20 mmHg

AoV: aortic valve; LV: left ventricle; MV: mitral valve.

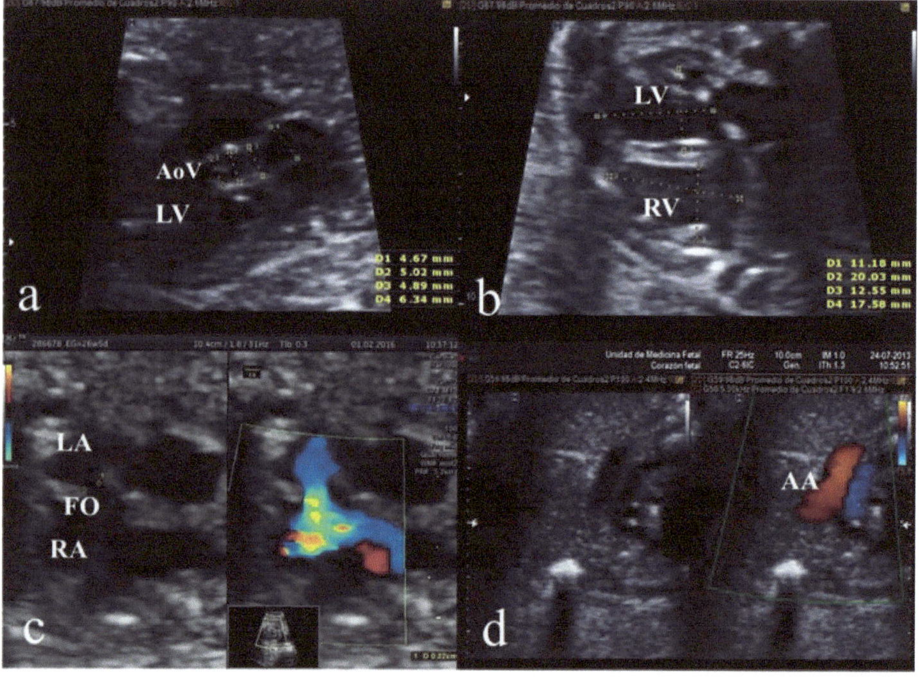

Fig. (2). Echocardiographic findings in fetus with aortic stenosis evolving to hypoplastic left heart syndrome. **a**, Aortic valve stenosis. **b**, Dilated left ventricle. **c**, left-to-right flow across the foramen ovale. **d**, retrograde flow across the aortic arch. AoV: aortic valve; LV: left ventricle; RV: right ventricle; LA: left atrium; RA: right atrium FO: foramen ovale; AA: aortic arch.

The optimal fetal position for aortic valvuloplasty is with the left side of the chest upwards. The needle is introduced in the fetal heart through the LV apex and progressed into the LV outlet and across the stenotic aortic valve, where the cannula is progressed, and the balloon inflated several times and ideally to a 1:1.2 valve annulus: balloon ratio [16]. If the procedure is technically successful antegrade flow across the valve increases, and in some cases, there is also antegrade flow across the aortic arch (Fig. **3**). Procedural success rates reported are in the 70 - 80% range, with 82% in Boston; 78.6% in Austria; and 75% in our center [14 - 16].

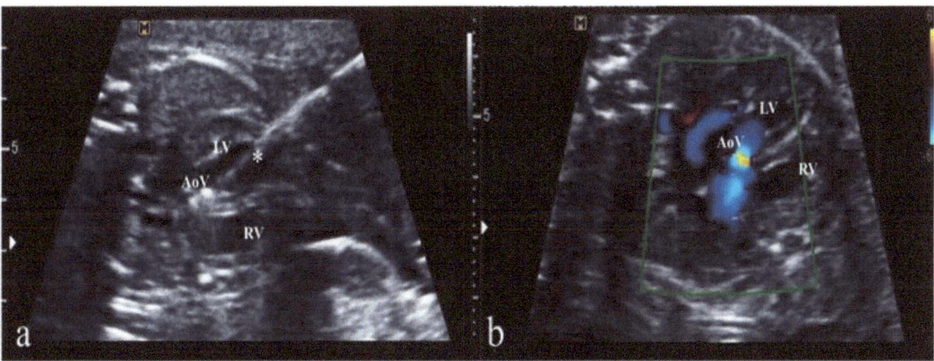

Fig. (3). a, Fetal aortic valvuloplasty: balloon dilatation of a severely stenotic aortic valve. Note the needle passing through the stenotic aortic valve (*). **b**, Antegrade aortic flow after fetal aortic valvuloplasty in a mid-trimester fetus. LV: left ventricle; RV: right ventricle; AoV: aortic valve.

Postnatal therapeutic strategies depend on the clinical status of the newborn and the particular cardiac anatomic and functional features and vary according to different medical centers. These interventions include different combinations of catheter-based and surgical treatment; such as transcatheter aortic valvuloplasty, surgical aortic valvotomy, surgical correction of aortic coarctation, neonatal Ross procedure, aortic or mitral valve repair or replacement, Damus-Kaye-Stansel procedure, Norwood procedure, Glenn operation and take-down strategies.

The group of Boston Children's Hospital has recently reported 59% (27/46) of live born patients who underwent a technically successful fetal aortic valvuloplasty and achieved a biventricular circulation postnatal [14, 15]. At Linz Hospital the biventricular circulation rate reached 66.7% (10/15), and from the IFCIR registry 42.8% (24/56) was reported [1, 16]. At Hospital Italiano de Buenos Aires there were 60% (6/10) patients with technically successful fetal interventions and a biventricular outcome.

HYPOPLASTIC LEFT HEART SYNDROME WITH SEVERELY RESTRICTIVE FORAMEN OVALE OR INTACT ATRIAL SEPTUM

A severely restrictive foramen ovale or an intact atrial septum (IAS), in patients with a hypoplastic left ventricle leads to an increase in left atrial pressure and to the dilatation of pulmonary veins and lymphatics, with varying degrees of arterialization of the pulmonary veins and postnatal development of pulmonary hypertension. At birth, a high-risk urgent decompression of the atrial septum is needed to avoid severe hypoxemia due to pulmonary venous return obstruction, with high associated neonatal mortality. A two centre study reported overall survival to stage 2 or transplantation of 85% in patients with HLHS with adequate interatrial communication, and 67% in those with HLHS with intact atrial septum requiring immediate transcatheter intervention [17].

An intact or highly restrictive atrial septum is suspected when a thick not freely mobile atrial septum with limited or absent shunting on color Doppler interrogation. In the pulsed-wave Doppler evaluation of pulmonary vein flow a forward (combined S and D waves) VTI (velocity-time integral): reverse (A wave) VTI ratio threshold of 3 or less allows the identification of fetuses with higher risk of requiring early atrial septostomy at birth, and selected as candidates for fetal cardiac intervention [18] (Fig. **4**).

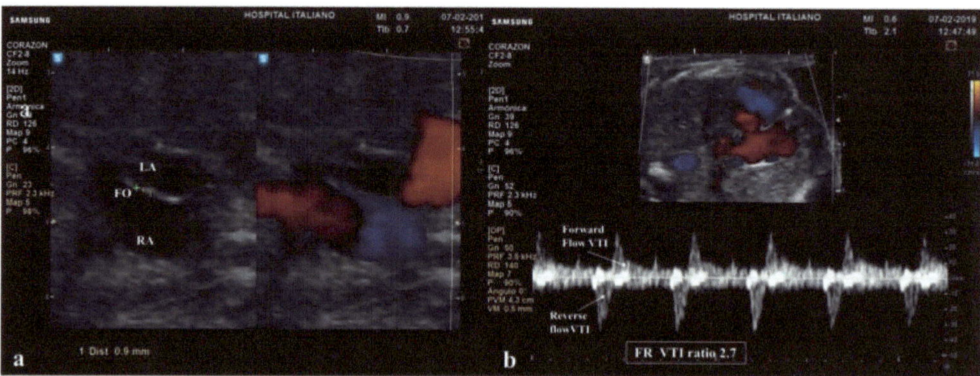

Fig. (4). Fetal echocardiographic findings in a 22-weeks of gestation fetus with hypoplastic left heart syndrome and restrictive foramen ovale. **a**, small, < 1mm, restrictive foramen ovale. **b**, pulsed-wave Doppler pulmonar vein flow pattern with VTI FR ratio 2.7. FO: foramen ovale; RA: right atrium; LA: left atrium; VTI: velocity-time integral; FR: forward reverse.

In these patients, the prenatal decompression of the restrictive atrial septum has the potential to prevent the progression to severe and irreversible damage of the pulmonary vasculature, and to improve oxygenation after birth, in some cases even sparing an urgent neonatal Rashkind procedure [19 - 21]. In a multicenter FICIR-based report atrial septal stent placement was better than atrial septoplasty (atrial perforation/balloon dilatation) in maintaining a nonrestrictive foramen ovale at delivery following procedurally success (75% *vs.* 39%, p=0.075) (Fig. **5**). Successful interventions were associated with reduced C-sections and improved neonatal stability at delivery, but no significant improvement in overall survival at discharge was observed [22]. Pulmonary vascular changes at autopsy of patients with successful *in utero* interventions suggest that interventions earlier in gestation might be needed to prevent pulmonary parenchymal damage, posing new technical challenges for achieving intervention in smaller hearts [23].

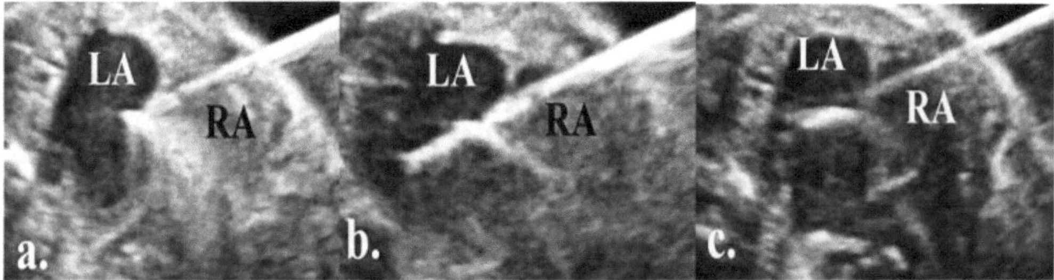

Fig. (5). Atrial septum stent placement in a fetus with aortic stenosis and restrictive atrial septum, **a**. the 19-G needle across the right atrium punctures the atrial septum, **b**. the cannula and guidewire across the atrial septum and into the left atrium, **c**. releasing the stent in the atrial septum. LA: left atrium; RA: right atrium.

AORTIC STENOSIS WITH SEVERE MITRAL INSUFFICIENCY, RESTRICTIVE FORAMEN OVALE AND SEVERELY DILATED LEFT ATRIUM

Severe aortic stenosis associated with an abnormal mitral valve with severe regurgitation and a severely restrictive or intact atrial septum produces severe left atrial dilatation and LV dysfunction and dilatation, which evolves with right chambers´ compression, low cardiac output and hydrops. Moreover, left atrial enlargement causes the compression of the esophagus and polyhydramnios, increasing the risk for premature birth. Thus, the prognosis is poor. Fetal cardiac intervention has been proposed for improving both prenatal and postnatal survival, ideally by a combination of a fetal aortic valvuloplasty and a fetal atrial septoplasty with an atrial septal stent placement in order to improve the fetal heart function and hemodynamics.

In the first reported experience 7/10 intervened patients survived to delivery and 2 of them were alive at the time of report. In only 1 fetus both aortic valvuloplasty and atrial septal opening procedures were performed. All 7 patients diagnosed in the neonatal period died soon after birth [8]. In our center, among 5 fetuses diagnosed, 2 were not intervened and died after birth, 2 were hydropic and died during fetal aortic valvuloplasty, and in 1 patient fetal aortic valvuloplasty and atrial stent placing were performed with a favorable outcome (neonatal Ross procedure, mitral operation at 6 months of age, currently alive 1-year old) (Fig. **6**).

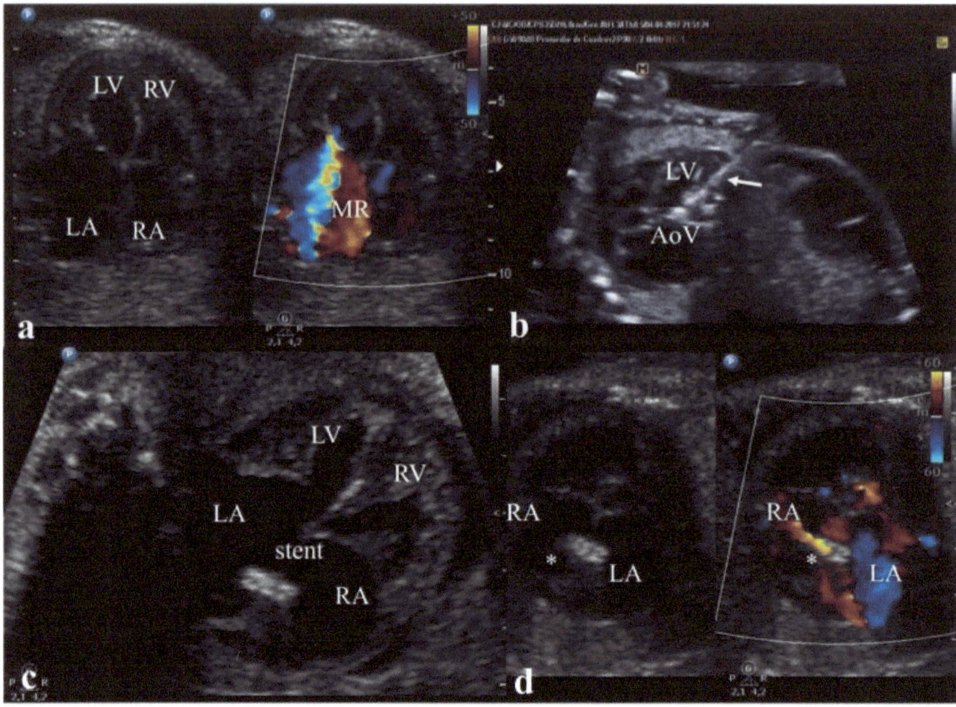

Fig. (6). A fetus with severe aortic stenosis, abnormal mitral valve, severely restrictive foramen ovale and severely dilated left atrium. **a**, severe mitral regurgitation. **b**, fetal aortic valvuloplasty (arrow), fetal ascites. **c**, stent in atrial septum. **d**, left-to-right flow across the stent (*). AoV: aortic valve; MR: mitral regurgitation; LV: left ventricle; RV: right ventricle; LA: left atrium; RA: right atrium.

PULMONARY ATRESIA WITH INTACT VENTRICULAR SEPTUM AND ECHOCARDIOGRAPHIC CRITERIA OF PROGRESSION TO HYPOPLASTIC RIGHT VENTRICLE AND SINGLE-VENTRICLE CIRCULATION

In some fetuses with pulmonary atresia or critical pulmonary stenosis with intact ventricular septum or very restrictive ventricular septal defect, right-side heart structures growth is impeded, evolving to right ventricular hypoplasia and univentricular heart [24]. Fetal pulmonary valvuloplasty has been proposed in this group of patients in order to augment antegrade pulmonary valve flow and favor the growth of the tricuspid and pulmonary valves, the right ventricle and the pulmonary trunk and branches; increasing the chance of candidacy for biventricular repair after birth [25].

There is significant variability in the reported morphological and functional fetal echocardiographic predictors of postnatal circulation and outcome, necessary for the identification of patients amenable to fetal cardiac intervention [26 - 32]. Thus, there is variability among different centers in their selection criteria for fetal pulmonary valvuloplasty [33 - 35] (Table **3**).

Table 3. Criteria for patient selection for fetal pulmonary valvuloplasty.

Study	Pulmonary Valve (PV)	Interventricular Septum	Tricuspid Valve (TV) Annulus	Tricuspid Regurgitation	Right Ventricle (RV)	Ductus Arteriosus	RV Sinusoids
Tworetzky *et al.* (2009)	Membranous PV atresia, with identifiable PV leaflets or membrane	Intact or highly restrictive ventricular septum	*Z* score of -2 or below	Not specified	Identifiable but small RV	Not specified	Not specified
Gómez-Montes *et al.* (2011)	Thin membranous PV atresia with an open outflow tract below the valve and with reasonable sized pulmonary arteries PV/AV ratio ≤ 0.75	Not specified	TV/MV ratio ≤ 0.83 Tricuspid inflow duration/cardiac cycle length ≤ 36.5%	Not specified	RV/LV length ratio ≤ 0.64	Not specified	Not specified
Arzt *et al.* (2018)	Membranous atresia or a critical stenosis of the PV with a recognizable RV outflow tract (exclusion if muscular atresia of PV)	Not specified	Not specified	Suprasystemic pressures as assessed by the velocity of the TR jet (exclusion if severe TR with low velocity <2.5m/s)	hypoplastic hypertrophic RV	retrograde flow	(exclusion if large RV sinusoids)

PV: pulmonary vale; TV: tricuspid valve; TR: tricuspid regurgitation; AV: aortic valve; RV: right ventricle; LV: left ventricle; MV: mitral valve.

The fetal pulmonary valvuloplasty is a technically difficult and challenging procedure, which implies an important learning curve. In fetuses with pulmonary atresia or critical stenosis, the right ventricle outlet is usually narrow; short; curved and hypertrophic; making the needle entry more difficult, as well as the visualization of the balloon during its inflation (Fig. **7**). As a consequence, a significant rate of fetal complications (60%) and of technically unsuccessful procedures have been reported (40%) [33]. In our center, the procedure could not be performed in three cases as a consequence of not achieving the correct fetal position after repeated fetal external version maneuvers.

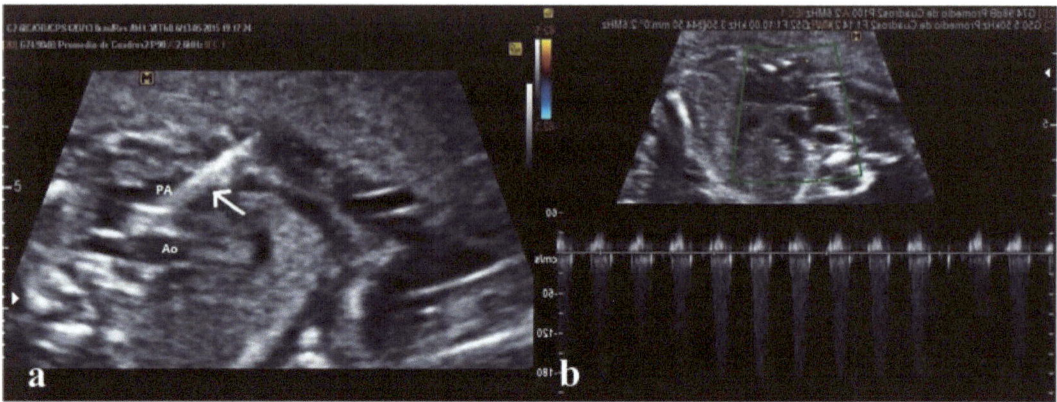

Fig. (7). Fetal pulmonary valvuloplasty: **a**, 18-gauge needle is positioned across the right ventricle outflow tract and severely stenotic pulmonary valve (arrow). **b**, Pulsed Doppler in the pulmonary artery shows increased flow across the pulmonary valve after fetal valvuloplasty. PA: pulmonary artery; Ao: aorta.

In the largest series, reported by the Linz Hospital group, 71.4% (15/21) of patients with a successful or partially successful procedure, became biventricular, 14.3% (3/21) had a one-and-a-half ventricle circulation and 14.3% (3/21) had an undetermined circulation [35]. The Boston Childrens´ Hospital reported 6 cases of live-borns who underwent successful fetal pulmonary valvuloplasty, 5 of which evolved with biventricular circulation and 1 with a single ventricle. In our group, 4 fetal pulmonary valvuloplasties were performed, with one periprocedural fetal demise and 3 technically successful procedures, and all 3 of them with a biventricular outcome [33]. Initial results seem promising but larger randomized studies are needed to evaluate efficacy and impact of this procedure.

SEVERE PERICARDIAL EFFUSION, GENERALLY SECONDARY TO HEART TUMORS

In the presence of cardiac diverticula, aneurysms or certain heart tumors, such as intrapericardial teratomas, a severe increase in pericardial effusion may occur and result in heart failure with hydrops fetalis and pulmonary hypoplasia, leading to fetal death. In these patients pericardiocentesis has been proposed to improve survival. Cardiac diverticula and aneurysms are rare malformations of the cardiac ventricular wall, most frequently found in the cardiac apex. Cardiac diverticula are finger-like appendices, with a narrow communication with the ventricular cavity. Whereas, cardiac aneurysms have a wider connection to the cardiac ventricle, are larger and may be diskinetic. Left ventricular aneurysms seem to have the highest rate of associated fetal demise among these defects [36]. Intrapericardial teratomas are a rare primary tumor of the pericardium with a high mortality due to cardiac tamponade and hydrops fetalis, which is seen in approximately 68% of cases detected antenatally [37].

Under, maternal and fetal anesthesia the pericardial effusion is drained with a 20-gauge needle (Fig. **8**). In cases of recurrent pericardial effusion serial pericardiocentesis, or placement of a pericardial amniotic shunt can be performed. Improvement in perinatal outcome has been reported, but this should be considered cautiously since there are only small series and case reports. In a systematic review of these studies, 24 studies reported fetal death following pericardiocentesis or pericardio-amniotic shunt placement, that is, 29% of a total sample size of 36 (95% CI, 18-41); $I^2 = 0\%$) [12].

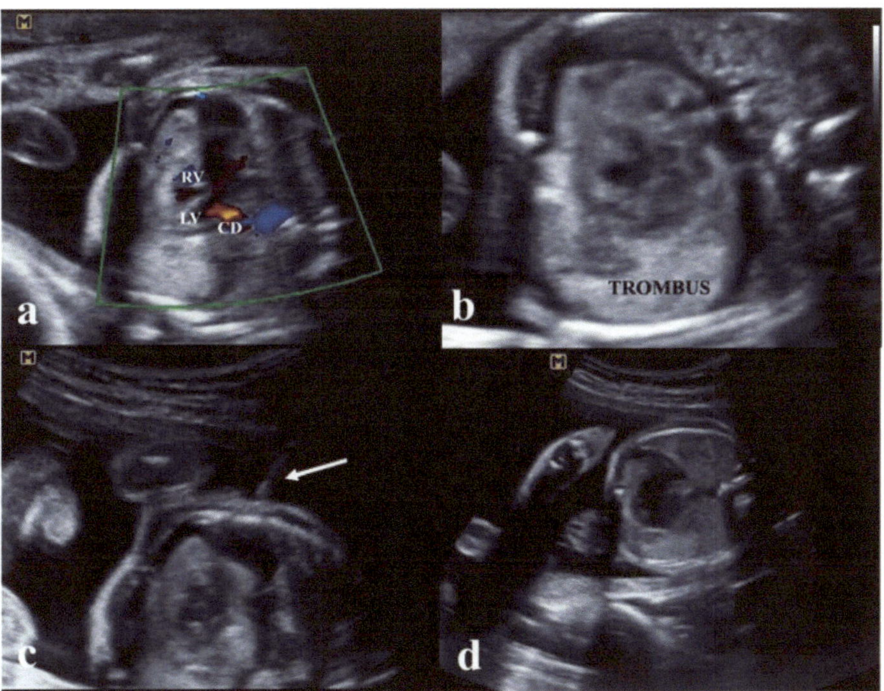

Fig. (8). a, Cardiac diverticulum in the left atrio-ventricular groove in a mid-trimester fetus. **b**, Rupture of the diverticulum with hemopericardium and pericardial thrombus formation. **c**, Fetal pericardiocentesis, the needle (arrow) for pericardial drainage across the fetal thorax. **d**, minimum pericardial effusion after the procedure. LV: left ventricle; RV: right ventricle; CD: cardiac diverticulum.

CONCLUSION

Fetal cardiac interventions for certain CHD have been developed. They are feasible yet technically challenging procedures; with low-maternal and high-fetal risks, that should be performed in highly selected cases and in specifically specialized tertiary centers by trained teams. In recent years higher rates of technical success and better clinical results have been reported, especially in terms of perinatal survival. Nevertheless, evidence is mostly based upon small series and case reports. International collaboration, through the international fetal cardiac intervention registry and ongoing multicenter studies; and ideally, future randomized controlled trials; will allow an improvement in the quality of available evidence that will probably bring further light upon the role of this unique field of fetal medicine.

CONSENT FOR PUBLICATION

Not applicable.

CONFLICT OF INTEREST

The authors confirm that the contents of this chapter have no conflict of interest.

ACKNOWLEDGEMENTS

Declare none.

REFERENCES

[1]　Moon-Grady AJ, Morris SA, Belfort M, *et al.* International fetal cardiac intervention registry. International fetal cardiac intervention registry: a worldwide collaborative description and preliminary outcomes. J Am Coll Cardiol 2015; 66(4): 388-99.
[http://dx.doi.org/10.1016/j.jacc.2015.05.037] [PMID: 26205597]

[2]　Mäkikallio K, McElhinney DB, Levine JC, *et al.* Fetal aortic valve stenosis and the evolution of hypoplastic left heart syndrome: Patient selection for fetal intervention. Circulation 2006; 113(11): 1401-5.
[http://dx.doi.org/10.1161/CIRCULATIONAHA.105.588194] [PMID: 16534003]

[3]　Matsui H, Gardiner H. Fetal intervention for cardiac disease: The cutting edge of perinatal care. Semin Fetal Neonatal Med 2007; 12(6): 482-9.
[http://dx.doi.org/10.1016/j.siny.2007.06.003] [PMID: 17827079]

[4]　Tulzer G, Arzt W. Fetal cardiac interventions: Rationale, risk and benefit. Semin Fetal Neonatal Med 2013; 18(5): 298-301.
[http://dx.doi.org/10.1016/j.siny.2013.04.002] [PMID: 23764271]

[5]　McElhinney DB, Marshall AC, Wilkins-Haug LE, *et al.* Predictors of technical success and postnatal biventricular outcome after *in utero* aortic valvuloplasty for aortic stenosis with evolving hypoplastic left heart syndrome. Circulation 2009; 120(15): 1482-90.
[http://dx.doi.org/10.1161/CIRCULATIONAHA.109.848994] [PMID: 19786635]

[6]　Tulzer A, Arzt W, Gitter R, *et al.* Immediate effects and outcome of *in-utero* pulmonary valvuloplasty in fetuses with pulmonary atresia with intact ventricular septum or critical pulmonary stenosis. Ultrasound Obstet Gynecol 2018; 52(2): 230-7.
[http://dx.doi.org/10.1002/uog.19047] [PMID: 29569770]

[7]　Gómez Montes E, Herraiz I, Mendoza A, Galindo A. Fetal intervention in right outflow tract obstructive disease: Selection of candidates and results. Cardiol Res Pract 2012; 2012592403

[http://dx.doi.org/10.1155/2012/592403] [PMID: 22928144]

[8]   Vogel M, McElhinney DB, Wilkins-Haug LE, *et al.* Aortic stenosis and severe mitral regurgitation in the fetus resulting in giant left atrium and hydrops: Pathophysiology, outcomes, and preliminary experience with pre-natal cardiac intervention. J Am Coll Cardiol 2011; 57(3): 348-55.
[http://dx.doi.org/10.1016/j.jacc.2010.08.636] [PMID: 21232673]

[9]   Kalish BT, Tworetzky W, Benson CB, *et al.* Technical challenges of atrial septal stent placement in fetuses with hypoplastic left heart syndrome and intact atrial septum. Catheter Cardiovasc Interv 2014; 84(1): 77-85.
[http://dx.doi.org/10.1002/ccd.25098] [PMID: 23804575]

[10]   Wohlmuth C, Tulzer G, Arzt W, Gitter R, Wertaschnigg D. Maternal aspects of fetal cardiac intervention. Ultrasound Obstet Gynecol 2014; 44(5): 532-7.
[http://dx.doi.org/10.1002/uog.13438] [PMID: 24920505]

[11]   Mizrahi-Arnaud A, Tworetzky W, Bulich LA, *et al.* Pathophysiology, management, and outcomes of fetal hemodynamic instability during prenatal cardiac intervention. Pediatr Res 2007; 62(3): 325-30.
[http://dx.doi.org/10.1203/PDR.0b013e318123fd3a] [PMID: 17622948]

[12]   Araujo Júnior E, Tonni G, Chung M, Ruano R, Martins WP. Perinatal outcomes and intrauterine complications following fetal intervention for congenital heart disease: Systematic review and meta-analysis of observational studies. Ultrasound Obstet Gynecol 2016; 48(4): 426-33.
[http://dx.doi.org/10.1002/uog.15867] [PMID: 26799734]

[13]   Marantz P, Grinenco S. Fetal intervention for critical aortic stenosis: Advances, research and postnatal follow-up. Curr Opin Cardiol 2015; 30(1): 89-94.
[http://dx.doi.org/10.1097/HCO.0000000000000128] [PMID: 25389651]

[14]   Freud LR, McElhinney DB, Marshall AC, *et al.* Fetal aortic valvuloplasty for evolving hypoplastic left heart syndrome: Postnatal outcomes of the first 100 patients. Circulation 2014; 130(8): 638-45.
[http://dx.doi.org/10.1161/CIRCULATIONAHA.114.009032] [PMID: 25052401]

[15]   Friedman KG, Sleeper LA, Freud LR, *et al.* Improved technical success, postnatal outcome and refined predictors of outcome for fetal aortic valvuloplasty. Ultrasound Obstet Gynecol 2018; 52(2): 212-20.
[http://dx.doi.org/10.1002/uog.17530] [PMID: 28543953]

[16]   Arzt W, Wertaschnigg D, Veit I, Klement F, Gitter R, Tulzer G. Intrauterine aortic valvuloplasty in fetuses with critical aortic stenosis: Experience and results of 24 procedures. Ultrasound Obstet Gynecol 2011; 37(6): 689-95.
[http://dx.doi.org/10.1002/uog.8927] [PMID: 21229549]

[17]   Sathanandam SK, Philip R, Gamboa D, *et al.* Management of hypoplastic left heart syndrome with intact atrial septum: A two-centre experience. Cardiol Young 2016; 26(6): 1072-81.
[http://dx.doi.org/10.1017/S1047951115001791] [PMID: 26346529]

[18]   Divanović A, Hor K, Cnota J, Hirsch R, Kinsel-Ziter M, Michelfelder E. Prediction and perinatal management of severely restrictive atrial septum in fetuses with critical left heart obstruction: Clinical experience using pulmonary venous Doppler analysis. J Thorac Cardiovasc Surg 2011; 141(4): 988-94.
[http://dx.doi.org/10.1016/j.jtcvs.2010.09.043] [PMID: 21130471]

[19]   Marshall AC, Levine J, Morash D, *et al.* Results of *in utero* atrial septoplasty in fetuses with hypoplastic left heart syndrome. Prenat Diagn 2008; 28(11): 1023-8.
[http://dx.doi.org/10.1002/pd.2114] [PMID: 18925607]

[20]   Chaturvedi RR, Ryan G, Seed M, van Arsdell G, Jaeggi ET. Fetal stenting of the atrial septum: Technique and initial results in cardiac lesions with left atrial hypertension. Int J Cardiol 2013; 168(3): 2029-36.
[http://dx.doi.org/10.1016/j.ijcard.2013.01.173] [PMID: 23481911]

[21]   Kalish BT, Tworetzky W, Benson CB, *et al.* Technical challenges of atrial septal stent placement in fetuses with hypoplastic left heart syndrome and intact atrial septum. Catheter Cardiovasc Interv 2014; 84(1): 77-85.
[http://dx.doi.org/10.1002/ccd.25098] [PMID: 23804575]

[22]   Jantzen DW, Moon-Grady AJ, Morris SA, *et al.* Hypoplastic left heart syndrome with intact or restrictive atrial septum: a report from the international fetal cardiac intervention registry. Circulation 2017; 136(14): 1346-9.
[http://dx.doi.org/10.1161/CIRCULATIONAHA.116.025873] [PMID: 28864444]

[23]   Mackesy MM, Kalish BT, Tworetzky W, *et al.* Sonographic pulmonary abnormalities in fetuses with hypoplastic left heart syndrome and intact atrial septum undergoing attempted atrial septostomy *in utero*. Ultrasound Q 2017; 33(1): 82-5.
[http://dx.doi.org/10.1097/RUQ.0000000000000247] [PMID: 27575842]

[24]   Todros T, Presbitero P, Gaglioti P, Demarie D. Pulmonary stenosis with intact ventricular septum: Documentation of development of the lesion echocardiographically during fetal life. Int J Cardiol 1988; 19(3): 355-62.
[http://dx.doi.org/10.1016/0167-5273(88)90240-9] [PMID: 3397198]

[25]   Tulzer G, Arzt W, Franklin RC, Loughna PV, Mair R, Gardiner HM. Fetal pulmonary valvuloplasty for critical pulmonary stenosis or atresia with intact septum. Lancet 2002; 360(9345): 1567-8.
[http://dx.doi.org/10.1016/S0140-6736(02)11531-5] [PMID: 12443597]

[26]   Cao L, Tian Z, Rychik J. Prenatal echocardiographic predictors of postnatal management strategy in the fetus with right ventricle hypoplasia and pulmonary atresia or stenosis. Pediatr Cardiol 2017; 38(8): 1562-8.
[http://dx.doi.org/10.1007/s00246-017-1696-4] [PMID: 28770306]

[27]   Daubeney PE, Sharland GK, Cook AC, Keeton BR, Anderson RH, Webber SA. UK and Eire Collaborative Study of Pulmonary Atresia with Intact Ventricular Septum. Pulmonary atresia with intact ventricular septum: Impact of fetal echocardiography on incidence at birth and postnatal outcome. Circulation 1998; 98(6): 562-6.
[http://dx.doi.org/10.1161/01.CIR.98.6.562] [PMID: 9714114]

[28]   Salvin JW, McElhinney DB, Colan SD, *et al.* Fetal tricuspid valve size and growth as predictors of outcome in pulmonary atresia with intact ventricular septum. Pediatrics 2006; 118(2): e415-20.
[http://dx.doi.org/10.1542/peds.2006-0428] [PMID: 16882782]

[29]   Roman KS, Fouron JC, Nii M, Smallhorn JF, Chaturvedi R, Jaeggi ET. Determinants of outcome in fetal pulmonary valve stenosis or atresia with intact ventricular septum. Am J Cardiol 2007; 99(5): 699-703.
[http://dx.doi.org/10.1016/j.amjcard.2006.09.120] [PMID: 17317375]

[30]   Gardiner HM, Belmar C, Tulzer G, *et al.* Morphologic and functional predictors of eventual circulation in the fetus with pulmonary atresia or critical pulmonary stenosis with intact septum. J Am Coll Cardiol 2008; 51(13): 1299-308.
[http://dx.doi.org/10.1016/j.jacc.2007.08.073] [PMID: 18371563]

[31]   Iacobelli R, Pasquini L, Toscano A, *et al.* Role of tricuspid regurgitation in fetal echocardiographic diagnosis of pulmonary atresia with intact ventricular septum. Ultrasound Obstet Gynecol 2008; 32(1): 31-5.
[http://dx.doi.org/10.1002/uog.5356] [PMID: 18570204]

[32]   Lowenthal A, Lemley B, Kipps AK, Brook MM, Moon-Grady AJ. Prenatal tricuspid valve size as a predictor of postnatal outcome in patients with severe pulmonary stenosis or pulmonary atresia with intact ventricular septum. Fetal Diagn Ther 2014; 35(2): 101-7.
[http://dx.doi.org/10.1159/000357429] [PMID: 24457468]

[33]   Tworetzky W, McElhinney DB, Marx GR, *et al.* In utero valvuloplasty for pulmonary atresia with hypoplastic right ventricle: Techniques and outcomes. Pediatrics 2009; 124(3): e510-8.

[http://dx.doi.org/10.1542/peds.2008-2014] [PMID: 19706566]

[34]   Gómez Montes E, Herraiz I, Mendoza A, Galindo A. Fetal intervention in right outflow tract obstructive disease: Selection of candidates and results. Cardiol Res Pract 2012; 2012592403
[http://dx.doi.org/10.1155/2012/592403] [PMID: 22928144]

[35]   Tulzer A, Arzt W, Gitter R, *et al.* Immediate effects and outcome of *in-utero* pulmonary valvuloplasty in fetuses with pulmonary atresia with intact ventricular septum or critical pulmonary stenosis. Ultrasound Obstet Gynecol 2018; 52(2): 230-7.
[http://dx.doi.org/10.1002/uog.19047] [PMID: 29569770]

[36]   Zeng S, Zhou Q, Zhang M, Zhou J, Peng Q. Features and outcome of fetal cardiac aneurysms and diverticula: A single center experience in China. Prenat Diagn 2016; 36(1): 68-73.
[http://dx.doi.org/10.1002/pd.4714] [PMID: 26517281]

[37]   Nassr AA, Shazly SA, Morris SA, *et al.* Prenatal management of fetal intrapericardial teratoma: A systematic review. Prenat Diagn 2017; 37(9): 849-63.
[http://dx.doi.org/10.1002/pd.5113] [PMID: 28695637]

CHAPTER 12

Clinical Management of Congenital Heart Diseases in Neonates

Célia Maria Camelo Silva[*] and **Ana Carolina Buso Faccinetto**

Discipline of Cardiology, Department of Medicine, Paulista School of Medicine Federal University of São Paulo (EPM-UNIFESP), São Paulo-SP, Brazil

Abstract: Management strategies for congenital heart disease (CHD) in the neonate have evolved significantly. Advances in surgical technique, medical technology, and perioperative care have resulted in excellent post-repair survival, even for complex types of CHD. Furthermore, with the increased availability and accuracy of prenatal diagnosis by fetal echocardiography, the postnatal management of these newborns can often be anticipated and planned. The prenatal diagnosis of CHD has been associated with decreased morbidity and mortality for some forms of major CHD. As most cases of major CHD are not identified prenatally, clinical examination of the newborn and pulse oximetry are also important means of identifying additional cases. In summary, to improve the outcomes of a neonate with CHD, surgical repair or catheter intervention may be offered. For this purpose, early recognition of a neonate with CHD is necessary for stabilization and timely intervention.

Keywords: Cardiac catheterization, Cardiac surgery, Cardiac surgical procedure, Congenital heart disease, Neonate, Prenatal diagnosis.

INTRODUCTION

Congenital heart disease (CHD) is the most common congenital disorder in neonates; its incidence ranges from 8 to 10 per 1,000 live births, ranging from complex heart diseases potentially fatal in the neonatal period to mild lesions that will remain asymptomatic throughout life [1]. Approximately 25% of those with CHD will require surgery or catheter-based intervention in the first year of life. Advances in surgical techniques have reduced the perioperative mortality of neonates with CHD substantially. In specialized centers, in-hospital mortality for complex surgery is now between 1% and 3%; therefore, the occurrence of death before cardiac surgery has taken on even greater significance. Second trimester screening for CHD has been contributed with decrease mortality and morbidity

[*] **Address for correspondence Célia Maria Camelo:** Discipline of Cardiology, Department of Medicine, Paulista School of Medicine - Federal University of São Paulo (EPM-UNIFESP), R. Sena Madureira, 1500 Vila Clementino, São Paulo-SP, Brazil, Zip code 04021-001, Tel: +55 11 55764321, E-mail: celiasilv@uol.com.br

Edward Araujo Júnior, Nathalie Jeanne M. Bravo-Valenzuela and Alberto Borges Peixoto (Eds.)

for some forms of major CHD. However, due to the lack of prenatal diagnosis of most cases of CHD, clinical examination and pulse oximetry of the newborn can help identify additional cases [2 - 6].

RECOGNITION, DIAGNOSIS, AND MANAGEMENT OF CONGENITAL HEART DISEASE

Early recognition of CHD, emergency stabilization, and transport to a cardiac care center with expertise in the management of CHD are important to ensure an optimal outcome. In this regard, fetal echocardiography plays an important role because, when complex CHD is diagnosed, the newborn has the advantage of being born in a specialized center [7]. Diagnosis of congenital cardiovascular malformations requires close observation during the neonatal period [8 - 12].

Special Considerations for an Appropriate Therapeutic Plan

Screening Programs for the Diagnosis of Congenital Heart Diseases During the Fetal and Neonatal Periods

Most cases of CHD are unexpected; therefore, early recognition is important. However, despite the effort devoted to the development of screening programs for the detection of CHD in prenatal and postnatal care, a great number of children with CHD remain undiagnosed, coming to the physician's attention only after the onset of symptoms and presenting as extremely ill. In order to increase its recognition, consultation and referral to a pediatric cardiologist should be done for infants with any of the following signs and symptoms indicative of critical CHD: shock unresponsive to volume resuscitation, cardiomegaly, cyanosis, pulmonary edema, or otherwise unexplained respiratory symptoms [4].

Two-dimensional echocardiogram is a necessary, fundamental, and definitive tool for the diagnosis of CHD, allowing an anatomical-morphological and functional definition [8, 13, 14].

Pulse Oximetry Screening

Pulse oximetry screening for critical CHD in neonates improves the identification of patients with critical CHD compared with physical examination [15, 16]. It consists of measuring oxygen saturation simultaneously in the upper right limb and in one of the lower limbs between 24 and 48 hours of life. Oxygen saturation below 95% or difference more than 3% between limbs requires investigation to rule out CHD. However, screening does not identify all critical CHDs, particularly noncyanotic lesions and some left heart obstructive lesions. All cases with positive pulse oximetry screening should be evaluated by a pediatric cardiologist and an echocardiogram done before hospital discharge to identify the etiology of the hypoxemia.

Hyperoxia Test

The hyperoxia test is used to help distinguish cardiac from pulmonary causes of cyanosis. However, with the advent of routine pulse oximetry screening for critical CHD and improved access to echocardiography, the hyperoxia test is usually not necessary. If the cause of cyanosis is cardiac, the arterial PaO2 will remain <100 mmHg, and these neonates should receive prostaglandin until the CHD is definitively diagnosed [17].

Electrocardiogram

An electrocardiogram (EKG) can be used to identify rhythm abnormalities and signs of atrial enlargement or ventricular hypertrophy, or QRS axis deviation.

Chest X-ray

A chest X-ray demonstrates the cardiac size and shape, pulmonary vascularity (normal pulmonary blood flow, pulmonary hypoflow, or pulmonary hyperflow). Certain chest x-ray findings can be helpful in the differential diagnosis of pulmonary and cardiac diseases (Figs. **1** to **3**).

Echocardiography

Color Doppler echocardiography is a noninvasive test to determine the presence of CHD, associated lesions and its hemodynamics status.

Additional Imaging Modalities

These include cardiac catheterization and angiography, magnetic resonance imaging (MRI), and computed tomography scanning, to further visualize of the cardiac anatomy.

Principles of Resuscitation and Stabilization of Symptomatic Neonates with Suspected Congenital Heart Disease

It is important that the critically ill neonate be stabilized in the hospital of origin while awaiting transfer to a referral center.

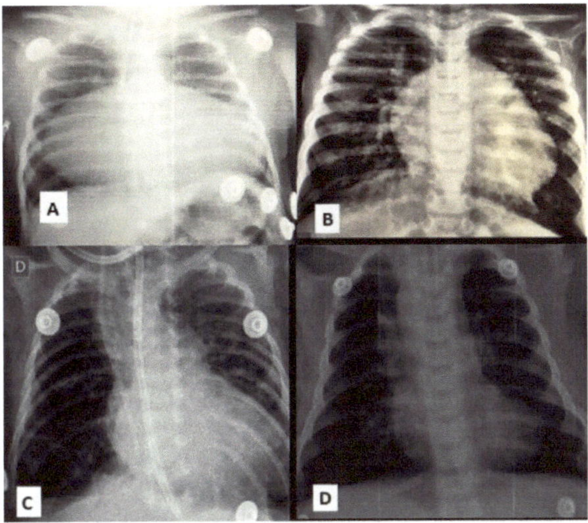

Fig. (1). Chest x-ray. A: Ebstein's anomaly; note the extreme cardiomegaly. B: from a patient with transposition of the great arteries with a ventricular septal defect; note the "egg-shaped" heart. C: from a newborn with truncus arteriosus type II showing an enlarged heart, particularly the left ventricle, and increased pulmonary vascular markings. D: from a newborn with tetralogy of Fallot; note the "boot-shaped" heart and oligemic lungs.

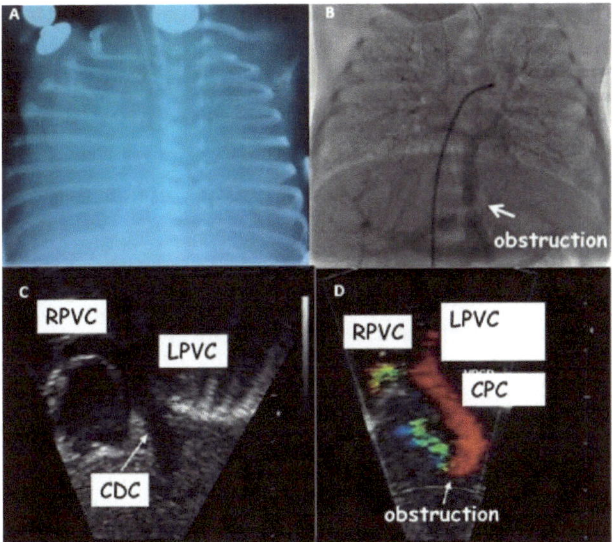

Fig. (2). Infradiaphragmatic total anomalous pulmonary venous drainage, obstructive type. **A:** Chest radiograph showing important bilateral pulmonary edema. **B:** Pulmonary arteriography; on the venous return it is observed that the right and left pulmonary veins join in a common downward collector. Significant obstruction of the collector (arrow) when entering the portal system. **C** and **D:** Subcostal echocardiographic sections showing the right and left pulmonary vein collectors and the common descending collecting vein. The Doppler study shows a mosaic that corresponds to an obstruction point (arrow) at the entrance of the portal system. RPVC: right pulmonary vein; LPVC: left pulmonary vein; CPC: common pulmonary collector vein.

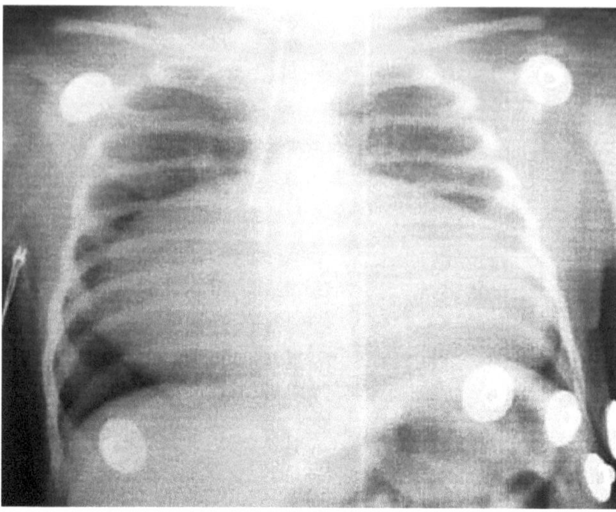

Fig. (3). Chest radiograph showing an Ebstein's anomaly case. Note the extreme cardiomegaly.

When to Prescribe Prostaglandin

In patients with ductal-dependent circulation, as closure of the ductus arteriosus within the first few days of life can precipitate rapid clinical deterioration with potentially life-threatening consequences. Prostaglandin (PG) E1 to reopen or maintain the ductus arteriosus can be life-saving in these patients and should be initiated as soon as CHD is suspected in symptomatic neonates. When the diagnosis is not yet established, the decision to start or not to start on PG should be made based on clinical findings. The decision process is based on the presence of cyanosis, with or without heart murmur, whereas in acyanotic neonates, pulse abnormality is an important indicator. A combination of clinical findings—cyanosis, murmur, and abnormal pulses—increases the probability of a CHD with ductus arteriosus-dependent circulation [18].

The dosage of PGE1 ranges from 0.05 to 0.1mcg/kg/minute continuous intravenous infusion (increasing the dose every 10 minutes until the desired effect is obtained). Subsequently, the PGE1's dose may be reduced to 0.01 mcg/kg/minute. The main PGE1's side effects are the following: apnea (12%), fever (14%), cutaneous flush (10%), bradycardia (7%), among other effects [19]. For these reasons, a cautions cardiorespiratory monitoring should be required during PGE1 infusion.

Special Situations

A Neonate with Congenital Heart Disease who is Unresponsive to Prostaglandin

1.Obstructed total anomalous pulmonary venous drainage. The PG's effect in neonates with obstructed total anomalous pulmonary venous drainage is to reduce pulmonary vascular resistance. However, by increasing pulmonary blood flow, PG may exacerbate venous congestion because of obstructed return. Neonates with transposition of the great arteries with an intact ventricular septum and a restrictive atrial septum will require emergency balloon atrioseptostomy (BAS) (Fig. **4**) [20 - 22].

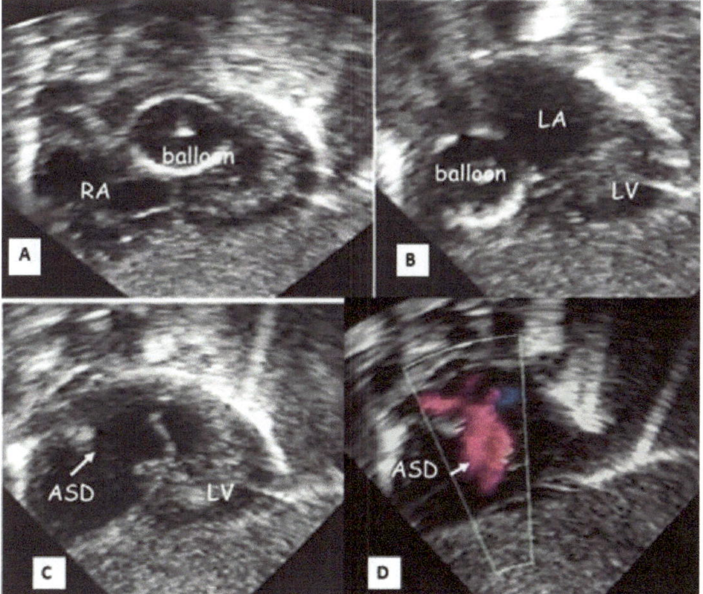

Fig. (4). Balloon atrioseptostomy in a neonate with transposition of the great arteries (A,B) and restrictive atrial septal defect (C,D). RA: right ventricle; LA: left atrium; LV: left ventricle; ASD: atrial septal defect.

Presentation of a Neonate with Congenital Heart Disease

Two conditions may influence the timing of presentation and severity of CHD in neonates: the severity and nature of the defect and the changes in cardiovascular physiology secondary to the effect of the transitional circulation.

CHD presenting as a cardiac emergency in the neonatal period can be broadly categorized as follows:

Ductal-dependent Circulation

Left-sided and right-sided obstructive defects require the patency of the ductus arteriosus to maintain systemic and pulmonary blood flow, respectively. The ductal-dependent CHDs are as follow:

A) Ductal- dependent systemic blood flow

• Critical aortic stenosis;

• Severe coarctation of the aorta or interruption of the aortic arch;

• Hypoplastic left heart syndrome;

• Complex CHD with severe systemic outflow obstruction.

B) Ductal- dependent pulmonary blood flow

• Critical pulmonary stenosis or pulmonary atresia;

• Severe form of tetralogy of Fallot ;

• Severe form Ebstein's anomaly of the tricuspid valve;

• Complex CHD with severe pulmonary stenosis or atresia.

C) CHD with parallel circulation

• Transposition of the great arteries (TGA).

Restricted Atrial Septal Defect

Large atrial communication is required to maintain adequate systemic output in some critical CHDs, such as:

A) To relieve pulmonary congestion in left heart obstruction defects, such as: hypoplastic left heart syndrome and mitral stenosis or atresia.

B) To relief right-sided congestion in right-sided heart obstruction defects: pulmonary atresia with intact septum; atresia of tricuspid valve and total anomalous pulmonary venous connection.

Neonate Presenting with Circulatory Collapse

The closure of the ductus arteriosus after birth can result in circulatory collapse (systemic hypoperfusion) in the following CHD: critical aortic stenosis, critical aorta coarctation, aortic arch interruption, hypoplastic left heart syndrome [23]. In such cases, the use of PG and additional care is required to keep the ductus arteriosus opened to maintain systemic blood flow.

Critical Aortic Valve Stenosis

Critical aortic valve stenosis is a severe left outflow obstruction accompanying left ventricular hypertrophy and endocardial fibroelastosis. After the postnatal ductus arteriosus closure, the LV cannot maintain the systemic blood flow. Severe dysfunction, clinical congestive heart failure or shock will become apparent.

Critical Aortic Coarctation

In patients with critical aortic coarctation, closure of the affects lower body circulation without significantly affecting upper body circulation. The severity of coarctation may increase with the closure of the ductus arteriosus, due to simultaneous contraction of the tissue surrounding the narrowing area of the aortic arch. The main cardiac abnormalities associated with aorta coarctation are the following: bicuspid aortic valve, and ventricular septal defect. The spectrum of severity varies; as with aortic stenosis, milder forms present later in life.

Aortic Arch Interruption

The complete interruption locations may occur between the left common carotid and left subclavian arteries, distal to the left subclavian artery or between the innominate artery and left common carotid artery. Aortic arch interruption is usually associated with a large, nonrestrictive malalignment-type ventricular septal defect. Surgical correction is required for both the arch obstruction and the ventricular septal defect.

Hypoplastic Left Heart Syndrome

In classic hypoplastic left heart syndrome, all the left-sided structures, are unable to maintain the entire systemic output due to the severity of own hypoplasia. Consequently, the right ventricle and the patency of the ductus arteriosus maintain the systemic output.

1. Physical examination

• Reduced peripheral pulses: all limbs critical aortic stenosis/hypoplastic left heart syndrome or reduced femoral pulses (asymmetrical pulses) - aorta coarctation/interrupted aortic arch;

• Mild cyanosis (HLHS);

• Single second heart sound.

2. Electrocardiography

• Hypertrophy of the right ventricle (in cases with coarctation of the aorta);

• Left ventricular hypertrophy (in critical aortic stenosis);

• Poor or absence of left ventricle forces (HLHS).

3. Chest X-Ray

• Cardiomegaly;

• Pulmonary venous hypertension;

• Increased pulmonary blood flow with HLHS.

4. Echocardiography

• It has an important role in establishing the diagnosis, its severity, the hemodynamic effect, pulmonary artery pressure, and ventricular dysfunction (Fig. **5**).

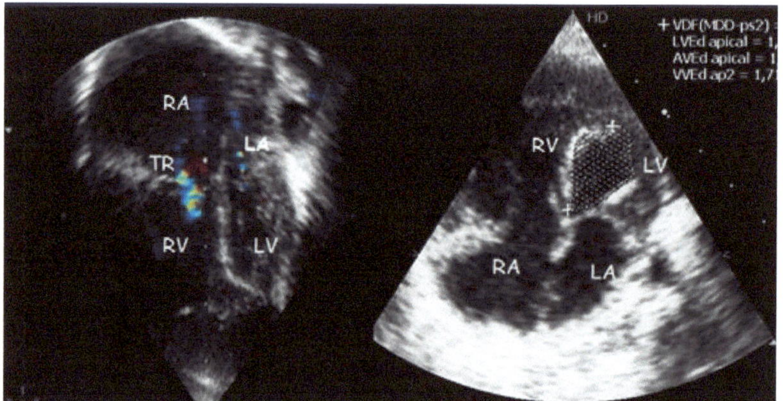

Fig. (5). Four-chamber view by echocardiogram showing enlarged right heart chambers, small left chambers, and mild tricuspid regurgitation. RA: right atrium; LA: left atrium; TR: tricuspid regurgitation; RV: right ventricle; LV: left ventricle.

5. Management

In neonates with cardiovascular collapse, the initial management includes shock treatment, to obtain a vascular access, attention to airway and breathing, and correction of metabolic acidosis. These neonates should be started on PGE1 infusion.

Subsequently, it is important to keep a balance between systemic and pulmonary blood flow by avoiding any manipulation that decreases pulmonary vascular resistance (avoidance: hyperventilation and excessive use of inotropes).

In critical aortic stenosis, after initial stabilization, neonatal echocardiography should be performed to assess left ventricle size to determine its viability to sustain the systemic circulation. If yes, balloon dilatation of the aortic valve is the main option of treatment [20, 24].

Balloon dilation is also an alternative, particularly in those with a high risk for cardiac surgery, with immediate good results, for neonates with aorta coarctation, when additional problems as sepsis and multiorgan dysfunction may be present, treatment. The risk of restenosis (>80%) is the main complication of balloon dilation. The surgery is the only treatment option for newborns with interruption of the aortic arch.

The surgical management for newborns with HLHS includes staged surgery (Norwood operation stages I, II and III) and in such cases cardiac transplantation [25 - 28].

Neonates Presenting with Cyanosis and Ductal-dependent Pulmonary Circulation

Cyanosis is an important sign in neonates with duct-dependent pulmonary circulation. If these conditions are not recognized on time, they may lead to severe hypoxemia, metabolic acidosis, and finally death. The ductal closure substantially influences the pulmonary blood flow and consequently the progression of the disease. Physical examination, chest radiography, and electrocardiogram can help to distinguish the more common forms of cyanotic CHD from each other and from other causes of central cyanosis. Echocardiography confirms the diagnosis and determines the underlying cardiac anatomy and function (Fig. **6**).

Pulmonary Atresia or Critical Stenosis of Pulmonary Blood Flow

In utero, the ductus arteriosus is patent with no hemodynamics instability in cases of pulmonary atresia or critical stenosis. After birth, with the ductal closure or restriction, the neonate becomes cyanosed, develops metabolic acidosis and, if this condition is left untreated, it may evolve with neonatal death.

i. Physical examination

• No hyperdynamic precordium;

• No significant murmur;

• Single second heart sound.

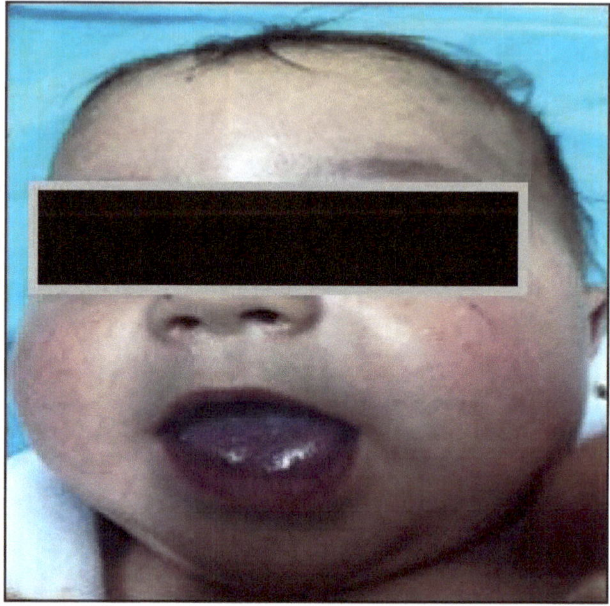

Fig. (6). Neonate with cyanosis.

ii. Chest X-Ray

• Normal heart size, except when there is associated valvar regurgitation, as a dysplastic tricuspid valve can have a marked cardiomegaly as in Ebstein's anomaly;

• Decreased pulmonary vascular markings –oligemic lung field.

iii. Electrocardiography

• Right axis deviation;

• Right ventricular forces *;

* in cases with tricuspid atresia with hypoplastic RV: there is left axis deviation with left ventricle hypertrophy

Echocardiography

This is a fundamental tool for diagnosis and definition of the basic anatomy and status of the ductus arteriosus. Depending on the dimensions of the right ventricle, the best options of treatment can be biventricular repair or univentricular repair.

iv. Cardiac catheterization may be necessary in the majority of cases for refining the anatomy and as a therapeutic interventional procedure.

v. Management

The guidelines for the management of a neonate with cyanosis are as follows:

• Temperature maintenance, and oxygen saturation should be kept between 80 to 85% the newborn should be started on PGE1 infusion;

• Inotropic agents are rarely required. Some routinely start a combination of renal doses of Dopamine (3–5 mcg/kg/min) to increase renal perfusion and Dobutamine (5 mcg/kg/min) as an inotrope to correct the myocardial depressant effect of severe metabolic acidosis;

• Feeding: the newborn should not be given oral feeding till stabilization.

vi. Treatment

a) Critical pulmonary stenosis

The main treatment of critical pulmonary stenosis is the balloon valvotomy. However, in some cases, arterial duct stenting is necessary [29 - 31].

b) Pulmonary atresia with an intact ventricular septum

Pulmonary atresia with an intact ventricular septum (PA/IVS) is characterized by complete obstruction of the right ventricular outflow with varying degrees of right ventricular and tricuspid valve hypoplasia. Blood is thus unable to flow from the right ventricle to the pulmonary artery and lungs, and an alternative source of pulmonary blood flow (*i.e.*, a PDA) is required for survival. The management of PA/IVS includes initial stabilization followed by corrective or palliative repair. Definitive treatment of pulmonary atresia depends upon the ventricle's dimension and whether or not the coronary circulation is right ventricle dependent. If the dimensions of the right ventricle are of adequate size, then opening of the outflow tract (RVOT) by surgery or catheter intervention is the main treatment (Fig. 7). In some cases, when the right ventricle is borderline, one needs an additional source of pulmonary blood flow in the form of a Blalock-Taussig shunt or ductal stenting after balloon dilatation of the pulmonary valve. In patients with a hypoplastic right ventricle or right ventricle coronary circulation, the newborn becomes a candidate for single ventricular physiology. The Blalock-Taussig (systemic-pulmonary shunt) procedure can be the first surgical procedure in cases of pulmonary atresia or critical pulmonary stenosis with a ventricular septal defect. Posteriorly, a second staged surgical correction can be planned at a later age.

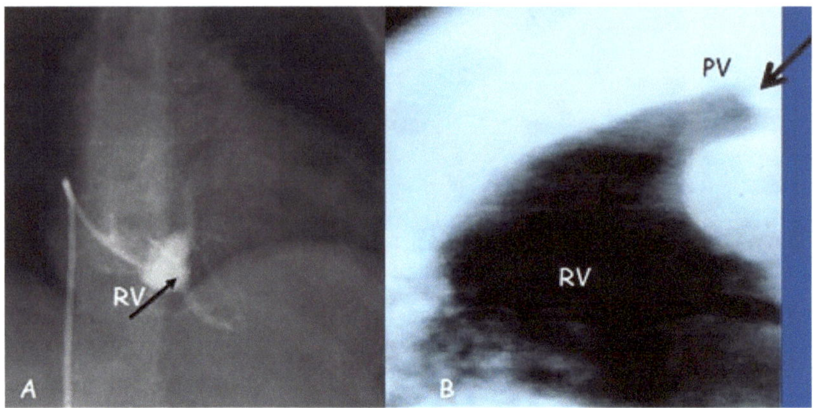

Fig. (7). Pulmonary atresia with an intact ventricular septum: A - a very small right ventricle (RV) (arrow) and B - a well-developed and dilated RV with a membranous pulmonary valve (arrow); PV: pulmonary vein.

Severe tricuspid regurgitation causes a reduction of blood flow through the pulmonary valve. In the neonatal period, as pulmonary artery pressure is high, the pulmonary valve fails to open, causing functional pulmonary atresia. As time goes by, with the decrease in pulmonary artery pressure and PVR, the pulmonary valve opens, maintaining forward flow and a decrease in tricuspid regurgitation, causing improvement in the clinical condition [32].

Chest X-Ray –extreme cardiomegaly (Ebstein's anomaly).

Ebstein's anomaly –Tall P wave, low voltage QRS complexes, conduction defects.

Neonates presenting with cyanosis and non-ductal-dependent lesions

Non-ductal-dependent congenital heart defects that cause cyanosis include

● Total anomalous pulmonary venous connection;

● Truncus arteriosus;

● Tetralogy of Fallot and tricuspid atresia may or may not be ductal-dependent, depending upon the degree of right ventricular outflow tract obstruction and the presence and size of a ventricular septal defect (VSD, in tricuspid atresia).

Connection of Total Anomalous Pulmonary Venous Connection

Total anomalous pulmonary venous connection (TAPVC) is a cyanotic congenital defect in which all four pulmonary veins fail to make their normal connection to the left atrium. This results in drainage of all pulmonary venous return into the systematic venous circulation.

In TAPVC the pulmonary veins can be connected to right side of the heart by superior vena cava, vertical vein, coronary sinus, or directly to right atrium, or by the inferior vena cava or a combination of these. In those cases, the only source of blood flow to left side is through the oval foramen. If the pathway from the pulmonary veins to the left atrium is unobstructed, the child presents with features of congestive heart failure (CHF) beyond the neonatal period with mild cyanosis. However, if there is an obstruction in this pathway, which is always with infradiaphragmatic TAPVC and, in about one third of cases, to the superior vena cava, the child presents on day 1 or 2 of life with cyanosis and respiratory distress (Fig. **8**). The obstruction of the pulmonary venous pathway causes pulmonary (arterial and venous) hypertension.

This is one cardiac emergency wherein prostaglandins will not benefit the neonate and may cause further deterioration of the condition.

i. Clinical scenario:

• Newborn with cyanosis, tachypnea and CHF.

ii. Physical examination

• Absence of cardiomegaly;

• Loud pulmonary second heart sound;

• Continuous or ejection systolic murmur.

iii. Arterial blood gases–metabolic acidosis, low pO_2, normal or elevated pCO_2, failure of 100% oxygen to increase pO_2 >100 mmHg.

iv. Chest X-ray:

• No cardiomegaly;

• Prominent main pulmonary artery;

• Pulmonary edema.

v. Electrocardiography: not specific.

• Right axis deviation with right ventricle forces;

• Right atrial enlargement may be present.

vi. Echocardiography –diagnostic tool that reveals the site of anomalous connection and level of obstruction. TAPVC should be suspected, every time that primary hypertension in the neonatal intensive care will be diagnosed

vii. Management: immediate surgical correction of the defect is the main treatment.

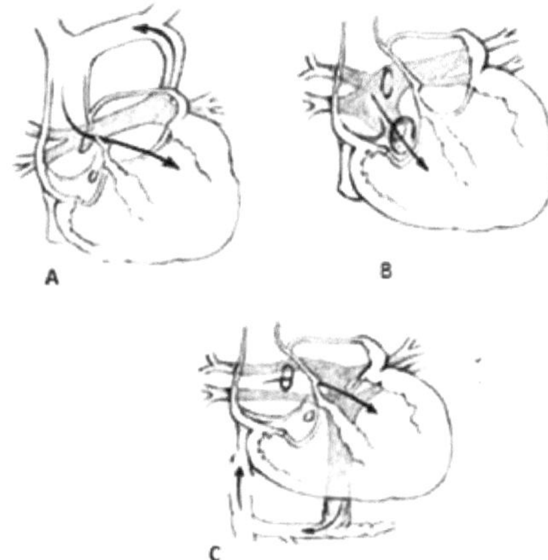

Fig. (8). Common types of total anomalous pulmonary drainage A. Supracardiac –The total anomalous supracardiac pulmonary venous drainage through the vertical vein that joins to the innominate vein that connects with the right superior vena cava and drains into the right atrium. B. Cardiac –The pulmonary veins meet behind the heart and then drain directly into the right atrium or through the coronary sinus. C. Infracardiac –The pulmonary veins attach behind the heart and then drain downward, connecting to the portal vein system. They then dissipate through the vascular bed of the liver and drain into the right atrium.

Truncus Arteriosus

Truncus arteriosus is a conotruncal anomaly with a single arterial trunk overriding the crest of the ventricular septum large subarterial VSD, through which a single valve is responsible for systemic, pulmonary, and coronary circulation.

Tetralogy of Fallot

Tetralogy of Fallot (TOF) is a conotruncal anomaly with the following major features:

• Right ventricular outflow tract obstruction;

• Large malalignment-type subaortic VSD;

• Overriding aorta artery;

• Concentric right ventricular hypertrophy.

TOF is a common cyanotic congenital heart defect affecting approximately 10% of all cases diagnosed intrauterine.

Medical Management

The need for medical intervention depends on the degree of RVOT obstruction. Patients with severe RVOT have inadequate pulmonary flow and usually present profound cyanosis in the immediate newborn period. These patients may need urgent therapy. Patients with moderate obstruction and balanced pulmonary and systemic flow typically come to clinical attention during elective evaluation for a murmur. These children may also present with hypercyanotic ("tet"). Patients with RVOT minimal obstruction may present with increased pulmonary blood flow and heart failure. In addition, some affected newborns will be detected by a failed oximetry-screening test. Neonates with severe RVOT obstruction present with profound hypoxemia and cyanosis. These patients may require intravenous PG therapy to keep ductal patency [33].

Surgical Management

Most patients with TOF undergo intracardiac repair as their initial intervention by one year of age typically after four months of age [34]. Pulmonary to systemic shunts such as Blalock-Taussig may be necessary due to severe RVOT obstruction in premature infants who are not initially acceptable for intracardiac repair, hypoplastic pulmonary arteries, or coronary artery anatomy. Although, as an alternative, a percutaneous procedure such as percutaneous implantation of stents in the RVOT or in the ductus arteriosus can be performed in order to reduce the complications of very early surgery (Figs. **9** to **11**).

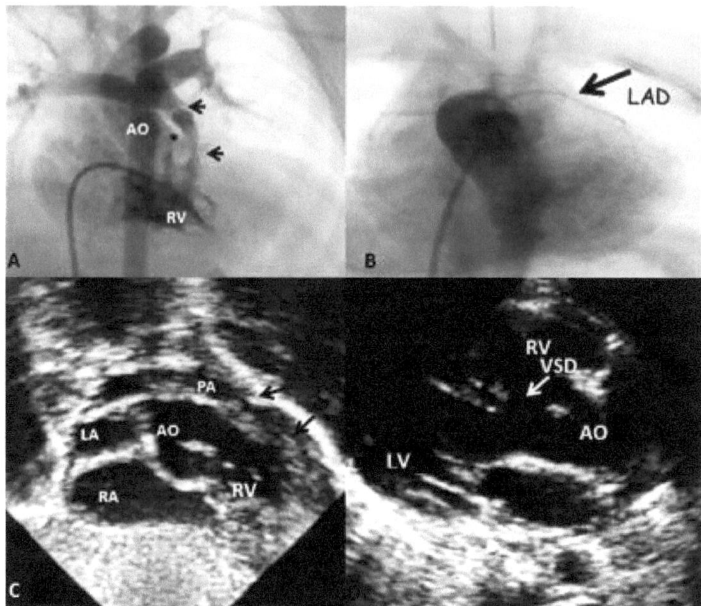

Fig. (9). A and **B:** Right ventricular angiography from a patient with tetralogy of Fallot and a single coronary artery arising from the left coronary sinus. **C** and **D:** Subcostal and long-axis parasternal views showing the features of tetralogy of Fallot. LA: left atrium; RA: right atrium; Ao: aorta; PA: pulmonary artery; RV: right ventricle; VSD: ventricular septal defect; LAD: descending coronary artery. LV: left ventricle.

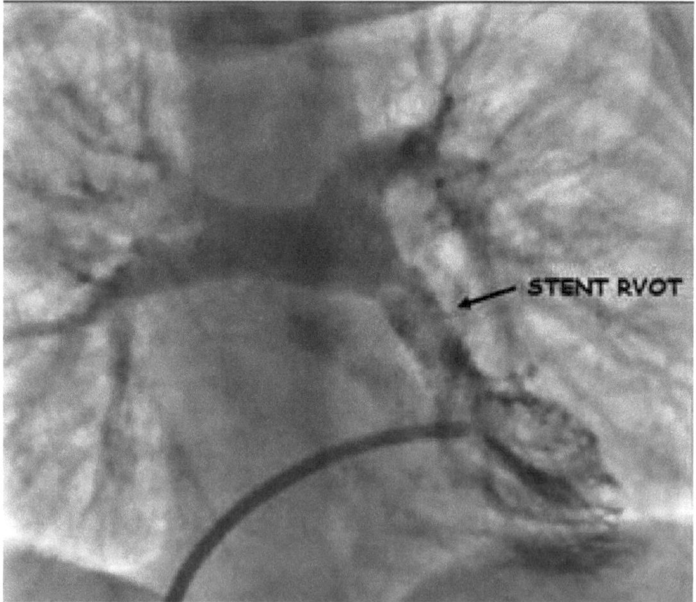

Fig. (10). Right ventricle angiography from a newborn with tetralogy of Fallot with cyanotic spells due to pneumonia who underwent stent implantation at its right ventricle outflow tract.

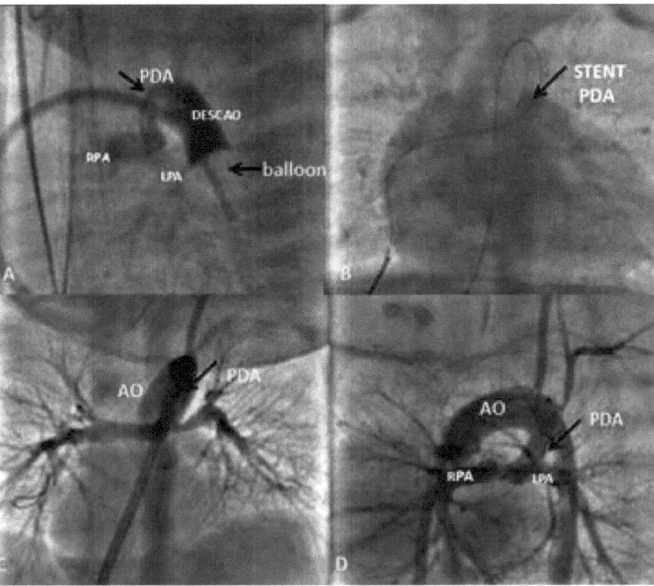

Fig. (11). Patent ductus arteriosus (PDA) stenting percutaneous procedure from a newborn with a pulmonary atresia and ventricular septal defect. AO: aorta; RPA: right pulmonary artery; LPA: left pulmonary artery.

Transposition of the Great Arteries

Transposition of the great arteries (TGA) is a CHD with concordant atrioventricular connection with a ventriculo-arterial discordant lesion in which the aorta arises from the RV and the pulmonary artery from the left ventricle. This creates two parallel circulations that result in cyanotic heart disease. The deoxygenated systemic venous blood arrives in the right atrium. During the diastole, the blood is sent to the systemic circulation by RV and aorta. The oxygenated pulmonary venous blood arrives in the left atrium and back to the pulmonary circulation by left ventricle and pulmonary artery. The parallel circulation does not cause any adverse effect in fetuses, but in neonates and infants, there must be adequate mixing between the intracardiac (atrial or ventricular septal defect/patent foramen ovale) and extra cardiac (PDA) circulation for survival. This mixing actually determines the clinical presentation, prognosis, and management:

a. TGA with Poor Mixing (Intact Ventricular Septum or Restrictive VSD with Small Septal Defect/FO)

Severe hypoxemia occurs after ductal closure. The atrial communication restrictive will not be able to maintain adequate mixing.

b. TGA with Adequate Mixing (with VSD /PDA)

Clinical presentation with CHF at 4–6 weeks with mild cyanosis. Large VSD/PDA enables adequate mixing with increased pulmonary flow. These patients are at high risk for early development of the pulmonary vascular disease. Similarly, TGA with large atrial septal defect (ASD) provides adequate mixing, however, without causing pulmonary hypertension (low-pressure site of mixing) and with a lower risk for CHF and pulmonary edema.

c. TGA with VSD/Pulmonary Stenosis

Neonates with TGA with VSD/pulmonary stenosis, usually has deeper cyanosis.

Features of TGA with large VSD/PDA:

• Physical examination: Quiet precordium; Single second heart sound (A2); no significant murmur; cyanosis.

• Arterial blood gas: metabolic acidosis, low pO_2, normal pCO_2, failure of 100% oxygen to increase pO_2 >100 mmHg.

i. Chest X-ray:

• "egg-shaped" heart (over a period of few days);

• Cardiomegaly with increased pulmonary blood flow in TGA with large VSD;

• Increased pulmonary blood flow in patients with d-TGA, VSD with restrictive atrial communication.

ii. Electrocardiography: Right axis deviation, right ventricle forces.

iii. Echocardiography: Important tool in non-invasive diagnosis of TGA, enabling the identification of the site of mixing and associated defects (Fig. **12**).

iv. Management:

• Initial stabilization with correction of metabolic disorder (acidosis, hypoglycemia) and temperature control;

• PG should be started as soon as the newborn is diagnosed with cyanotic CHD or high suspicion of congenital cyanotic cardiac defect;

• Newborns with restrictive FO with an intact ventricular septum, should be treated by balloon atrial septostomy. In neonates with VSD, a balloon atriosseptostomy is not an emergency procedure although it can be helpful to reduce left atrial pressure and pulmonary venous congestion;

• Atrial septostomy: when it is successful, infusion of PG, can be reduced or even stopped.

Surgical treatment: Jatene's procedure (arterial switch) is the operation of choice and should be performed preferably in the first two weeks of life of age [35]. In late presenters, beyond 4 weeks of age, a two-staged Jatene surgical repair can be performed with a preparatory surgery using pulmonary artery banding and cases with severe pulmonary stenosis may require initial palliation with Blalock-Taussig shunt can be an option. After a few months or in such cases, the atrial switch operation (Senning and Mustard) can be the switch operation of choice [36, 37].

Neonatal Cardiac Heart Failure

Some neonates present with features of CHF in an insidious manner. Causes of neonatal CHF may be CHD or acquired: truncus arteriosus (large left-to-right shunt.), large VSD (complete atrioventricular canal defect with valve regurgitation); large PDA/aorto-pulmonary window and arteriovenous malformations (vein of Galen malformation).

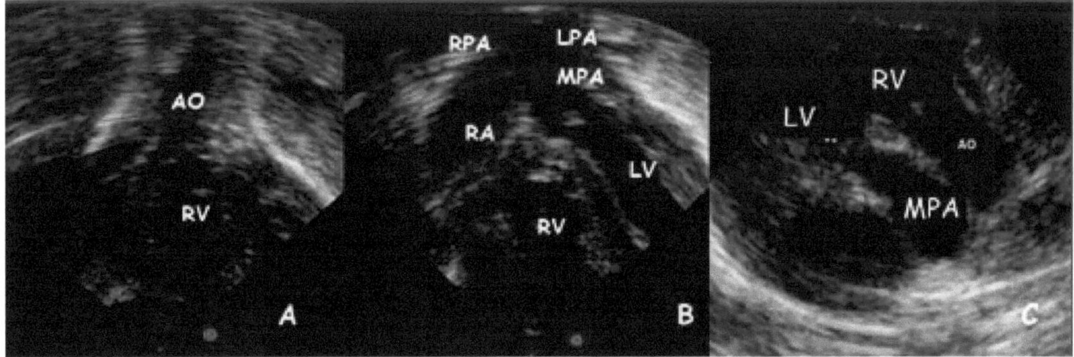

Fig. (12). Echocardiogram of transposition of the great arteries. Subcostal view shows A) the aorta arising from the RV with B) concordant atrioventricular connection (4-chamber view). C) Parasternal long-axis view demonstrates discordant ventriculoarterial connection with the great arteries in a parallel relationship. AO: aorta; RA: right atrium; RV: right ventricle; LV: left ventricle; MPA: main pulmonary artery; RPA: right pulmonary artery; LPA: left pulmonary artery.

Left Ventricular Dysfunction

Anomalous Origin of the Left Coronary Artery from the Pulmonary Artery

Neonate with septal defects usually presents between 2-8 weeks of age with CHF due to pulmonary over-circulation as there is fall in pulmonary vascular resistance causing increase in pulmonary blood flow, rarely there can be an early presentation as in preterm child where precipitous fall in pulmonary vascular resistance occurs causing large left to right shunt. In any newborn presenting with CHF, one should always look for other causes contributing to heart failure in addition to septal defects (Figs. **13** and **14**).

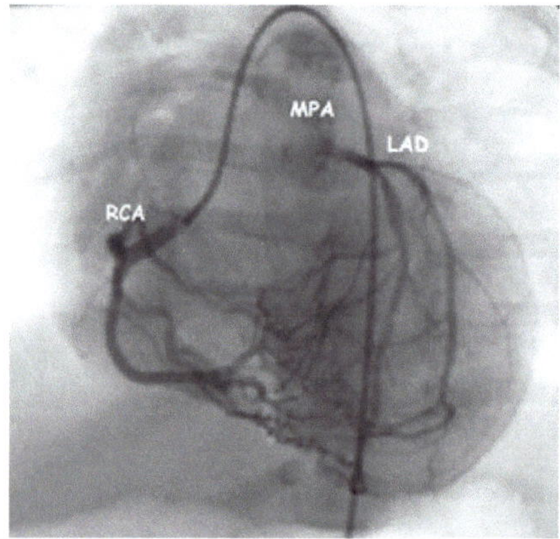

Fig. (13). Right coronarography showing the LAD arising from the main pulmonary artery. RCA: right coronary artery, LAD: left anterior descending artery, MPA: main pulmonary artery.

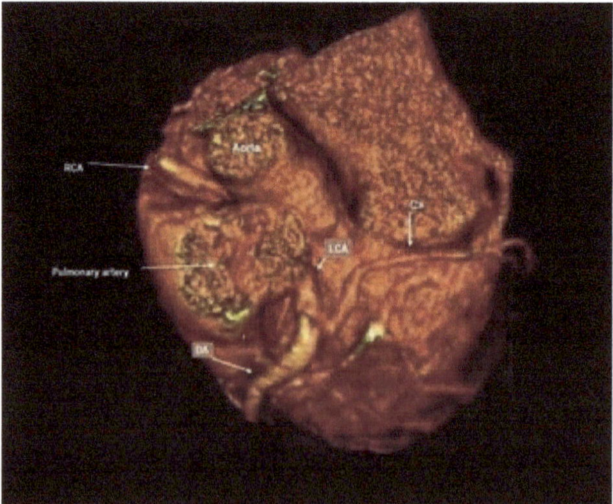

Fig. (14). Coronary angiotomography showing the left coronary artery arising from the main pulmonary trunk. RCA: right coronary artery; LCA: left coronary artery; DA: ductus arteriosus.

Acquired Ventricular Dysfunction (Myocarditis, Septicemia, Dilated Cardiomyopathy, Perinatal Asphyxia, Arrhythmias)

Arrhythmia

Arrhythmias, though rare, are not uncommon in fetuses and newborns. Evaluation of the electrocardiogram is essential, especially because many of these electrocardiograms may be casually interpreted as sinus tachycardia, which is commonly associated with left ventricular dysfunction. In all neonates with suspected CHD, 12-lead electrocardiogram should be performed routinely. Arrhythmias, for example, congenital complete heart block or tachyarrhythmias, can be caused by CHD (Ebstein's anomaly, congenitally corrected TGA, and others) or intracardiac tumors, but the majority of them occur in the neonate with a structurally normal heart [38 - 40].

The key features to establish when examining a neonatal electrocardiogram are that there is a regular narrow QRS complex, with a rate of 100–150, each complex being preceded by a P wave, which is upright in lead DI and AVF. Of course, these guidelines are not absolute, as sinus rates exceeding these levels may be encountered in the sick neonate. Neonatal bradyarrhythmia or tachyarrhythmia can present with shock, with clinical signs and symptoms similar to those of a critically obstructed systemic circulation. One potential clinical manifestation of prolonged (in other words *in utero*) arrhythmias may be the presence of hydrops, which carries with it a poor prognosis. All neonates with an arrhythmia require echocardiography to exclude associated intracardiac defects, but prompt diagnosis and treatment of a tachyarrhythmia can often rapidly reverse a spiraling clinical situation and should not be delayed. A diagnosis of complete heart block in the neonate with a low cardiac output should prompt the neonatologist to seek early advice from a pediatric cardiologist. The treatment may require isoprenaline or dopamine, and urgent transfer for the insertion of a pacemaker [41, 42].

Suspicion is aroused when

a. The heart rate shows no variability and is fixed between 150 and 180 beats per minute (bpm);
b. there is an abnormal P wave axis; c) there is atrioventricular dissociation.

Tachyarrhythmia

Classified into two groups: narrow QRS tachycardia and wide QRS tachycardia.

<u>Narrow QRS Tachycardia</u>

Paroxysmal supraventricular tachycardia (SVT) is the most common where the reentry node tachycardia is the main mechanism during the neonatal period. Structural heart defects are uncommon in this group of tachycardia. The much rarer type of sustained supraventricular tachycardia is the junctional ectopic tachycardia which is more often associated to heart failure because of its sustained nature is most seen in postoperative period. Atrial arrhythmias, like atrial flutter or atrial fibrillation, are very rarely seen in pediatric practice and are even rarer in the neonate.

<u>Wide QRS Tachycardia</u>

Wide QRS tachycardia is rare in neonates and usually associated with myocarditis, and cardiac tumor.

<u>Management</u>

Early management: initial management, based on the guidelines of the advanced pediatric life support group, depends on the general condition of the infant.

a) With circulatory collapse with a tachycardia (with narrow or wide QRS), requires cardioversion, which should be synchronized;

b) Without circulatory collapse, the adenosine is the first option of treatment.

c) In the infant with a narrow complex tachycardia who is not compromised, facial immersion can be attempted. With the infant wrapped in a towel and connected to an electrocardiogram, the face is immersed for approximately 5 seconds into a bowl of cold water. It is safe and effective. Ocular pressure is not recommended at any age, and carotid massage does not work in neonates and infants and compresses the airway.

Adenosine (200 mcg/kg) can be given rapidly intravenously. Failure of adenosine to terminate the tachycardia may be due to

1. Inadequate dosage or administration (too slow) of the drug;

2. The mechanism being atrial tachycardia or atrial flutter; as adenosine blocks the atrioventricular node make possible to recognize them;

3. The mechanism being ventricular tachycardia (VT).

In the case of transient termination of the arrythmia, additional antiarrhythmic treatment is required. Intravenous amiodarone is increasingly used to SVT [43 -

45].

Maintenance Therapy

Commonly used medications used in the management of neonatal tachycardias are: beta blockers, amiodarone, flecainide, and sotalol. Digoxin is sometimes used as adjunctive treatment to provide some atrioventricular block in combination with another agent, (flecainide or sotalol or amiodarone). The natural history of SVT presenting in the neonate suggests that spontaneous resolution usually occurs in the first year of life [46].

Bradyarrhythmia

Bradyarrhythmia (the commonest being complete heart block) can cause heart failure even in fetal life (Fig. **15**). Careful and regular follow-up of those neonates is crucial. The current recommendations for a permanent cardiac pacemaker in neonates are:

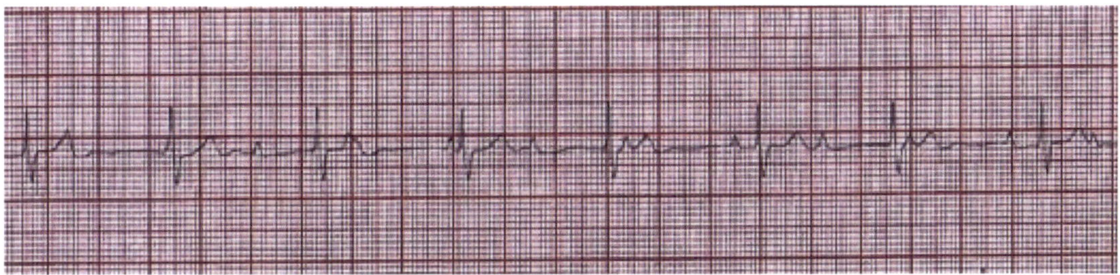

Fig. (15). Electrocardiogram from a newborn with complete atrioventricular heart block.

• Symptoms –most commonly heart failure and circulatory collapse, mainly when the heart rate is less than 55 bpm in normal heart and and less than 70 bpm in structural heart defects;

• Left ventricular dysfunction on echocardiography.

CONSENT FOR PUBLICATION

Not applicable.

CONFLICT OF INTEREST

The authors confirm that the contents of this chapter have no conflict of interest.

ACKNOWLEDGEMENTS

Declare none.

REFERENCES

[1]   Hoffman JI, Kaplan S. The incidence of congenital heart disease. J Am Coll Cardiol 2002; 39(12): 1890-900.
[http://dx.doi.org/10.1016/S0735-1097(02)01886-7] [PMID: 12084585]

[2]   Tennant PW, Pearce MS, Bythell M, Rankin J. 20-year survival of children born with congenital anomalies: a population-based study. Lancet 2010; 375(9715): 649-56.
[http://dx.doi.org/10.1016/S0140-6736(09)61922-X] [PMID: 20092884]

[3]   Bird TM, Hobbs CA, Cleves MA, Tilford JM, Robbins JM. National rates of birth defects among hospitalized newborns. Birth Defects Res A Clin Mol Teratol 2006; 76(11): 762-9.
[http://dx.doi.org/10.1002/bdra.20323] [PMID: 17063529]

[4]   Wren C, Reinhardt Z, Khawaja K. Twenty-year trends in diagnosis of life-threatening neonatal cardiovascular malformations. Arch Dis Child Fetal Neonatal Ed 2008; 93(1): F33-5.
[http://dx.doi.org/10.1136/adc.2007.119032] [PMID: 17556383]

[5]   Khoshnood B, Lelong N, Houyel L, *et al.* EPICARD Study Group. Prevalence, timing of diagnosis and mortality of newborns with congenital heart defects: a population-based study. Heart 2012; 98(22): 1667-73.
[http://dx.doi.org/10.1136/heartjnl-2012-302543] [PMID: 22888161]

[6]   Pruetz JD, Carroll C, Trento LU, *et al.* Outcomes of critical congenital heart disease requiring emergent neonatal cardiac intervention. Prenat Diagn 2014; 34(12): 1127-32.
[http://dx.doi.org/10.1002/pd.4438] [PMID: 24947130]

[7]   Morris SA, Ethen MK, Penny DJ, *et al.* Prenatal diagnosis, birth location, surgical center, and neonatal mortality in infants with hypoplastic left heart syndrome. Circulation 2014; 129(3): 285-92.
[http://dx.doi.org/10.1161/CIRCULATIONAHA.113.003711] [PMID: 24135071]

[8]   Kuehl KS, Loffredo CA, Ferencz C. Failure to diagnose congenital heart disease in infancy. Pediatrics 1999; 103(4 Pt 1): 743-7.
[http://dx.doi.org/10.1542/peds.103.4.743] [PMID: 10103296]

[9]   Mellander M. Diagnosis and management of life-threatening cardiac malformations in the newborn. Semin Fetal Neonatal Med 2013; 18(5): 302-10.
[http://dx.doi.org/10.1016/j.siny.2013.04.007] [PMID: 23688937]

[10]   Changlani TD, Jose A, Sudhakar A, Rojal R, Kunjikutty R, Vaidyanathan B. Outcomes of infants with prenatally diagnosed congenital heart disease delivered in a tertiary-care pediatric cardiac facility. Indian Pediatr 2015; 52(10): 852-6.
[http://dx.doi.org/10.1007/s13312-015-0731-x] [PMID: 26499008]

[11]   Colaco SM, Karande T, Bobhate PR, Jiyani R, Rao SG, Kulkarni S. Neonates with critical congenital heart defects: Impact of fetal diagnosis on immediate and short-term outcomes. Ann Pediatr Cardiol 2017; 10(2): 126-30.
[http://dx.doi.org/10.4103/apc.APC_125_16] [PMID: 28566819]

[12]   Dorfman AT, Marino BS, Wernovsky G, *et al.* Critical heart disease in the neonate: presentation and outcome at a tertiary care center. Pediatr Crit Care Med 2008; 9(2): 193-202.
[http://dx.doi.org/10.1097/PCC.0b013e318166eda5] [PMID: 18477933]

[13]   Schultz AH, Localio AR, Clark BJ, Ravishankar C, Videon N, Kimmel SE. Epidemiologic features of the presentation of critical congenital heart disease: implications for screening. Pediatrics 2008; 121(4): 751-7.
[http://dx.doi.org/10.1542/peds.2007-0421] [PMID: 18381540]

[14]   Desai K, Rabinowitz EJ, Epstein S. Physiologic diagnosis of congenital heart disease in cyanotic neonates. Curr Opin Pediatr 2019; 31(2): 274-83.
[http://dx.doi.org/10.1097/MOP.0000000000000742] [PMID: 30730315]

[15] Peterson C, Ailes E, Riehle-Colarusso T, *et al*. Late detection of critical congenital heart disease among US infants: estimation of the potential impact of proposed universal screening using pulse oximetry. JAMA Pediatr 2014; 168(4): 361-70.
[http://dx.doi.org/10.1001/jamapediatrics.2013.4779] [PMID: 24493342]

[16] Ewer AK, Middleton LJ, Furmston AT, *et al*. PulseOx Study Group. Pulse oximetry screening for congenital heart defects in newborn infants (PulseOx): a test accuracy study. Lancet 2011; 378(9793): 785-94.
[http://dx.doi.org/10.1016/S0140-6736(11)60753-8] [PMID: 21820732]

[17] Gardner TH. Cardiac emergencies in the newborn period. Radiol Clin North Am 1971; 9(3): 385-96.
[PMID: 4256916]

[18] Danford DA, Gutgesell HP, McNamara DG. Application of information theory to decision analysis in potentially prostaglandin-responsive neonates. J Am Coll Cardiol 1986; 8(5): 1125-30.
[http://dx.doi.org/10.1016/S0735-1097(86)80391-6] [PMID: 3760386]

[19] Coceani F. Prostaglandins and the central nervous system. Arch Intern Med 1974; 133(1): 119-29.
[http://dx.doi.org/10.1001/archinte.1974.00320130121010] [PMID: 4357265]

[20] Penny DJ, Shekerdemian LS. Management of the neonate with symptomatic congenital heart disease. Arch Dis Child Fetal Neonatal Ed 2001; 84(3): F141-5.
[http://dx.doi.org/10.1136/fn.84.3.F141] [PMID: 11320036]

[21] McGovern E, Sands AJ. Perinatal management of major congenital heart disease. Ulster Med J 2014; 83(3): 135-9.
[PMID: 25484461]

[22] Tomar M. Neonatal cardiac emergencies: evaluation and management. J Intensive Crit Care 2016; 2: 1.
[http://dx.doi.org/10.21767/2471-8505.100021]

[23] Schamberger MS. Cardiac emergencies in children. Pediatr Ann 1996; 25(6): 339-44.
[http://dx.doi.org/10.3928/0090-4481-19960601-09] [PMID: 8793920]

[24] Lee C, Mason LJ. Pediatric cardiac emergencies. Anesthesiol Clin North America 2001; 19(2): 287-308.
[http://dx.doi.org/10.1016/S0889-8537(05)70230-3] [PMID: 11469066]

[25] Forbess JM, Cook N, Roth SJ, Serraf A, Mayer JE Jr, Jonas RA. Ten-year institutional experience with palliative surgery for hypoplastic left heart syndrome. Risk factors related to stage I mortality. Circulation 1995; 92(9) (Suppl.): II262-6.
[http://dx.doi.org/10.1161/01.CIR.92.9.262] [PMID: 7586421]

[26] Stasik CN, Gelehrter S, Goldberg CS, Bove EL, Devaney EJ, Ohye RG. Current outcomes and risk factors for the Norwood procedure. J Thorac Cardiovasc Surg 2006; 131(2): 412-7.
[http://dx.doi.org/10.1016/j.jtcvs.2005.09.030] [PMID: 16434272]

[27] Gordon BM, Rodriguez S, Lee M, Chang RK. Decreasing number of deaths of infants with hypoplastic left heart syndrome. J Pediatr 2008; 153(3): 354-8.
[http://dx.doi.org/10.1016/j.jpeds.2008.03.009] [PMID: 18534240]

[28] Karamlou T, Diggs BS, Ungerleider RM, Welke KF. Evolution of treatment options and outcomes for hypoplastic left heart syndrome over an 18-year period. J Thorac Cardiovasc Surg 2010; 139(1): 119-26.
[http://dx.doi.org/10.1016/j.jtcvs.2009.04.061] [PMID: 19909991]

[29] Colli AM, Perry SB, Lock JE, Keane JF. Balloon dilation of critical valvar pulmonary stenosis in the first month of life. Cathet Cardiovasc Diagn 1995; 34(1): 23-8.
[http://dx.doi.org/10.1002/ccd.1810340307] [PMID: 7728847]

[30] Justo RN, Nykanen DG, Williams WG, Freedom RM, Benson LN. Transcatheter perforation of the

right ventricular outflow tract as initial therapy for pulmonary valve atresia and intact ventricular septum in the newborn. Cathet Cardiovasc Diagn 1997; 40(4): 408-13.
[http://dx.doi.org/10.1002/(SICI)1097-0304(199704)40:4<408::AID-CCD21>3.0.CO;2-H] [PMID: 9096947]

[31] Schranz D, Michel-Behnke I, Heyer R, *et al.* Stent implantation of the arterial duct in newborns with a truly duct-dependent pulmonary circulation: a single-center experience with emphasis on aspects of the interventional technique. J Interv Cardiol 2010; 23(6): 581-8.
[http://dx.doi.org/10.1111/j.1540-8183.2010.00576.x] [PMID: 20642476]

[32] Rosenthal E, Qureshi SA, Tynan M. Percutaneous pulmonary valvotomy and arterial duct stenting in neonates with right ventricular hypoplasia. Am J Cardiol 1994; 74(3): 304-6.
[http://dx.doi.org/10.1016/0002-9149(94)90385-9] [PMID: 8037148]

[33] Abe K, Shimada Y, Takezawa J, Oka N, Yoshiya I. Long-term administration of prostaglandin E1: report of two cases with tetralogy of Fallot and esophageal atresia. Crit Care Med 1982; 10(3): 155-8.
[http://dx.doi.org/10.1097/00003246-198203000-00003] [PMID: 7199417]

[34] Tsze DS, Vitberg YM, Berezow J, Starc TJ, Dayan PS. Treatment of tetralogy of Fallot hypoxic spell with intranasal fentanyl. Pediatrics 2014; 134(1): e266-9.
[http://dx.doi.org/10.1542/peds.2013-3183] [PMID: 24936003]

[35] Idriss FS, Ilbawi MN, DeLeon SY, *et al.* Arterial switch in simple and complex transposition of the great arteries. J Thorac Cardiovasc Surg 1988; 95(1): 29-36.
[http://dx.doi.org/10.1016/S0022-5223(19)35383-8] [PMID: 3336233]

[36] Jonas RA, Giglia TM, Sanders SP, *et al.* Rapid, two-stage arterial switch for transposition of the great arteries and intact ventricular septum beyond the neonatal period. Circulation 1989; 80(3 Pt 1): I203-8.
[PMID: 2766528]

[37] Bisoi AK, Sharma P, Chauhan S, *et al.* Primary arterial switch operation in children presenting late with d-transposition of great arteries and intact ventricular septum. When is it too late for a primary arterial switch operation? Eur J Cardiothorac Surg 2010; 38(6): 707-13.
[http://dx.doi.org/10.1016/j.ejcts.2010.03.037] [PMID: 20663683]

[38] Mas C, Penny DJ, Menahem S. Pre-excitation syndrome secondary to cardiac rhabdomyomas in tuberous sclerosis. J Paediatr Child Health 2000; 36(1): 84-6.
[http://dx.doi.org/10.1046/j.1440-1754.2000.00443.x] [PMID: 10723700]

[39] Deal BJ, Keane JF, Gillette PC, Garson A Jr. Wolff-Parkinson-White syndrome and supraventricular tachycardia during infancy: management and follow-up. J Am Coll Cardiol 1985; 5(1): 130-5.
[http://dx.doi.org/10.1016/S0735-1097(85)80095-4] [PMID: 3964800]

[40] Eronen M, Sirèn MK, Ekblad H, Tikanoja T, Julkunen H, Paavilainen T. Short- and long-term outcome of children with congenital complete heart block diagnosed *in utero* or as a newborn. Pediatrics 2000; 106(1 Pt 1): 86-91.
[http://dx.doi.org/10.1542/peds.106.1.86] [PMID: 10878154]

[41] Eronen M. Outcome of fetuses with heart disease diagnosed *in utero* . Arch Dis Child Fetal Neonatal Ed 1997; 77(1): F41-6.
[http://dx.doi.org/10.1136/fn.77.1.F41] [PMID: 9279182]

[42] Palmisano JM, Moler FW, Custer JR, Meliones JN, Snedecor S, Revesz SM. Unsuspected congenital heart disease in neonates receiving extracorporeal life support: a review of ninety-five cases from the Extracorporeal Life Support Organization Registry. J Pediatr 1992; 121(1): 115-7.
[http://dx.doi.org/10.1016/S0022-3476(05)82555-7] [PMID: 1625068]

[43] Stacy AS. Killen and frank a. fish. fetal and neonatal arrhythmias. Neoreviews 2008; 9(6): e242-52.
[http://dx.doi.org/10.1542/neo.9-6-e242]

[44] Chu PY, Hill KD, Clark RH, Smith PB, Hornik CP. Treatment of supraventricular tachycardia in infants: Analysis of a large multicenter database. Early Hum Dev 2015; 91(6): 345-50.

[http://dx.doi.org/10.1016/j.earlhumdev.2015.04.001] [PMID: 25933212]

[45]   Dixon J, Foster K, Wyllie J, Wren C. Guidelines and adenosine dosing in supraventricular tachycardia. Arch Dis Child 2005; 90(11): 1190-1.
[http://dx.doi.org/10.1136/adc.2005.077636] [PMID: 16243875]

[46]   van Engelen AD, Weijtens O, Brenner JI, *et al.* Management outcome and follow-up of fetal tachycardia. J Am Coll Cardiol 1994; 24(5): 1371-5.
[http://dx.doi.org/10.1016/0735-1097(94)90122-8] [PMID: 7930263]

CHAPTER 13

Postnatal Surgical Approach of Congenital Heart Disease

Jose Pedro Da Silva[*] and **Luciana Da Fonseca Da Silva**

Department of Cardiothoracic Surgery, UPMC Children's Hospital of Pittsburgh, PA,United States of America

Abstract: The advances in neonatal care and pediatric cardiac surgery have allowed repairing of complex congenital heart disease in the newborn and young infants with excellent results. The most common congenital heart defects that may need early surgical treatment are tetralogy of Fallot (TOF), transposition of the great arteries (TGA), univentricular heart, total anomalous pulmonary veins connection, hypoplastic left heart syndrome, critical aortic stenosis, and truncus arteriosus. TGA, characterized by atrioventricular concordance with ventriculoarterial discordance, is the most common cyanogenic cardiopathy, which requires treatment in the neonatal period. Atrioseptostomy with Raskind balloon must be performed in the newborn with TGA, who presents significant hypoxia and restrictive atrial septal defect. Surgical treatment of TGA depends on the gestational age diagnosis, associated defects and evaluation of the left ventricle anatomy and function. TOF is the cyanogenic cardiopathy that requires therapy more frequently within the first year of life. Those newborns with TOF who present severe cyanoses and or hypoxic crises may become ductus dependent, requiring surgical shunting procedure, percutaneous ductal stenting or total repair. Currently, there is a trend to perform neonatal total surgical repair in the centers of excellence, based in the low surgical risk. In univentricular hearts, medical decision depends on some anatomical aspects. While in case of significant pulmonary flow obstruction, it will require shunting procedure, in case of pulmonary overflow, it may need pulmonary banding. Total anomalous pulmonary venous return, critical aortic valve stenosis, and pulmonary atresia patients will require surgical or interventional heart catheterization procedures as a newborn. While, newborns with Ebstein's anomaly have about 60% chance of requiring early surgical intervention.

Keywords: Ballon atrioseptostomy, Congenital heart disease, Neonatal cardiac surgery.

---

[*] **Address Correspondence Jose Pedro Da Silva:** Department of Cardiothoracic Surgery, UPMC Children's Hospital of Pittsburgh, 4401 Penn Avenue, Cardiothoracic Surgery, Faculty Pavilion, 5th Floor, Pittsburgh, PA 15224, USA, Tel: 412-692-5319/ Fax: 412-692-5817; E-mail: dasilvajp@upmc.ed

Edward Araujo Júnior, Nathalie Jeanne M. Bravo-Valenzuela and Alberto Borges Peixoto (Eds.)

INTRODUCTION

The advances in fetal medicine and neonatal care have improved the diagnosis and chances of survival of neonates with congenital heart disease in the recent years. Consequently, the number of newborns that would benefit neonatal surgical treatment has increased. The development of fetal echocardiographic diagnosis allowed the anticipation of immediate need for clinical or surgical intervention in the first hours or days of life. However, a large population of neonates with heart defects remains undiagnosed until after developing serious manifestations [1, 2].

Fortunately, the pharmacology and technology applied for the clinical and the surgical treatment have improved, as well as the surgical techniques have advanced in the recent decades, allowing good surgical results even in very small neonates with complex congenital heart diseases [3, 4].

Congenital heart diseases range from mild to severe, with variable clinical presentations. The symptoms in the neonate may be vague, so it is very important to have a high index of suspicion, identifying the need for rapid cardiac evaluation to rule out a serious congenital cardiac problem that needs early intervention [5].

In isolated critical congenital heart diseases, physical examination might not detect cyanosis or other clinical signs before transitions from fetal circulation are completed, which can occur after nursery discharge. Newborn screening for heart defects has progressed in the recent years, aiming to decrease infant mortality [1]

Neonatologists must be aware that some patients will need maneuvers in the preoperative period to improve the clinical condition, such as:

-Immediate use of prostaglandin E (PGE) to improve lung perfusion (pulmonary atresia and other ductal dependent pulmonary circulation) or to keep adequate systemic output in ductal-dependent systemic circulation (hypoplastic left heart syndrome - HLHS, interrupted aortic arch and others);

-Clinical maneuvers to decrease the pulmonary blood flow, like the addition of nitrogen in room air in cases of HLHS;

-Opening of atrial septal defect (ASD) to decompress the pulmonary venous system (HLHS with restrictive ASD), to improve the venous arterial blood mixing (transposition of the great arteries - TGA with low saturation) or to increase the systemic cardiac output (tricuspid atresia, pulmonary/tricuspid valve hypoplasia with hypoplastic right ventricle, total anomalous pulmonary venous return).

The life-threatening conditions will dictate the need for surgical treatment in the neonatal period [6, 7]. This chapter will address the main congenital heart diseases with emphasis on those that often require early surgical intervention.

TETRALOGY OF FALLOT

Tetralogy of Fallot (TOF) is characterized by ventricular septal defect, aortic overriding of the interventricular septal crest, right ventricular outflow tract obstruction, and right ventricle hypertrophy. TOF is the most common cyanogenic congenital heart disease, representing 10% of all congenital heart diseases. TOF occurs in equal frequency in both sexes. It is a heart disease that regularly requires surgery during the first year of life. When the newborn presents with severe cyanosis and are ductal dependent, they require either a shunting procedure or total repair as a newborn.

ANATOMY AND MORPHOLOGY

The ventricular septal defect (VSD) is usually single, wide and localized in the subaortic region (misaligned conoventricular VSD). The right ventricular outflow tract (RVO) obstruction occurs at various levels and may be infundibular, valvular (pulmonary valve stenosis), supravalvular and pulmonary artery branches. The RVOT obstruction is the more constant feature of TOF, and the infundibular anatomical and dynamic obstruction is regarded as the main characteristic of TOF. It results from anterior and upward deviation of the infundibular septum. The hypertrophy of the muscular bands of the RVOT pathway may accentuate the pulmonary subvalvar obstruction. The pulmonary valve annulus is usually hypoplastic but may be normal in some cases. The pulmonary valve is often stenotic, and often bicuspid. In extreme cases, the RVOT may be completely obstructed (pulmonary atresia), not allowing anterograde flow from the right ventricle to the pulmonary artery. In this situation, the pulmonary flow depends on the ductus arteriosus, on aortopulmonary collateral arteries or on both. In the case of supravalvular stenosis, the obstruction may occur in the pulmonary trunk and branches. The pulmonary artery hypoplasia may be diffuse or focal, as often occurs in the left pulmonary artery, at the ductus arteriosus insertion site. The aortic overriding of the ventricular septal crest is variable and may be between 10 and 50% (Fig. **1**). The cases in which the aorta overrides the ventricular septum more than 50%, are defined as double right ventricular outflow tract.

Fig. (1). Tetralogy of Fallot echocardiogram shows the ventricular septum overriding the aorta in about 50% diastole **(A)**, and systole **(B,C)**. Right ventricle outflow tract with muscular obstruction and mild hypoplasia of the pulmonary valve **(D)**. RV: right ventricle, VS: ventricular septum, LV: left ventricle, LA: left atrium, Ao: aorta, RVOT: right ventricle outflow tract, PV: pulmonary valve, AV: aortic valve, PA: pulmonary artery.

ASSOCIATED MALFORMATIONS

The ascending aorta is usually dilated, and approximately 25% of cases have a right aortic arch. Coronary artery anomalies can be found in 5 to 10% of cases, with the origin of the anterior descending coronary artery from the right coronary artery, which is the most frequent coronary anomaly. When a coronary artery branch crosses the outlet right ventricle, it can cause difficulty in corrective surgery [8, 9]. Other heart diseases associated with heart defects, such as patent ductus arteriosus (PDA), multiple VSDs, atrioventricular septal defect, and aortopulmonary collaterals arteries may be present and must be recognized before the surgical correction. TOF with pulmonary atresia and aortopulmonary multiple collaterals is the most extreme variant form of TOF. The pulmonary atresia may be limited to the valve itself, known as membranous atresia, or involve the infundibulum (muscle atresia). Both ways result in the absence of anterograde flow from the right ventricle to the pulmonary artery. The alternate source of pulmonary flow can be through the ductus arteriosus or aortopulmonary collateral arteries.

PATHOPHYSIOLOGY

With the aorta riding the septum, this gets the blood coming from the left ventricle saturated and unsaturated coming from the right ventricle. The degree of mixture depends on the degree of obstruction of the outlet of the right ventricle. As the VSD is large, systolic pressure of both ventricles is usually equal; however, the more serious is the degree of the infundibular obstruction with pulmonary stenosis, which regulates the pulmonary blood flow and, consequently, the hypoxia. The hypoxemia stimulates the bone marrow, producing polycythemia. The extended cyanosis can lead to complications such as blood hyperviscosity, thromboembolic phenomena and brain abscess.

CLINICAL PRESENTATION

The clinical presentation depends on the degree of pulmonary stenosis. With mild stenosis (pink Fallot), the symptoms appear later in the childhood, and may lack symptoms at 4 to 6 weeks of age. However, in severe pulmonary stenosis, cyanosis occurs earlier, even in neonates. More often, the child is acyanotic in the neonatal period and develops cyanosis between 2 and 6 months of life. Cyanotic spell is a sudden event seen in infants with TOF, associated with progressive cyanosis, hyperpnea (increased rate and depth of breathing) and disappearance of heart murmur. If not treated on time, it may ultimately lead to altered sensorium, neurological complications and death. The infundibular spasm, precipitated by the sudden rise in the level of endogenous catecholamines, is regarded as the most likely mechanism [9, 10].

ECHOCARDIOGRAPHY, CARDIAC CATHETERIZATION, MAGNETIC RESONANCE IMAGING AND/OR COMPUTED TOMOGRAPHY

Although echocardiogram provides important information regarding the anatomy of TOF, in some circumstances there is a need for additional study methods to clarify the anatomical structures that are not properly defined in the echocardiogram. Therefore, cardiac catheterization, magnetic resonance imaging and/or computed tomography may be indicated to clarify pulmonary branches details, coronary arteries anatomy, systemic-pulmonary arterial collaterals and presence of multiple VSDs.

TREATMENT

The treatment of hypoxic spells consists of sedation, adequate IV hydration, beta-blockers (propranolol), knee chest position, morphine (IV, IM or SC), NaHCO$_3$, oxygen, phenylephrine hydrochloride, mechanical ventilation if necessary. Surgery is ultimately indicated in all cases. The need for surgery earlier in life depends on different variables, which includes early symptoms, age of onset and the associated lesions [11].

SURGICAL TREATMENT

There are two types of surgical treatments: total repair and palliative operation. Possible advantages of total repair in the neonate are: 1- early normalization of the flow and pressure in every heart chamber; 2- interruption of the process of right ventricular hypertrophy that occurs when this cavity works in the presence of pulmonary stenosis; 3- need for less extensive resection of the infundibulum during repair, which can reduce the incidence of ventricular arrhythmias in the late postoperative period; 4- early normalization of arterial oxygen saturation, thus avoiding the deleterious effects of chronic hypoxemia on the heart, the brain and other organs; 5- avoid complications of shunt operations, especially distortion of pulmonary arteries and pulmonary hypertension development; 6- psychosocial and economic advantages, especially in hypoxemic and acidotic newborns, who requires intravenous prostaglandin for stabilization. Although there are controversies about the best treatment in the first few months of life, there is a tendency to prefer the total repair. Two risk factors that contraindicates the correction in the first year are marked hypoplasia of the pulmonary arteries and anomalous origin of anterior descending artery right coronary artery. More recent studies have shown that the best survival and physiological result are obtained between 3 and 11 months [11 - 14]. However, institutions of excellence prefer to approach newborns who require intervention with total repair. Palliation through interventionist heart catheterization seems to be preferred instead of surgical shunting in ductus dependent newborns [14 - 16]. Total repair with pulmonary valve-sparing technique is our preferred strategy whenever possible, regardless of children's age. In cases of TOF with pulmonary atresia presenting good pulmonary artery anatomy, can undergo the standard procedure for total repair [17, 18]. Regarding the patients with pulmonary atresia (PA) with VSD and major aortopulmonary collateral arteries (MAPCAs) and absent pulmonary arteries, they can undergo complete single-stage repair with satisfactory postoperative hemodynamics. The unifocalization of MAPCAs can provide a reasonable pulmonary vascular bed in the absence of intrapericardial pulmonary arteries [19].

THERAPEUTIC CARDIAC CATHETERIZATION

Interventionist cardiac catheterization is an attractive alternative to palliative surgery (systemic-pulmonary shunt), in the treatment of TOF and other cyanotic heart diseases dependent on the ductus arteriosus. For TOF, there are two alternatives for the percutaneous treatment: in the ductus arteriosus stenting or right ventricle outlet stenting. Such procedures promote improved oxygen saturation and stimulate the growth of pulmonary arteries [17 - 19].

TRANSPOSITION OF THE GREAT ARTERIES

The transposition of the great arteries (TGA) is a congenital cardiopathy consisting of concordant atrioventricular connection and discordant arterial-ventricle connection. Therefore, the aorta originates from the right ventricle and the pulmonary artery from the left ventricle. The aorta is usually positioned anterior and a little to the right (Fig. **2**). Its embryology is unclear, but there is a hypothesis that the bilateral abnormal growth and development of the sub arterial conus result in the arterial ventricular discordance. It has a higher incidence in children from diabetic mothers, in males and is rarely associated with abnormal extracardiac and genetic syndromes. The TGA represents 3% of all congenital heart diseases and 20% of cyanotic congenital cardiopathies [20].

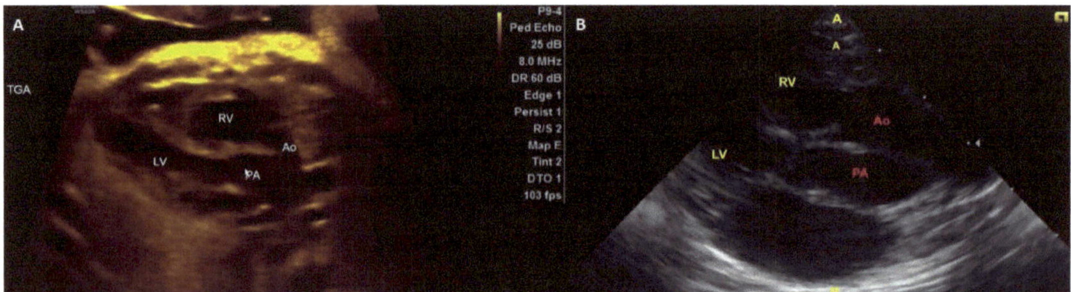

Fig. (2). Echocardiographic diagnosis of transposition of the great arteries (TGA). **A:** Fetal echocardiogram and **B:** Postnatal echocardiogram (parasternal longitudinal view) shows the vessels of the base in parallel – anterior course of the aorta in relation to the pulmonary artery. Note the ventriculoarterial discordance (transposed great arteries). Ao: Aorta; PA: pulmonary artery; RV: right ventricle; LV: left ventricle; A: anterior; P: posterior.

ANATOMY

There are two anatomical types of TGA: 1. TGA with intact ventricular septum (IVS), known as simple TGA, and this is the most frequent type; 2. TGA with VSD, associated or not with left ventricle outflow tract obstruction (LVOT).

PATHOPHYSIOLOGY

The circulation in these cases is in parallel and not in series, as in the normal heart. That is why the blood that reaches the heart through the vena cava does not become oxygenated and the blood of the pulmonary venous return does not reach the body and returns to the lungs. Survival depends on the existence of an intercirculatory shunting, either by atrial septal defect (ASD), VSD, PDA or multiple sources. It is a cardiopathy of high mortality in the first months of life and, when not corrected, the probability of death is 90% at the end of the first year of life. Children with wide VSD tend to present pulmonary overflow and higher systemic saturation, resulting in heart failure and mild cyanosis. The presence of fixed pulmonary stenosis, usually subvalvar, is more common in the presence of VSD and it modifies the balance between systemic and pulmonary circulations. In TGA, the pulmonary vascular disease is more frequent and precocious, mainly in patients with VSD.

CLINICAL MANIFESTATIONS

Children born with TGA present, in their majority, normal birth weight. Cyanosis observed on the first day of life suggests the possibility of TGA and, if the ventricular septum is intact, the child becomes very cyanotic in the first days of life. Tachypnea in general is present, without prominent chest retraction. Children with small VSD can follow a course like those with intact ventricular septum. If a large VSD is present, cyanosis can be absent or minimal and respiratory distress gradually progresses from minimal to severe. In the TGA with VSD and LVOT, the presentation is variable, and the cyanosis is directly proportional to the degree of LVOT/pulmonary stenosis.

PHYSICAL EXAMINATION

Usually, the newborn is visibly cyanotic and comfortably tachypneic. Murmur is not an important finding, unless there is LVOT. The second heart sound may be unique, due to the anterior position of the aortic valve in relation to the pulmonary valve. In the presence of VSD, a systolic murmur may be present within a few days after the birth, followed by signs of heart failure.

ELECTROCARDIOGRAM

In most newborns the electrocardiogram is within the limits of normality and subsequently manifested with right ventricular overload.

CHEST RADIOGRAPHY

A chest X-ray is virtually normal in the first few days of life. Even in the simple TGA the pulmonary flow is normal or increased. In those with large VSD, cardiomegaly and pulmonary overflow are present and sometimes present a characteristic heart silhouette, with a narrow pedicle as a result of the position of the great arteries, similar to a "lying egg".

ECHOCARDIOGRAPHY

Echocardiography is the main diagnostic method. Prenatal ultrasonography studies one performed as screening for congenital heart disease, focusing only on the four-chamber view, may not diagnose heart disease, when there is no discrepancy in the size of the ventricles. The accuracy of the test becomes greater when the outflow tracts are evaluated to verify that the large arteries intersect normally or not. Children diagnosed prenatally improve cognitive skills in the long term, as compared with children with postnatal diagnosis. In the newborn, the subcostal view and the longitudinal parasternal view demonstrate that the pulmonary artery (posterior) emerges from the left ventricle, while the aorta is seen anteriorly emerging from the right ventricle. The echocardiogram should systematically delineate atrioventricular and ventriculoarterial connections and detect other associated lesions, such as coronary anomalies, aortic arch obstruction and VSD, in addition to verifying the presence and size of the ASD and evaluation of the PDA, its size and degree of shunt. The interatrial shunt is easily demonstrated using color Doppler. A restrictive ASD is suspected when it is < 3 mm, presents septum deviation to the right atrium, as well as by the pressure gradient between the atria. Causes of LVOT obstruction include posterior misalignment of the infundibular septum, bulging of the interventricular septum (obstruction due to subvalvar pulmonary stenosis, subvalvar membrane, accessory tissue of the atrioventricular valve and muscle hypertrophy). Accurate identification of the anatomy of the arteries and coronary arteries is fundamental in TGA; therefore, they must be evaluated from multiple echocardiographic views, before surgery.

CARDIAC CATHETERIZATION

Little information is needed beyond those provided by echocardiography. Catheterization is indicated to perform balloon atrioseptostomy (Rashkind procedure) and to confirm the anatomy of the coronary arteries before the arterial switch operation, when necessary. Balloon atrioseptostomy which was introduced by Rashkind and Miller, is the standard method to enlarge the ASD in a newborn. In the TGA, it is indicated to increase the mixture between the two circulations [21]. It can be performed under fluoroscopy or just guided by the echocardiogram and thus can be performed at bedside.

COMPUTED TOMOGRAPHY ANGIOGRAPHY

Computed tomography angiography (CTA) may be necessary to clarify the anatomy of the coronary arteries or obstruction of the aortic arch.

TREATMENT

In case of fetal TGA diagnosis, the best treatment includes the birth in a reference center for pediatric cardiac surgery. In newborns diagnosed with TGA and intact ventricular septum, prostaglandin can be initiated at the initial dose of 0.05 to 0.1 mg/kg/min and maintenance of 0.01 to 0.4 m/kg/min. The child should be transferred to intensive care unit and a postnatal echocardiogram should be performed. With the introduction of the Jatene's operation, the atrioseptostomy, performed routinely in the past, has become more selectively indicated [21, 22]. Currently, atrioseptostomy is used in cases of severe hypoxemia and restrictive ASD, and in those patients with no prediction for surgery in the next few days.

SURGICAL TREATMENT

The anatomical correction of TGA was introduced by Adib Jatene in 1975 [23]. Since then, it has gradually become the procedure of choice for the treatment of simple TGA and TGA with VSD. The Jatene's operation or arterial switch operation (ASO) consists of transection of the great arteries just above the associated valve and then are switched to their usual position. Next, the coronary arteries are transferred and reattached to the new aorta. With this technique, the ascending aorta is reconnected to the morphologically left ventricle. If any septal defects are present, they are closed during the same surgery. Indicated in newborns with TGA with intact ventricular septum, or TGA with VSD without pulmonary stenosis. This operation, that results in the left ventricle pumping to the systemic circulation, is indicated in the first 3 weeks of life.

INDICATIONS FOR OPERATION

In general, the surgical repair of simple TGA with the Jatene's ASO should be performed in the first days of life in full term babies. Ideally, at ages between three and ten days. The patient should be stable, and free of infection or severe pulmonary hypertension or severe cyanosis. Premature babies with simple TGA are generally maintained on intensive care taking IV PGE until completing gestation age of 37 weeks. This treatment protocol seems to optimize the results of surgical treatment of patients with simple TGA. In cases of TGA with VSD the Jatene's operation can be delayed for a few days but should be performed within three weeks of age. Early ASO contributes for a low mortality, improves neurological outcome, and reduces the treatment cost. The expected hospital stay after the ASO is approximately 2 weeks. This can vary depending on how sick the patient is prior to surgery, time to full feeds postoperatively, and any other issues that may delay discharge. Single or intramural coronary arteries may be risk factors for operation [22, 24].

LATE SURGICAL INDICATIONS OF ARTERIAL SWITCH OPERATION

Patients who had lost the best time window for the ASO have to be studied regarding the left ventricle adequacy for the anatomical repair. The morphologically left ventricle, in subpulmonary valve position, needs to have the adequate muscle mass required to maintain the systemic circulation after anatomical repair. This evaluation is performed by the echocardiogram, which classifies the left ventricle in the following types: 1. IVS is bulging into the right ventricle; 2. Rectified IVS; 3. IVS is bulging to the left ventricle (banana-shape). The left ventricle type 3 is considered inadequate to support the systemic circulation, consequently for the anatomical repair. Therefore, patients diagnosed with TGA without VSD having more than one month of life and presenting left ventricle type 3 need to undergo left ventricle retraining by pulmonary banding and Blalock-Taussig (BT) shunt. After this left ventricle preparation, the Jatene's operation can be performed, safely.

ATRIAL CORRECTION OF TRANSPOSITION OF THE GREAT ARTERIES

The atrial and physiological correction of TGA were developed by Mustard and Senning by the creation of two completely different surgical techniques to repair TGA at the atrial level [23]. These operations redirect the systemic venous return to the left ventricle (pulmonary ventricle) and the pulmonary venous return to the right ventricle (systemic ventricle). Therefore, they correct the atrial discordance, keeping the ventriculoarterial discordance. The baby turns pink but the right ventricle continues the systemic pump with its known disadvantages in the long-term.

INDICATIONS FOR SENNING/MUSTARD OPERATIONS

The fact that the Senning and Mustard techniques for TGA repair result in the right ventricle as the systemic ventricle has limited its indication. Currently, it can be considered in: 1- TGA without VSD with more than one month of life, presenting type 3 left ventricle, who fails in left ventricle retraining procedure for the Jatene's operation. 2- Neonates with TGA and inadequate coronary arteries for the arterial switch operation (< 1% of cases). 3- Patients with TGA, intact ventricular septum and severe LVOT obstruction. The Mustard and Senning procedures are also used as part of the double switch procedure for congenitally corrected TGA.

SURGICAL OPTIONS FOR TRANSPOSITION OF THE GREAT ARTERIES WITH VENTRICULAR SEPTAL DEFECT AND OBSTRUCTION OF THE LEFT VENTRICLE OUTFLOW TRACT

Patients with TGA, VSD and LVOT obstruction are not candidates for the ASO due to the pulmonary valve that cannot be transformed in the systemic valve. These patients usually do not require surgery in the newborn period, since the pulmonary flow is controlled by the LVOT. If the newborn presents severe cyanosis, a BT shunt can be indicated to increase pulmonary flow, performing the corrective surgery within the next six months. Currently, several surgical options are available. Optimal surgical treatment of patients with TGA with VSD and LVOT obstruction remains a matter of debate. The Rastelli operation published in 1969 [25] presented high incidence of reoperation due to complications of the right ventricle to pulmonary artery conduit and also to obstruction of the LVOT in the long-term follow-up [26]. The complications reported in the initial publications on the Rastelli operation have stimulated the development of other techniques as follows: REV (Réparation à l'Etage Ventriculaire) or Lecompte procedure (1981) [27, 28] and aortic translocation (1984) [29] which revived an idea proposed by Bex, Lecompte and Baillot (1980) [30] for TGA with intact ventricular septum. In the Rastelli operation, the left ventricle blood flow is redirected for the aorta through the VSD; with the creation of a left ventricle-aorta tunnel, the pulmonary artery is sectioned and its stump in the left ventricle is sutured to a conduit placed to connect the right ventricle and the pulmonary artery. Reoperations are required by tube stenosis, mainly in children operated under the age of 4 years. In addition, obstruction in the left ventricle outflow pathway may also occur in the long term. In the Lecompte operation (Réparation à l'Etage Ventriculaire – REV) [27, 28], the VSD is enlarged, a patch used to close the VSD diverts the blood flow from left ventricle to the aorta. The pulmonary artery, without valve, is anastomosed to the RVOT, being enlarged with a monocuspid. The Lecompte maneuver (anteriorization of the pulmonary trunk in relation to the aorta) is often associated. The pulmonary insufficiency in the long term may lead to the failure of the right ventricle. Initial mortality reported is 12% and reoperations are required in 20% of patients in ten years.

In 1994, we began to use the pulmonary root translocation (PRT) with the aim of overcoming the limitations related to the previous operations and attempting to assure pulmonary valve competency, since we do not discard the pulmonary native valve. We have PRT as an alternative surgical approach for TGA with VSD and RVOT obstruction and for selected cases of double-outlet right ventricle with subpulmonary VSD. More recently, we extended its use as part of the double switch procedure in patients with congenitally corrected TGA, PS, and VSD [31, 32]. In the PRT (Fig. **3**), the pulmonary root is harvested from the left ventricle with caution not to damage the pulmonary valve and coronary arteries. The resulting LVOT orifice is closed with autologous pericardium. A right ventriculotomy is performed, the position of the VSD is confirmed, and the conal septum is resected, whenever necessary to clear the LVOT. A VSD to aorta tunnel is constructed, applying a patch, fashioned to divert the left ventricle blood flow to the aorta. The RVOT is reconstructed with the anastomosis of the pulmonary trunk, with the pulmonary valve being the right ventriculotomy. A monocuspid is used to complete the pulmonary valve only when the valve annulus persists very small after the dissection and dilation. The Lecompte maneuver is not used in this technique.

From April 1994 to November 2009, we employed this technique in 70 patients. Thirteen of them had corrected TGA (c-TGA) with VSD and pulmonary ventricle outflow obstruction. In c-TGA repair, the Senning procedure was used for the atrial switch [32]. A long-term follow-up has shown growth of the pulmonary annulus in all patients, and absence of without valvular insufficiency in most patients. The serial echocardiographic study of a patient operated at five years of age demonstrated that she had a good and permanent solution for her heart malformation with the PRP procedure (Fig. **4**).

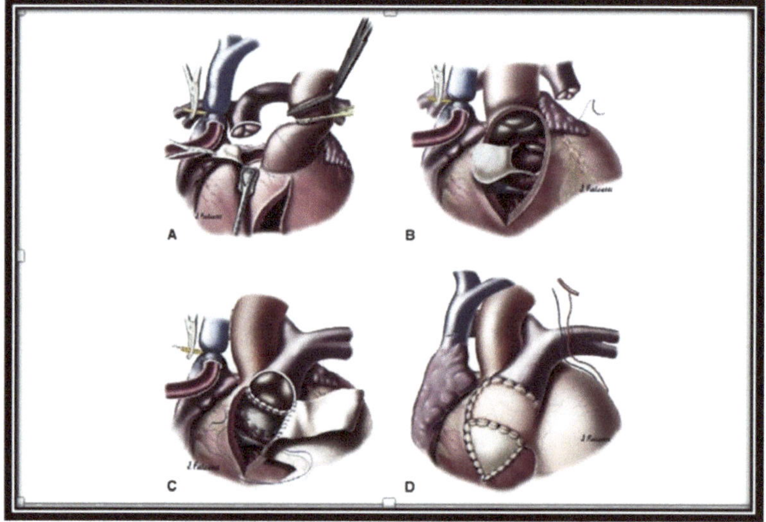

Fig. (3). Pulmonary root translocation. The pulmonary root is dissected out and its origin is closed using a glutaraldehyde-treated autologous pericardial patch **(A)**. After partial resection of the conal septum, a Dracon patch is used to create a tunnel from the left ventricle to the aorta **(B)**. The pulmonary root is sutured to the right ventricle with a running 6-0 polydioxanone suture, and the right ventricular outflow tract is completed using an in situ pericardial patch combined with a glutaraldehyde-treated autologous pericardial patch **(C)**. The final appearance after the procedure **(D)**.

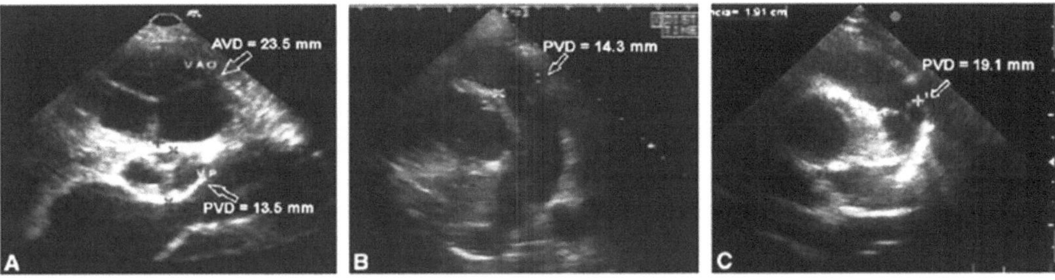

Fig. (4). Echocardiographic follow-up from a girl who underwent pulmonary root translocation surgery at 5 years old: preoperative cross-sectional view of the aortic and pulmonary valves **(A)**, and postoperative views of the translocated pulmonary valve after 3 years **(B)** and 8.5 years **(C)** of follow-up. AVD: aortic valve; PVD: pulmonary valve.

In the Nikaidoh procedure (aortic translocation), the aortic root is removed from the right ventricle, obstruction of LVOT is alleviated with the division of the septum and excision of the pulmonary valve, rebuilding the LVOT with the aortic root translocated and the VSD patch, and the RVOT with a patch of pericardium. Modifications of the original technique include individual transfer of coronary arteries during the translocation (to avoid the possibility of ischemia), use of Lecompte maneuver and reconstruction of the RVOT with a pulmonary homologous graft or direct anastomosis of the pulmonary artery in the right ventricle. Although technically challenging, the aortic translocation combines elements of surgical techniques commonly carried out, including the procedures of Ross, Konno and Jatene [29].

In 1980, Bex *et al.* [30] were the first to introduce the concept of aortic translocation in the treatment of TGA, but it was Nikaidoh in 1984, who popularized the technique for the treatment of TGA with VSD [29]. This technique is particularly useful in the presence of restrictive VSD or of the inlet, hypoplastic right ventricle, in the straddling atrioventricular valve and/or anomalous coronary anatomy interfering in the RVOT incision. It allows for better alignment of right ventricle and LVOT. In addition, the RVOT is less likely to be compressed by the sternum, a major problem associated with the Rastelli operation [26]. However, the extracardiac tube is incapable of growth and calcifies and reoperations are needed.

In the double aortic and pulmonary translocation, the ascending aorta and the pulmonary trunk are transected above the sinotubular junction. The coronary arteries are mobilized and disinserted from the aorta. The aortic root and the pulmonary root, including the semilunar valves are sectioned just below the level of the valvar annulus and removed from the ventricles. The conal septum is resected to prevent LVOT obstruction and the VSD is closed with synthetic material. Subsequently, the aortic root is translocated and the coronary arteries are reimplanted. The Lecompte maneuver is done. The pulmonary root is then translocated anteriorly to the RVOT. The pulmonary root is incised in its anterior wall and a monocuspid patch of bovine jugular vein is used to enlarge the RVOT. The native pulmonary valve is preserved, trying to avoid insufficiency and stenosis in the long term.

UNIVENTRICULAR HEART

An univentricular atrioventricular connection is characterized by atresia of one of the atrioventricular valves (mitral or tricuspid atresia) or by the two atrioventricular valves or one and more than 50% of the other emptying into the same ventricular chamber (double inlet ventricle). In this situation, there is one dominant ventricle and one hypoplastic, or just a ventricular cavity ('The true single ventricle') [33]. The diagnosis and early treatment of univentricular cardiopathies are essential to prevent prolonged period of cyanosis and in some situations, to avoid pulmonary hypertension and protect the dominant ventricle of cardiomyopathy due to volume or pressure overload.

ANATOMY

The dominant ventricular chamber can be recognized as left or right, by the presence or absence of characteristics of the trabecular portion, as well as the position (anterior or posterior) and anatomy of the atrioventricular valves accompanying it. The most common type is the morphological left ventricle dominant with malposition of the great arteries, with aorta emerging of the hypoplastic right ventricle. The pulmonary artery and the mitral valve are on the right and the tricuspid valve on the left, observed in 74% of autopsy series and 70% of clinical series. In some cases, the VSD (bulboventricular foramen) becomes restrictive during the child development, producing functional subaortic stenosis. Pulmonary stenosis or atresia occurs in 50% of patients.

PHYSIOPATHOLOGY AND CLINICAL MANIFESTATIONS

The amount of pulmonary flow determines the clinical presentation of children with single ventricle, having factors determining the presence or absence of pulmonary stenosis and the degree of pulmonary vascular resistance. Most children with single ventricle whose diagnosis was not performed by fetal echocardiography, are diagnosed in the first weeks of life. In the absence of pulmonary stenosis, and the fall of the pulmonary vascular resistance of newborn, pulmonary flow gradually increases. Unobstructed pulmonary blood flow causes a left-to-right shunt, resulting in congestive heart failure with a relative decrease in systemic perfusion as seen in double-inlet left ventricles with ventriculoarterial discordance. These patients are at risk of developing irreversible pulmonary vascular disease.

Neonates may be cyanotic if pulmonary obstruction is severe, as seen in patients with valvular and subvalvar pulmonary stenosis or in double-inlet left ventricle with ventriculoarterial concordance and a severely restrictive ventricular septal defect. Children with moderate pulmonary stenosis usually evolve well, despite cyanotic. Patients with balanced pulmonary and systemic circulation, moderate to severe pulmonary stenosis, and unobstructed systemic blood flow often survive well beyond the neonatal period and have the best overall long-term prognosis. Such patients may present quite late, with minimal cyanosis and a long ejection systolic heart murmur due to pulmonary stenosis. Children with single ventricle and pulmonary atresia are cyanotic since birth. The degree of cyanosis is determined by the amount of pulmonary flow supplied by the ductus arteriosus, systemic-pulmonary collateral arteries or bronchial circulation [34].

Coexisting aortic coarctation, arch hypoplasia or interruption, aortic or subaortic obstruction, result in more severe cardiac disease and earlier presentation. When suspected, continuous infusion of prostaglandin IV should be initiated without delay and confirmation with additional exams may be required (echocardiogram, CTA, magnetic resonance imaging - MRI or cardiac catheterization).

PHYSICAL EXAMINATION

In patients with pulmonary stenosis an ejection systolic murmur can be auscultated on the sternal border. Right and left atrioventricular valve insufficiency can be expressed as a holosystolic murmur. Peripheric cyanosis and signs of heart failure are variable, depending on the associated lesions. Poor systemic perfusion can be a sign of ductal dependent associated disease or restrictive ASD (in diseases like tricuspid atresia).

CHEST RADIOGRAPHY

If there is no pulmonary stenosis, the chest X-ray cardiomegaly and pulmonary overflow are observed. In pulmonary stenosis, the cardiac area is normal or slightly increased and the pulmonary flow is normal or decreased.

ECHOCARDIOGRAM

The echocardiogram can show in detail the anatomy of the defect. Given the countless possibilities and variations, examination should be performed with sequential analysis and in a systematic way. Further anatomic definition may be determined by MRI, whereas additional hemodynamic data can be obtained from cardiac catheterization.

TREATMENT

It is important to emphasize that there is no anatomical correction to univentricular heart, but only palliative treatment. The ultimate treatment of the single ventricle is the complete deviation of the systemic venous return to the pulmonary arteries, directly, passively and without interposition of contractile chamber (Fontan operation or total cavopulmonary connection) [35]. Usually, this treatment is achieved following stages, during different periods in life:

In the Neonatal Period

- Blalock-Taussig shunt: when there is significant obstruction to the pulmonary flow, the creation of a systemic-pulmonary anastomosis or shunt BT is necessary [36];

- Clinical treatment: patients with moderate pulmonary stenosis may not require shunt in neonatal period, because they are naturally balanced;

- Pulmonary artery banding: single ventricle hearts without obstruction to the pulmonary flow will present pulmonary overflow and will be managed with a pulmonary banding as initial procedure in the first month of life [36];

- Norwood procedure: Patients presenting with univentricular heart + hypoplastic aortic arch and aortic atresia or valvar or subvalvar stenosis (HLHS and variants). The Norwood procedure involves atrial septectomy and transection and ligation of the distal main pulmonary artery. The proximal pulmonary artery is then connected to the hypoplastic aortic arch, while the aortic arch is enlarged with a homologous patch or autologous pericardium, glutaraldehyde treated. The pulmonary arteries are detached from the pulmonary artery trunk and a BT shunt or a right ventricle – pulmonary artery conduit is interposed to provide pulmonary blood flow [36 - 38];

- Hybrid procedure: patients presenting with univentricular heart + hypoplastic aortic arch and aortic atresia or valvar or subvalvar stenosis (HLHS and variants). The hybrid procedure involves balloon atrial septostomy if needed, the PDA receives a stent to keep it opened and the pulmonary arteries are bilaterally banded. The second stage in this case will be the comprehensive surgery (Norwood + Glenn) [36, 39];

- Damus-Kaye-Stansel procedure: similar to the Norwood procedure, except that the aortic arch does not need to be enlarged [36, 40].

At Age 3 Months to 6 Months of Life

- The superior cavopulmonary connection (bidirectional Glenn procedure or hemi-Fontan): the superior vena cava is anastomosed to right pulmonary artery. The azygous vein is ligated, to avoid flow from the superior vena cava (SVC) to the inferior vena cava (IVC) in the postoperative care (the pressure in SVC after Glenn equals the pressure of pulmonary artery and the IVC pressure continues normal) [36].

- Kawashima procedure: it is applied in some complex cases, with absent inferior vena cava and great azygous vein draining the inferior part of the body. It consists of the same anastomose of SVC to right pulmonary artery, without closure of azygous vein. In this special situation, only the suprahepatic veins will continue draining in the atrium [36].

At Age ≥ 1,5 Years

- Total cavopulmonary connection, extracardiac Fontan procedure: in this procedure, the remaining blood of systemic venous return is diverted directly to the pulmonary arteries. A PTFE tube, usually 16- or 18-mm graft, is interposed between the inferior vena cava and suprahepatic veins (after Glenn procedure) or the supra-hepatic veins (after the Kawashima procedure) and the pulmonary artery. Usually, a fenestration is created in the PTFE tube, allowing the blood to flow from the tube to the atrium, decompressing the Fontan circuit in situations where the pulmonary artery pressure is elevated. In the recent era, an extracardiac position is the more usual way to place the tube, avoiding the arrhythmias due to distension of the R atrium in the long term [36]. The Fontan operation results in profound hemodynamic disturbances to the whole body attributed in large part to an elevated systemic venous pressure. Therefore, patients with univentricular heart physiology can present complications in the long-term follow-up, such as protein losing enteropathy, plastic bronchitis, thromboembolic events, arrhythmias, systemic-pulmonary collaterals and arteriovenous connections (especially before the total cavopulmonary completion), ventricular dysfunction, valve regurgitation *etc.* [41] The need for anticoagulation in the long term is controversial [42].

TOTAL ANOMALOUS PULMONARY VENOUS RETURN

Total anomalous pulmonary venous return (TAPVR) is the absence of connection between pulmonary veins and the left atrium. Therefore, all four pulmonary veins drain anomalously in a systemic venous structure, not directly in the left atrium. It occurs due to failure of all the pulmonary veins to divide from the splanchnic venous system. Patients presenting with TAPVR require interatrial communication for survival. Its incidence varies between 0.7 and 1.5% of all congenital heart diseases 1.23 or 1:17,000 births.

CLASSIFICATION

The TAPVR are classified into four types, depending on their anomalous connection with the systemic venous system: supracardiac (43-49%), cardiac (16-18%), infracardiac (26-27%), and mixed (9-12%) [43, 44].

SUPRACARDIAC

In this type of drainage, pulmonary veins come together behind the heart to a common collecting chamber that drains upward into the innominate vein through the vertical vein, and then into the SVC and the right atrium (Fig. **5**). Sometimes, it drains directly into the SVC. The site of the obstruction may be caused by adjacent structures, for example, the vertical vein can be compressed by the left bronchus and the pulmonary artery.

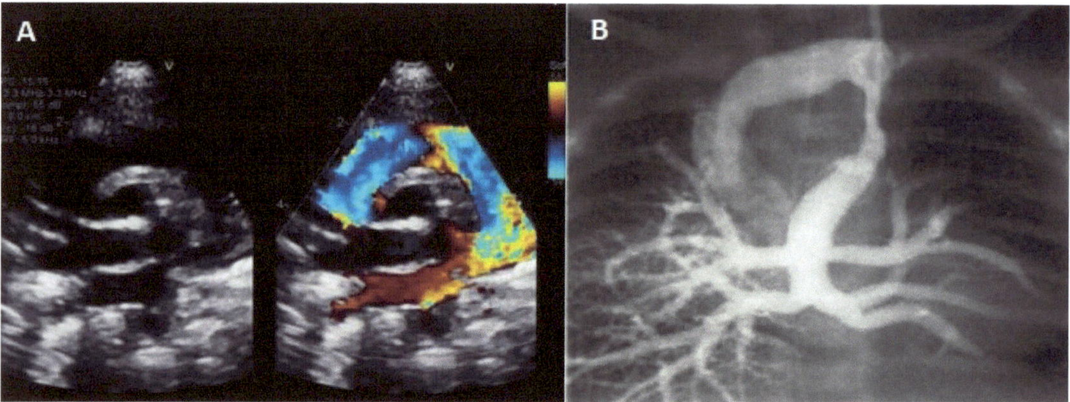

Fig. (5). Total anomalous pulmonary veins return in the innominate vein – supracardiac obstructive form. A- Echocardiogram shows supracardiac non-obstructive total anomalous pulmonary venous return to the innominate vein, by vertical vein. **B-** Pulmonary arteriography shows the pulmonary veins right and left joining in a common collector that returns to the innominate vein by vertical vein, with important obstruction of the vertical vein when entering the innominate vein.

CARDIAC

The pulmonary veins gather behind the heart into the collecting chamber, that drains into the coronary sinus, which occurs more often, or drains directly into the right atrium. They are rarely obstructive. When stenosis occurs, it is due to stenosis at the level of the coronary sinus.

INFRACARDIAC

In this type of venous connection, the pulmonary veins unite into common vein behind left atrium, then pass down retro-cardiac through esophageal hiatus and connect to portal/hepatic veins or directly to inferior vena cava. Infracardiac drainage may be obstructed in the level of the diaphragm, by the ligament of the ductus venosus, or by the hepatic sinusoids' resistance.

MIXED

The four veins drain anomalously in more than one of the venous structures described above.

PATHOPHYSIOLOGY

All pulmonary venous flow returns to the systemic circulation, occurring the mixture of systemic and pulmonary venous returns. The pulmonary blood flow in TAPVC is determined by the degree of pulmonary arteriolar resistance and obstruction of the pulmonary veins. Regarding the pulmonary vein obstruction, they can present a wide spectrum that goes from severe obstruction to without obstruction. In non-obstructive or minimal obstruction forms, the pulmonary overflow is intense, and the child presents with heart failure, and no apparent cyanosis, since oxygen saturation is usually > 90%. In the obstructive form, pulmonary venous hypertension with consequent pulmonary edema is observed.

CLINICAL PRESENTATION

In TAPVR, the clinical presentation is variable and depends on the presence and degree of venous obstruction. In the obstructive form, the clinical expression is severe, characterized by cyanosis and respiratory distress that occurs early in the neonatal period. The newborn progresses with tachypnea and intercostal retraction, which are indicative signs of pulmonary edema. The differential diagnosis with acute respiratory distress syndrome (ARDS) of the newborn is difficult. However, the starting time of symptoms is different. While in ARDS, the occurrence of symptoms starts shortly after birth, in the TAPVC, the symptoms usually appear after 12 hours of life [43]. In the non-obstructive form, in general, the child appears well. The clinical manifestation is usually later, and consists of heart failure secondary to pulmonary overflow, such as, tachypnea, fatigue at the breast feeding, and low weight gain. The clinical diagnosis is made from finding a heart murmur, fixed split of second heart sound or mild cyanosis. Cyanosis appears at birth, which can be detected in the screening test by pulse oximetry. Subsequently, they present symptoms related to pulmonary overflow.

PHYSICAL EXAMINATION

In the obstructive form, the child appears to be a carrier of a severe disease and has important cyanosis, tachypnea, and hepatomegaly. It is common not to detect a heart murmur. The only abnormality of auscultation is a loud second heart sound. You can hear continuous murmur over the obstruction area. In the non-obstructive form, in general, the child is well. Cardiac auscultation is similar to that of ASD, with fixed-split of the second heart sound, ejective systolic soft murmur on high left sternal edge. Sometimes, auscultation of a diastolic murmur due to tricuspid valve increased flow (relative stenosis). Tachypnea and hepatomegaly and varying degrees of cyanosis can also be observed.

ELECTROCARDIOGRAM

It shows right ventricular overload and often right atrium overload.

CHEST RADIOGRAPHY

In the obstructive form, the cardiac area is of normal size. There is evidence of pulmonary edema, with an appearance of ground glass in severe cases (Fig. **6A**). In the non-obstructive form, the cardiac area is mildly increased, there is dilatation of the pulmonary artery and its branches. There are signs of pulmonary overflow, without pulmonary congestion.

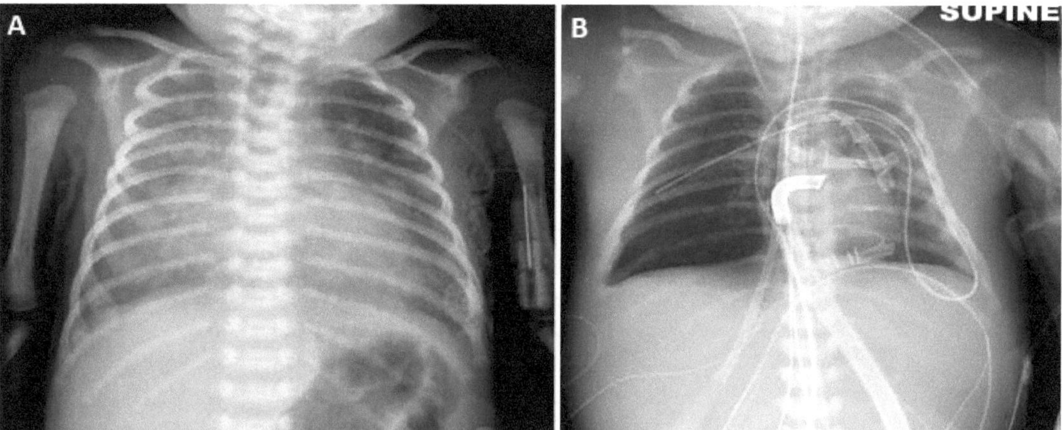

Fig. (6). Total anomalous pulmonary venous return, supracardiac obstructive type – Chest X-ray showing: **A** - Significant bilateral pulmonary congestion, and **B** - Central extracorporeal membrane oxygenation cannulation to treat postoperative low cardiac output related to pulmonary hypertension.

ECHOCARDIOGRAM

The echocardiographic diagnosis of TAPVR is based on a set of findings, which include: 1- inability to demonstrate the normal connection of pulmonary veins in the left atrium; 2- demonstration of ascending vertical vein and dilatation.

MAGNETIC RESONANCE IMAGING AND COMPUTED TOMOGRAPHY ANGIOGRAPHY

MRI and CT exams are excellent for evaluating the anatomy of the pulmonary veins and their connections, providing great details.

CARDIAC CATHETERIZATION

Cardiac catheterization is rarely necessary for anatomical definition. It can be indicated for performing balloon atrial septostomy, as a palliative procedure for clinical stabilization of a child with restrictive ASD.

TREATMENT

TAPVR requires surgical correction. The time of surgery depends on the degree of pulmonary venous obstruction and the patient clinical condition. In newborns with severe obstructive form, the surgical repair should be indicated immediately. In non-obstructive form, the surgery can be postponed, with close follow-up of the child, since the early age for surgery is an independent predictor for early death [44, 45]. The surgery is performed under cardiopulmonary bypass and, sometimes, a short period of hypothermic circulatory arrest is applied, which allows good visualization of the structures. The confluence of the veins, posterior to the left atrium, is opened and sutured to an opening in the posterior wall of the left atrium. A sutureless technique can be applied, especially in small children with small pulmonary veins, aiming to reduce the incidence of restenosis in the long-term follow-up but the benefits are unclear [45, 46].

POSTOPERATIVE OUTCOME

Most of it evolves very well. However, some patients will require extracorporeal membrane oxygenator (ECMO) support to overcome severe pulmonary hypertension or low cardiac output (Fig. **6B**). In the mid-term follow-up, the main postoperative complication is the obstruction of one or more pulmonary veins, which can occur in up to 10% of the patients and who may need reoperation, balloon dilatation or stent placement. New medications, such as Imatinib, can be used in cases of recurrent pulmonary vein stenosis [47].

AORTIC VALVE STENOSIS

Aortic valve stenosis (AS) is described as a restriction of blood flow through the aortic valve. It may present throughout life, but if expressing clinically in the early newborn period it is physiologically and morphologically at the severe end of the spectrum. Stenotic aortic valve looks small and dysplastic and often bicuspid. Left ventricle may be markedly dilated with poor contraction or be hypertrophied when the systolic function is preserved. In some cases, left ventricle is poorly developed, similar to the borderline spectrum of HLHS. Clinical symptoms depend entirely on the severity of the obstruction and associated abnormalities such as subaortic stenosis or coarctation of the aorta (CoA). Severity of the disease is correlated with the earlier presentation. Management also depends on the severity. Severe heart failure or other symptoms all require palliation by valvotomy through surgery or transcatheter methods. Early recognition before deterioration will inevitably lead to an improved outcome.

COARCTATION OF THE AORTA

Coarctation of the aorta (CoA) represents 8% to 10% of congenital heart disease. Major malformation is narrowing of distal part of the aortic arch commonly near the ductus arteriosus, and it is often accompanied by hypoplasia or diffuse narrowing of the aortic arch. In this case usually the lower half of the body is a ductus dependent and the symptoms will develop as it starts to close. About 40% of infants have other cardiac malformations and most of them present during the newborn period. The most commonly associated malformation is VSD or bicuspid aortic valve, AS, other left sided obstructive lesions and more complex anomalies are also common. Severe CoA may present with acidosis, congestive heart failure, renal impairment, cardiovascular collapse or even death. If the 'differential saturation' (feet saturations being significantly lower than the arms) is present, this highly suggests that legs are ductus dependent, which includes critical CoA/interrupted aortic arch - IAA, where the poorly saturated pulmonary arterial blood flow to the lower part of the body through the PDA. In this situation, differential diagnosis included persistent pulmonary hypertension of the newborn (PPHN). If there is a difference in blood pressure between arms and legs (right arm pressure being significantly higher than the feet), arch obstructive lesions are highly suggestive. If the baby is in a significant shock, pressures can be weakened in all extremities. If ductal dependent clinical presentations are detected early, infants can survive with PGE_1 treatment.

Surgical repair is the standard of care in infants and young children with native CoA. It was first described in 1944 and since then many modifications have been developed depending on the anatomy. The types of surgical repair include: 1. Resection with end-to-end anastomosis, preferred repair in neonates and infants; 2. Patch aortoplasty, for older patients; 3. Bypass graft insertion across the area of coarctation when the distance to be bridged is too long for an end-to-end repair; 4. Subclavian flap aortoplasty, good option for neonates and infants with long segment of aortic coarctation.

If the aortic arch is hypoplastic, a median sternotomy approach is applied, and the arch is also enlarged, usually with homograft patch or glutaraldehyde treated autologous pericardium. Balloon angioplasty is the standard of care postop recurrent coarctation in the young. While stent implantation is the preferred approach for older children and adults. Operative mortality of simple CoA repair is low but overall outcome depends on associated cardiac malformations. Surgical repair is also possible in preterm infants with birth weights less than 2.5 kg, with an overall survival rate of 76 percent one year after initial repair [48, 49].

PULMONARY ATRESIA

The main anatomical feature of PA is the absence of a direct connection between the right ventricle and the lungs. Two main types are:

1. Pulmonary Atresia with Intact Ventricular Septum

In the PA/IVS, tricuspid valve and right ventricle are usually underdeveloped, but pulmonary arteries are relatively well developed and supplied by the PDA. Infants with PA/IVS - a typical form of 'ductus-dependent pulmonary circulation' - become more cyanotic and aggravated as the ductal closes, and will collapse within a first few days of life, so prostaglandin infusion is needed in the neonatal period. In most patients, the pulmonary valve can be opened, either in the heart catheterization lab or surgically. With the surgical treatment, the pulmonary valve can be recovered, particularly, when the surgeon can view the commissures, like in membranous pulmonary atresia. Otherwise, the association of a monocuspid patch may be necessary. The RVOT should also be approached with resection of myocardial bands and patch enlargement. A BT shunt or a central aorto-pulmonary shunt is associated, to improve the oxygenation in the immediate postoperative stage, when usually the right ventricle is hypertrophied with a small cavity. Within weeks, the right ventricle hypertrophy decreases, and the right ventricle cavity becomes capable to keep a good forward flow to the pulmonary artery.

The right ventricle can be treated in the neonatal period; however, this can also be deferred but the pulmonary blood flow must be secured, preferentially by ductal stenting. The goal of two-ventricle repair can still be achieved, later. Some patients with PA/IVS and very small tricuspid valve anulus will be treated as functional single ventricular physiology, and the surgical goal will be 'Fontan' type operation. Early surgical palliation involves shunt such as BT shunt. However, the boundary to biventricular repair should always be challenged.

2. Pulmonary Atresia with Ventricular Septal Defect

In PA/VSD, also known as TOF with pulmonary atresia ('extreme form of TOF'), there are usually favorable sized two ventricles with large subaortic VSD and variable source of pulmonary blood flow supply. Some patients have only a PDA as pulmonary source, but more commonly, MAPCAs arising from the descending aorta are present. As ductal is less dependent than PA/IVS, the natural course of PA/VSD depends on the pulmonary blood supply and other variables. Affected infant may present cyanosis in the early life, but some can survive into adult life, even without any intervention if the various pulmonary supplies are appropriate, however elevated pulmonary resistance will develop. Management of PA/VSD depends on the pulmonary blood supply. About half of those will be suitable for corrective surgery with VSD closure and connect the right ventricle to the pulmonary arteries using the conduit placement. BT shunt or unifocalization of the collaterals can be needed as an initial treatment in the neonatal age. Most patients with PA/VSD/MAPCAs and absent pulmonary arteries, can undergo complete single-stage repair with satisfactory postoperative hemodynamics. The unifocalization of MAPCAs can provide a reasonable pulmonary vascular bed in the absence of intrapericardial pulmonary arteries [19]. Pulmonary atresia can also be part of more complex cardiac malformations such as, heterotaxy syndrome, congenitally corrected TGA or single ventricle.

EBSTEIN'S ANOMALY

Ebstein's anomaly is a congenital heart defect involving the tricuspid valve and the right ventricle. Its main features are downward displacement of the septal and inferior tricuspid valve leaflets, redundant anterior leaflet with a sail-like appearance, dilation of the true right atrioventricular annulus, tricuspid valve regurgitation, and right atrial and right ventricular dilation. Tricuspid regurgitation is mainly due to severe restriction of tricuspid leaflet tissue, particularly involving the septal and posterior leaflets. There is also annular dilation; the available mobile anterior leaflet tissue is insufficient to cover the orifice during systole. Displacement of the septal and posterior leaflet divides the right ventricle in two chambers: the atrialized right ventricle, which is positioned between the normal atrioventricular junction and the displaced tricuspid valve, and the functional right ventricle located distal to the tricuspid valve. The small capacitance of the functional right ventricle also plays an important role in the pathophysiology of Ebstein's anomaly. The echocardiographic morphology of Ebstein's anomaly is depicted in Fig. (7).

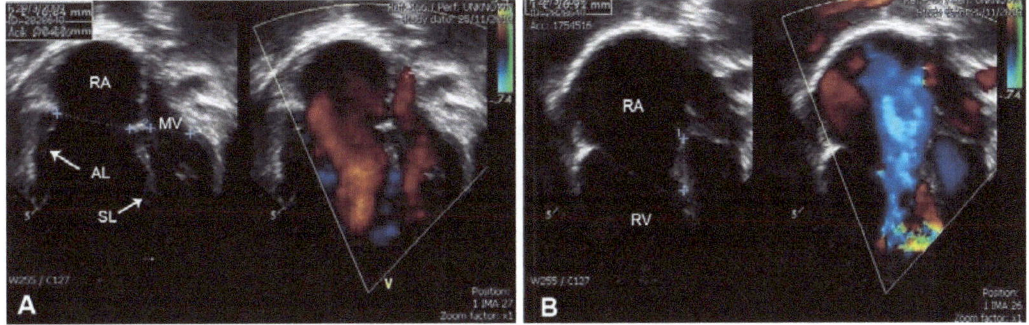

Fig. (7). Echocardiogram in four-chamber view of an Ebstein's anomaly patient showing: severe displacement of the septal leaflet of tricuspid valve, dilation of the right atrium and right ventricle. The color flow Doppler reveals good blood inflow in diastole **(A)** and severe tricuspid regurgitation in systole **(B)** mainly due to coaptation failure between the anterior and septal leaflets. AL: anterior leaflet; SL: septal leaflet; RA: right atrium; RV: right ventricle; MV: mitral valve.

CLINICAL PRESENTATION

Symptomatic presentation of Ebstein's anomaly of the tricuspid valve in the newborn period represents the most severe spectrum for this condition, commonly associated with significant morbidity and mortality. Neonates with severe Ebstein's anomaly need neonatal intensive care. About 40% of them will improve with medical management with slow PGE1 weaning, use of pulmonary vessel dilators, diuretics, and inotropic drugs. If the improvement is not enough to discharge the patient home, surgical intervention is usually warranted to eliminate or reduce the tricuspid regurgitation and provide adequate pulmonary blood flow with or without the contribution of the right ventricle.

SURGICAL OPTIONS IN NEONATAL PERIOD

- The Starnes procedure consists of single-ventricle palliation excluding the right ventricle, using a fenestrated tricuspid patch, which is important to prevent right ventricular distention, and placement of a systemic-to-pulmonary artery shunt [50, 51].

- Tricuspid valve repair as an attempt to achieve a biventricular circulation, being the Cone procedure is considered the "anatomical repair" for this malformation [52, 53].

- Initial BT shunt or ductal stenting may be adequate, especially in cases with pulmonary atresia and small right ventricle [51].

When considering biventricular management, the higher pulmonary vascular resistance seen in neonates mandates more valvar competency after repair and makes the use of a superior cavopulmonary connection contraindicated due to high pulmonary vascular resistance. Cone reconstruction of the tricuspid valve provides circumferential leaflet coverage around the perimeter of the remodeled tricuspid annulus (Fig. **8**), leading to improved coaptation and sustained competency of the valve during the follow-up [52].

The Cone reconstruction of the tricuspid valve can be applied in the neonatal period when the right ventricle presents a good function (Fig. **9**). The reverse remodeling of the heart usually happens very quickly after the cone repair in newborns (Fig. **10**). It can also be done some months after Starnes procedure. In cases of Ebstein's anomaly associated with pulmonary vein stenosis or atresia, the cone technique can be performed associated with pulmonary valve repair. In this situation, annular augmentation with a monocuspid patch, can be sometimes needed [53].

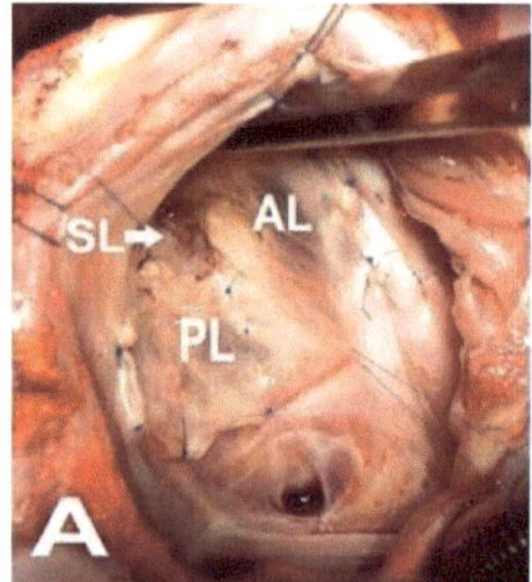

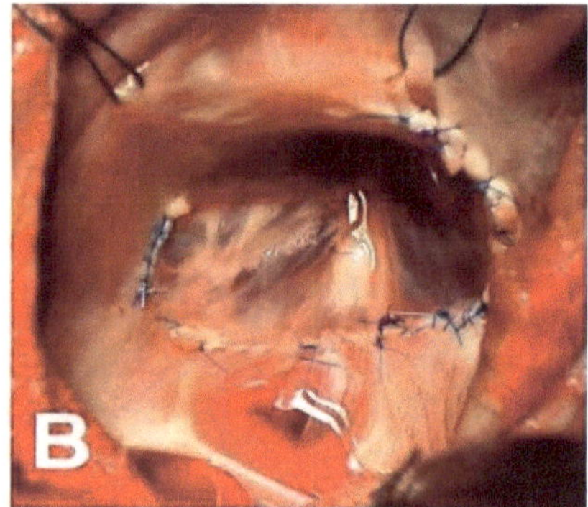

Fig. (8). Cone construction done by rotation of the posterior leaflet, which was combined with the septal leaflet **(A)**. The cone attached to the true tricuspid annulus, resulting in a competent tricuspid valve **(B)**. AL: anterior leaflet; PL: inferior leaflet; SL: septal leaflet.

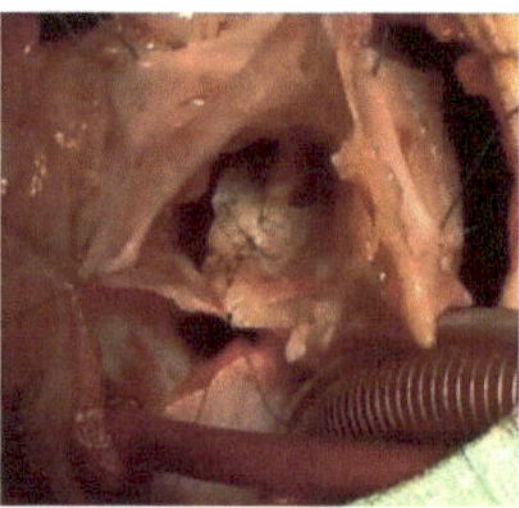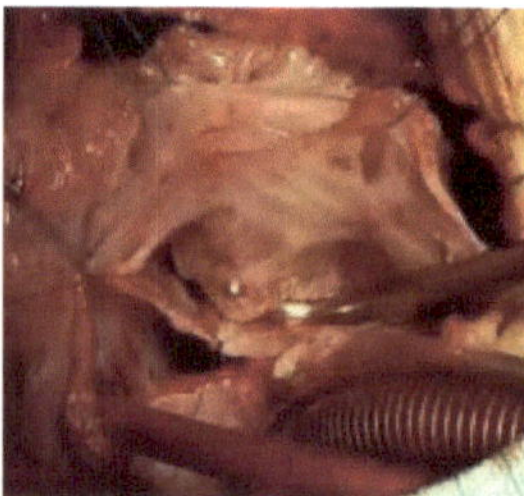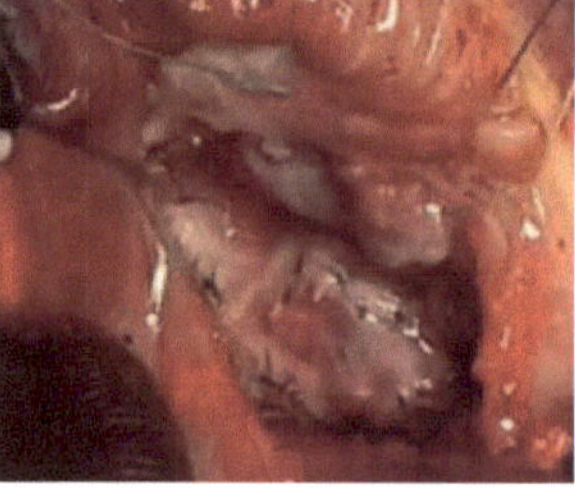

Fig. (9). Intraoperative pictures depict the Cone procedure in a newborn, yielding an excellent result.

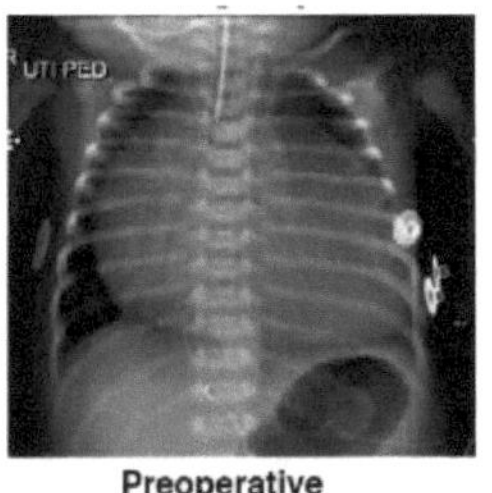
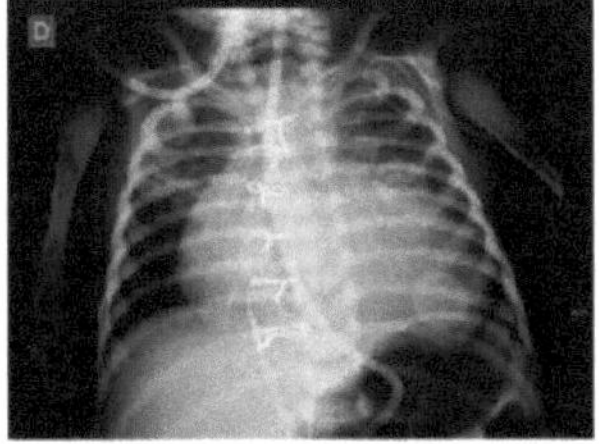
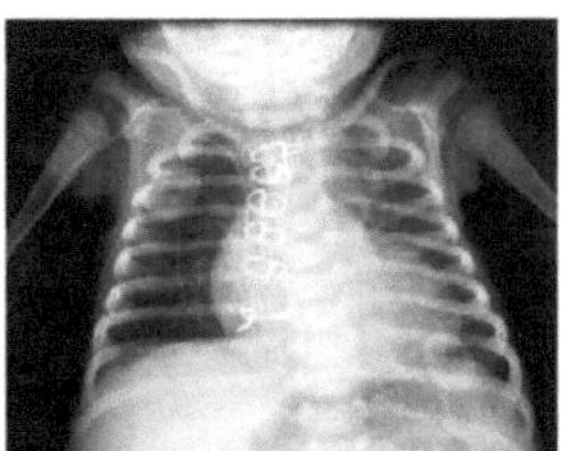

Fig. (10). Chest X-ray sequence of a neonate with Ebstein's anomaly, who underwent the cone repair at 3 days old. The preoperative cardiothoracic index (CTI) had a significant decrease in only 17 days.

Our experience with the treatment of neonates with Ebstein's anomaly encompasses 17 cases, 14 with the cone technique and 3 with the Starnes procedure. There were three yearly deaths and no late deaths. The early deaths occurred in the total repair group.

CONSENT FOR PUBLICATION

Not applicable.

CONFLICT OF INTEREST

The authors confirm that the contents of this chapter have no conflict of interest.

ACKNOWLEDGEMENTS

Declare none.

REFERENCES

[1]   Olney RS, Ailes EC, Sontag MK. Detection of critical congenital heart defects: Review of contributions from prenatal and newborn screening. Semin Perinatol 2015; 39(3): 230-7.
[http://dx.doi.org/10.1053/j.semperi.2015.03.007] [PMID: 25979782]

[2]   Knowles R, Griebsch I, Dezateux C, Brown J, Bull C, Wren C. Newborn screening for congenital heart defects: a systematic review and cost-effectiveness analysis. Health Technol Assess 2005; 9(44): 1-152, iii-iv.
[http://dx.doi.org/10.3310/hta9440] [PMID: 16297355]

[3]   Sadowski SL. Congenital cardiac disease in the newborn infant: past, present, and future. Crit Care Nurs Clin North Am 2009; 21(1): 37-48, vi.
[http://dx.doi.org/10.1016/j.ccell.2008.10.001] [PMID: 19237042]

[4]   Dorfman AT, Marino BS, Wernovsky G, *et al.* Critical heart disease in the neonate: presentation and outcome at a tertiary care center. Pediatr Crit Care Med 2008; 9(2): 193-202.
[http://dx.doi.org/10.1097/PCC.0b013e318166eda5] [PMID: 18477933]

[5]   Chang RK, Gurvitz M, Rodriguez S. Missed diagnosis of critical congenital heart disease. Arch Pediatr Adolesc Med 2008; 162(10): 969-74.

[http://dx.doi.org/10.1001/archpedi.162.10.969] [PMID: 18838650]

[6] Yee L. Cardiac emergencies in the first year of life. Emerg Med Clin North Am 2007; 25(4): 981-1008, vi.
[http://dx.doi.org/10.1016/j.emc.2007.08.001] [PMID: 17950133]

[7] Penny DJ, Shekerdemian LS. Management of the neonate with symptomatic congenital heart disease. Arch Dis Child Fetal Neonatal Ed 2001; 84(3): F141-5.
[http://dx.doi.org/10.1136/fn.84.3.F141] [PMID: 11320036]

[8] Dabizzi RP, Caprioli G, Aiazzi L, *et al.* Distribution and anomalies of coronary arteries in tetralogy of fallot. Circulation 1980; 61(1): 95-102.
[http://dx.doi.org/10.1161/01.CIR.61.1.95] [PMID: 7349946]

[9] Breitbart RE, Fyler DC. Tetralogy of Fallot. Nadas' Pediatric Cardiology. 2nd ed. Philadelphia: PA: Saunders Elsevier 2006; pp. 559-72.

[10] Waldman JD, Wernly JA. Cyanotic congenital heart disease with decreased pulmonary blood flow in children. Pediatr Clin North Am 1999; 46(2): 385-404.
[http://dx.doi.org/10.1016/S0031-3955(05)70125-5] [PMID: 10218082]

[11] Reddy VM, Liddicoat JR, McElhinney DB, Brook MM, Stanger P, Hanley FL. Routine primary repair of tetralogy of Fallot in neonates and infants less than three months of age. Ann Thorac Surg 1995; 60(6) (Suppl.): S592-6.
[http://dx.doi.org/10.1016/0003-4975(95)00732-6] [PMID: 8604943]

[12] Hennein HA, Mosca RS, Urcelay G, Crowley DC, Bove EL. Intermediate results after complete repair of tetralogy of Fallot in neonates. J Thorac Cardiovasc Surg 1995; 109(2): 332-42.
[http://dx.doi.org/10.1016/S0022-5223(95)70395-0] [PMID: 7531798]

[13] Pigula FA, Khalil PN, Mayer JE, del Nido PJ, Jonas RA. Repair of tetralogy of Fallot in neonates and young infants. Circulation 1999; 100(19) (Suppl.): II157-61.
[http://dx.doi.org/10.1161/01.CIR.100.suppl_2.II-157] [PMID: 10567296]

[14] Martins IF, Doles IC, Bravo-Valenzuela NJM, Santos AORD, Varella MSP. When is the Best Time for Corrective Surgery in Patients with Tetralogy of Fallot between 0 and 12 Months of Age? Rev Bras Cir Cardiovasc 2018; 33(5): 505-10.
[http://dx.doi.org/10.21470/1678-9741-2018-0019] [PMID: 30517260]

[15] Wilder TJ, Van Arsdell GS, Benson L, *et al.* Young infants with severe tetralogy of Fallot: Early primary surgery *versus* transcatheter palliation. J Thorac Cardiovasc Surg 2017; 154(5): 1692-1700.e2.
[http://dx.doi.org/10.1016/j.jtcvs.2017.05.042] [PMID: 28666664]

[16] Dohlen G, Chaturvedi RR, Benson LN, *et al.* Stenting of the right ventricular outflow tract in the symptomatic infant with tetralogy of Fallot. Heart 2009; 95(2): 142-7.
[http://dx.doi.org/10.1136/hrt.2007.135723] [PMID: 18332061]

[17] Kaza AK, Lim HG, Dibardino DJ, *et al.* Long-term results of right ventricular outflow tract reconstruction in neonatal cardiac surgery: options and outcomes. J Thorac Cardiovasc Surg 2009; 138(4): 911-6.
[http://dx.doi.org/10.1016/j.jtcvs.2008.10.058] [PMID: 19660342]

[18] Stewart RD, Backer CL, Young L, Mavroudis C. Tetralogy of Fallot: results of a pulmonary valve-sparing strategy. Ann Thorac Surg 2005; 80(4): 1431-8.
[http://dx.doi.org/10.1016/j.athoracsur.2005.04.016] [PMID: 16181883]

[19] Carrillo SA, Mainwaring RD, Patrick WL, *et al.* Surgical repair of pulmonary atresia with ventricular septal defect and major aortopulmonary collaterals with absent intrapericardial pulmonary arteries. Ann Thorac Surg 2015; 100(2): 606-14.
[http://dx.doi.org/10.1016/j.athoracsur.2015.03.110] [PMID: 26138766]

[20] Huhta JC, Edwards WD, Feldt RH, Puga FJ. Left ventricular wall thickness in complete transposition of the great arteries. J Thorac Cardiovasc Surg 1982; 84(1): 97-101.

[http://dx.doi.org/10.1016/S0022-5223(19)39522-4] [PMID: 7087546]

[21] Rashkind WJ, Miller WW. Transposition of the great arteries. Results of palliation by balloon atrioseptostomy in thirty-one infants. Circulation 1968; 38(3): 453-62.
[http://dx.doi.org/10.1161/01.CIR.38.3.453] [PMID: 5673596]

[22] Villafañe J, Lantin-Hermoso MR, Bhatt AB, *et al*. American College of Cardiology's Adult Congenital and Pediatric Cardiology Council. D-transposition of the great arteries: the current era of the arterial switch operation. J Am Coll Cardiol 2014; 64(5): 498-511.
[http://dx.doi.org/10.1016/j.jacc.2014.06.1150] [PMID: 25082585]

[23] Marathe SP, Talwar S. Surgery for transposition of great arteries: A historical perspective. Ann Pediatr Cardiol 2015; 8(2): 122-8.
[http://dx.doi.org/10.4103/0974-2069.157025] [PMID: 26085763]

[24] Khairy P, Clair M, Fernandes SM, *et al*. Cardiovascular outcomes after the arterial switch operation for D-transposition of the great arteries. Circulation 2013; 127(3): 331-9.
[http://dx.doi.org/10.1161/CIRCULATIONAHA.112.135046] [PMID: 23239839]

[25] Rastelli GC. A new approach to "anatomic" repair of transposition of the great arteries. Mayo Clin Proc 1969; 44(1): 1-12.
[PMID: 5767147]

[26] Kreutzer C, De Vive J, Oppido G, *et al*. Twenty-five-year experience with rastelli repair for transposition of the great arteries. J Thorac Cardiovasc Surg 2000; 120(2): 211-23.
[http://dx.doi.org/10.1067/mtc.2000.108163] [PMID: 10917934]

[27] Lecompte Y, Zannini L, Hazan E, *et al*. Anatomic correction of transposition of the great arteries. J Thorac Cardiovasc Surg 1981; 82(4): 629-31.
[http://dx.doi.org/10.1016/S0022-5223(19)39303-1] [PMID: 7278356]

[28] Di Carlo D, Lecompte Y, Tomasco B, *et al*. Surgery for malposition of the great arteries: the REV procedure. Multimed Man Cardiothorac Surg 2009; 2009:mmcts.2007.003046
[http://dx.doi.org/10.1510/mmcts.2007.003046]

[29] Nikaidoh H. Aortic translocation and biventricular outflow tract reconstruction. A new surgical repair for transposition of the great arteries associated with ventricular septal defect and pulmonary stenosis. J Thorac Cardiovasc Surg 1984; 88(3): 365-72.
[http://dx.doi.org/10.1016/S0022-5223(19)38323-0] [PMID: 6471887]

[30] Bex JP, Lecompte Y, Baillot F, Hazan E. Anatomical correction of transposition of the great arteries. Ann Thorac Surg 1980; 29(1): 86-8.
[http://dx.doi.org/10.1016/S0003-4975(10)61636-0] [PMID: 7356814]

[31] da Silva JP, Baumgratz JF, da Fonseca L. Pulmonary root translocation in transposition of great arteries repair. Ann Thorac Surg 2000; 69(2): 643-5.
[http://dx.doi.org/10.1016/S0003-4975(99)01387-9] [PMID: 10735726]

[32] Silva JP, Fonseca L. Pulmonary root translocation. Oper Tech Thorac Cardiovasc Surg 2009; 14: 23-34.
[http://dx.doi.org/10.1053/j.optechstcvs.2009.01.003]

[33] Hu SS, Li SJ, Wang X, *et al*. Pulmonary and aortic root translocation in the management of transposition of the great arteries with ventricular septal defect and left ventricular outflow tract obstruction. J Thorac Cardiovasc Surg 2007; 133(4): 1090-2.
[http://dx.doi.org/10.1016/j.jtcvs.2006.04.058] [PMID: 17382660]

[34] Anderson RH, Cook AC. Morphology of the functionally univentricular heart. Cardiol Young 2004; 14 (Suppl. 1): 3-12.
[http://dx.doi.org/10.1017/S1047951104006237] [PMID: 15244133]

[35] Kaulitz R, Hofbeck M. Current treatment and prognosis in children with functionally univentricular hearts. Arch Dis Child 2005; 90(7): 757-62.

[http://dx.doi.org/10.1136/adc.2003.034090] [PMID: 15970622]

[36] Davies RR, Pizarro C. Decision-making for surgery in the management of patients with univentricular heart. Front Pediatr 2015; 3: 61.
[http://dx.doi.org/10.3389/fped.2015.00061] [PMID: 26284226]

[37] Sano S, Kawada M, Yoshida H, *et al.* [Norwood procedure to hypoplastic left heart syndrome]. Jpn J Thorac Cardiovasc Surg 1998; 46(12): 1311-6.
[http://dx.doi.org/10.1007/BF03217921] [PMID: 10037841]

[38] Silva JP, Fonseca Ld, Baumgratz JF, *et al.* Hypoplastic left heart syndrome: the report of a surgical strategy and comparative results of Norwood x Norwood-Sano approach. Rev Bras Cir Cardiovasc 2007; 22(2): 160-8.
[PMID: 17992320]

[39] Gibbs JL, Wren C, Watterson KG, Hunter S, Hamilton JR. Stenting of the arterial duct combined with banding of the pulmonary arteries and atrial septectomy or septostomy: a new approach to palliation for the hypoplastic left heart syndrome. Br Heart J 1993; 69(6): 551-5.
[http://dx.doi.org/10.1136/hrt.69.6.551] [PMID: 7688231]

[40] Brawn WJ, Sethia B, Jagtap R, *et al.* Univentricular heart with systemic outflow obstruction: palliation by primary Damus procedure. Ann Thorac Surg 1995; 59(6): 1441-7.
[http://dx.doi.org/10.1016/0003-4975(95)00147-D] [PMID: 7539607]

[41] Rychik J. Forty years of the Fontan operation: a failed strategy. Semin Thorac Cardiovasc Surg Pediatr Card Surg Annu 2010; 13(1): 96-100.
[http://dx.doi.org/10.1053/j.pcsu.2010.02.006] [PMID: 20307870]

[42] Marrone C, Galasso G, Piccolo R, *et al.* Antiplatelet *versus* anticoagulation therapy after extracardiac conduit Fontan: a systematic review and meta-analysis. Pediatr Cardiol 2011; 32(1): 32-9.
[http://dx.doi.org/10.1007/s00246-010-9808-4] [PMID: 20967441]

[43] Geva T, Van Praagh S. Anomalies of the pulmonary veins.Moss and Adams' heart disease in infants, children, and adolescents: including the fetus and young adult. 8th ed. Philadelphia, PA: Lippincott Williams & Wilkins 2008; pp. 809-39.

[44] Seale AN, Uemura H, Webber SA, *et al.* British Congenital Cardiac Association. Total anomalous pulmonary venous connection: morphology and outcome from an international population-based study. Circulation 2010; 122(25): 2718-26.
[http://dx.doi.org/10.1161/CIRCULATIONAHA.110.940825] [PMID: 21135364]

[45] Yong MS, Yaftian N, Griffiths S, *et al.* Long-Term Outcomes of Total Anomalous Pulmonary Venous Drainage Repair in Neonates and Infants. Ann Thorac Surg 2018; 105(4): 1232-8.
[http://dx.doi.org/10.1016/j.athoracsur.2017.10.048] [PMID: 29452997]

[46] Zhu Y, Qi H, Jin Y. Comparison of conventional and primary sutureless surgery for repairing supracardiac total anomalous pulmonary venous drainage. J Cardiothorac Surg 2019; 14(1): 34.
[http://dx.doi.org/10.1186/s13019-019-0853-7] [PMID: 30736816]

[47] Overbeek MJ, van Nieuw Amerongen GP, Boonstra A, Smit EF, Vonk-Noordegraaf A. Possible role of imatinib in clinical pulmonary veno-occlusive disease. Eur Respir J 2008; 32(1): 232-5.
[http://dx.doi.org/10.1183/09031936.00054407] [PMID: 18591341]

[48] Seirafi PA, Warner KG, Geggel RL, Payne DD, Cleveland RJ. Repair of coarctation of the aorta during infancy minimizes the risk of late hypertension. Ann Thorac Surg 1998; 66(4): 1378-82.
[http://dx.doi.org/10.1016/S0003-4975(98)00595-5] [PMID: 9800836]

[49] Karamlou T, Bernasconi A, Jaeggi E, *et al.* Factors associated with arch reintervention and growth of the aortic arch after coarctation repair in neonates weighing less than 2.5 kg. J Thorac Cardiovasc Surg 2009; 137(5): 1163-7.
[http://dx.doi.org/10.1016/j.jtcvs.2008.07.065] [PMID: 19379984]

[50] Starnes VA, Pitlick PT, Bernstein D, Griffin ML, Choy M, Shumway NE. Ebstein's anomaly

appearing in the neonate. A new surgical approach. J Thorac Cardiovasc Surg 1991; 101(6): 1082-7.
[http://dx.doi.org/10.1016/S0022-5223(19)36627-9] [PMID: 2038202]

[51]   Kumar TKS, Boston US, Knott-Craig CJ. Neonatal Ebstein Anomaly. Semin Thorac Cardiovasc Surg 2017; 29(3): 331-7.
[http://dx.doi.org/10.1053/j.semtcvs.2017.09.006] [PMID: 28958645]

[52]   da Silva JP, Baumgratz JF, da Fonseca L, *et al.* The cone reconstruction of the tricuspid valve in Ebstein's anomaly. The operation: early and midterm results. J Thorac Cardiovasc Surg 2007; 133(1): 215-23.
[http://dx.doi.org/10.1016/j.jtcvs.2006.09.018] [PMID: 17198815]

[53]   Pizarro C, Bhat MA, Temple J. Cone reconstruction and ventricular septal. defect closure for neonatal Ebstein's anomaly. Multimed Man Cardiothorac Surg 2012; 2012: mms014.
[http://dx.doi.org/10.1093/mmcts/mms014] [PMID: 24414717]

SUBJECT INDEX

A

Abnormalities 2, 5, 45, 80, 88, 97, 98, 118, 119, 120, 121, 122, 123, 125, 128, 134, 135, 147, 154, 156, 197
  abdominal wall 118
  arterial 154
  cerebellar 156
  conduction 6
  congenital 156
  dental 121
  digestive system 118
  fetal gene 119
  genetic 118
  genital 118, 121, 147
  isolated valve 197
  musculoskeletal 134
  ocular 156
  palate 118
  relaxation 80
  renal 121, 135
  single umbilical artery 125
  skeletal 123, 128
Acute respiratory distress syndrome (ARDS) 272
Additional imaging modalities 227
Agenesis 25, 134, 135, 137, 200
  complete 134, 200
  corpus callosum 137
  renal 137
  venous duct 135
Agent 70, 71, 156, 248
  causal 70
  etiological 71
  known teratogenic 156
Akinesis 40
Alcohol 85, 155, 164, 175, 176, 182
  consumption 155, 175
  ingestion 155
  injection 85
Aldosterone 86
Alterations 25, 26, 31, 57, 59, 118, 125, 196
  fetal 196

fetal morphological 196
hemodynamic 31, 59
neuromuscular 26
numerical chromosome 118
Amalgamation 98
Anastomosis 10, 11, 12, 86, 87, 88, 265, 266, 269, 270
  direct 266
  placental 87
  surgical 10
  systemic-pulmonary 269
  veno-venous 88
Anatomical 86, 137
  continuity, complete 137
  rationale 86
Anemia 26, 81, 82, 84, 109, 110
  severe 81
Aneuploidies 131, 132, 135
Aneurysms 32, 82, 209, 219
  cardiac 219
Angiotensin 110, 170
  converting enzyme (ACE) 110, 170
  system blocker use 170
Anomalies 1, 2, 7, 16, 23, 37, 39, 78, 88, 118, 120, 121, 123, 125, 126, 131, 137, 138, 146, 147, 158, 159, 181, 200, 211, 239, 256, 261
  anatomical 78
  body stalk 120
  conotruncal 7, 123, 125, 239
  conotruncal rotation 131
  coronary 261
  coronary artery 256
  frequent coronary 256
  functional echocardiographic 39
  non-chromosomal origin 120
  preaxial limb 147
  rare cardiac 2, 200
  rare developmental 88
  renal 125, 137
  single 37
  skeletal 118, 137, 138
  structural 23, 158
  venous 181